Obstetric Anesthesia for Co-morbid Conditions

Berrin Gunaydin · Samina Ismail
Editors

Obstetric Anesthesia
for Co-morbid Conditions

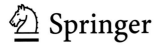 Springer

Editors
Berrin Gunaydin
Department of Anesthesiology
Gazi University School of Medicine
Ankara
Turkey

Samina Ismail
Department of Anaesthesiology
Aga Khan University
Karachi
Pakistan

ISBN 978-3-319-93162-3   ISBN 978-3-319-93163-0   (eBook)
https://doi.org/10.1007/978-3-319-93163-0

Library of Congress Control Number: 2018955195

This Springer imprint is published by the registered company Springer Nature Switzerland AG
The registered company address is: Gewerbestrasse 11, 6330 Cham, Switzerland

Foreword

Women with congenital and acquired disorders are able to enjoy longer and higher quality lives, which commonly now extend into the childbearing years. Once there, by design or by chance, these women are becoming pregnant; globally, there has been a significant increase in the prevalence of pregnant women with preexisting medical conditions.

For the anesthesiologist, these comorbidities have increased the complexity of care, the need for multidisciplinary consultations and conferences, and the consideration of additional lines, monitors, and tests. During and after the delivery, women remain at risk of decompensation, as the physiologic and anatomic demands associated with the disorder and pregnancy respond to the labor, birth, and other interventions. Continued and close observation, sometimes in a higher acuity setting (critical care, telemetry, or observation unit), is sometimes necessary.

These issues highlight the importance of this current, evidence-based textbook. The respected editors Berrin Gunaydin and Samina Ismail have assembled a global team of experts to guide us. Further, they assigned them to examine and expose disease conditions that we will likely see. In doing so, they have created a resource that is at once global, timely, and applicable. I fully anticipate that the anesthesia providers who use this textbook, and the women and fetuses for whom they care, will benefit greatly.

Lawrence C. Tsen
Department of Anesthesia and Pain Management
Faculty Development and Education
Center for Reproductive Medicine
Harvard Medical School
Brigham and Women's Hospital
Boston, MA, USA

Preface

Advancements in medical sciences have resulted in increased life span and better quality of life for women suffering from severe systemic diseases. As a result, more of these women are reaching childbearing age and are able to fulfill their dreams of becoming pregnant with a reasonable chance of carrying the child into the third trimester.

Therefore, providing safe obstetric anesthesia and analgesia to these obstetric patients has become an integral part of everyday anesthesia care. Extensive research and education on obstetric patients with comorbid conditions have led to tremendous improved outcomes in the management of these high-risk patients. Considering the importance of this topic, all obstetric anesthesia-related books have a dedicated section on this subject. Therefore, one would wonder the need for a separate book dedicated to obstetric anesthesia for comorbid conditions. What makes this book unique is relevant coverage of specific disorders that may be encountered in daily anesthesia practice but are often missed in most other competitive textbooks. It is designed to provide targeted information particularly on the anesthetic considerations and management of not only non-obstetric diseases during pregnancy but also pregnancy-induced diseases. In addition, it is believed that this book can serve as an introductory source of information and as a reference guide, therefore making it equally valuable to a trainee and to an established experienced anesthesiologist. We acknowledge the important role of all the outstanding anesthesiologists for their scientific contribution. We are extremely grateful to Springer International Publishing AG and to Ms. Kripa Guruprasad the project coordinator, Ms. Suganya Selvaraj the project manager and Ellen Blasig. Finally, we would like to thank the readers for their zest for knowledge for provision of safe and compassionate care for obstetric patients suffering from comorbid conditions for the better outcome of both mothers and the newborns.

Ankara, Turkey   Berrin Gunaydin
Karachi, Pakistan   Samina Ismail

Acknowledgements

I am very thankful to Professor Berrin Gunaydin, who had approached me to edit this book with her and had been the driving force behind the completion of this book.

Samina Ismail

It has been a privilege to work with Professor Samina Ismail; I appreciate her great contribution and motivation to share my dedication and ambition in this project.

Berrin Gunaydin

Contents

Anesthesia for Pregnancy Induced Liver Disease

1

Berrin Gunaydin

1.1   Introduction

Pregnancy induced liver diseases according to the frequency of reported incidence are hyperemesis gravidarum (HG), intrahepatic cholestasis of pregnancy (IHCP), hemolysis, elevated liver enzymes and low platelets (HELLP) syndrome, and acute fatty liver of pregnancy (AFLP). The IHCP, HELLP, and AFLP are very challenging for the anesthesiologists in case of need for urgent delivery, while HG which occurs in the first trimester is challenging for mostly obstetricians [1–4]. Therefore, in this chapter, after brief overview of the physiologic changes and alterations related to liver during pregnancy, anesthetic management and specific considerations in pregnant women undergoing either non-obstetric surgery or delivery are addressed based on the current literature.

The physiologic changes and/or abnormalities associated with pregnancy induced liver diseases are summarized.

Physiologic changes and markers of liver dysfunction during pregnancy are indicated below [3, 5]:

- Maternal plasma volume increases approximately 50% by the end of 34 weeks gestation resulting in a physiologic anemia because red blood cell volume increases more than plasma volume.
- Leukocyte count increases progressively but platelet count decreases or does not change.
- Cardiac output rises by 35–40% above baseline towards the end of first trimester.

B. Gunaydin
Department of Anesthesiology, Gazi University School of Medicine, Ankara, Turkey
e-mail: gunaydin@gazi.edu.tr

© Springer International Publishing AG, part of Springer Nature 2018
B. Gunaydin, S. Ismail (eds.), *Obstetric Anesthesia for Co-morbid Conditions*,
https://doi.org/10.1007/978-3-319-93163-0_1

- Alkaline Phosphatase (AP) which is found in biliary tract cells normally increases due to placental and fetal production but an elevated level of gamma glutamyl transferase (GGT) is suggestive of liver disease.
- Due to hepatocyte injury, release of alanine and aspartate aminotransferases (ALT and AST) increase which is called transaminitis.
- Coagulation factors I, VII, VIII, IX, X, and XII increase resulting in a physiologic hypercoagulable state, prothrombin time (PT) is unchanged and antithrombin III concentrations decreases whereas fibrinopeptide A, plasminogen, and fibrin degradation products (FDP) increase. Thus, increased PT/INR and/or PTT are indicators of liver disease.
- Progesterone inhibits contractility of gastrointestinal smooth muscle leading to gallbladder hypomotility and biliary stasis. Resulting increased bile secretion and cholesterol may increase the risk of gallstones during pregnancy.
- Albumin and total serum protein levels decrease.

However, there are no physiologic changes in the liver size, morphology, and blood flow in otherwise healthy parturients. Therefore, determining any hepatomegaly and/or increased serum bilirubin or bile acid levels are abnormal during pregnancy and regarded as supportive evidences for a pregnancy induced liver disease. Regarding aminotransferases, ALT is more specific than AST in liver diseases because ALT does not elevate due to tissue injury like AST [6].

1.2   Intrahepatic Cholestasis of Pregnancy

1.2.1   Incidence and Risk Factors

The incidence of IHCP is between 0.1% and 1.5% in Central Western Europe and North America but it may rise up to 4% in Chile and Bolivia [7]. The common risk factors are advanced maternal age, multiparity, family history, preexisting liver disease, or history of cholestasis while taking oral contraceptives [8, 9]. Pregnancy induced liver diseases except HG usually manifest either in the second or third trimester and reported incidences of these disorders are presented in Table 1.1.

Table 1.1 Incidences of unique liver diseases during pregnancy

	Incidence	Trimester
HG	<2%	First
IHCP	0.1–1.5%	Second or third
HELLP syndrome	0.1–0.6%	Third
AFLP	1:7000–1:16000	Third

HG hyperemesis gravidarum, *IHCP* intrahepatic cholestasis of pregnancy, *HELLP* hemolysis, elevated liver enzymes and low platelets, *AFLP* acute fatty liver of pregnancy

1.2.2 Diagnosis

The diagnosis is made by clinical signs and laboratory tests. Most of the parturients suffer from unbearable pruritis depending on the severity of the disease. Jaundice may develop in 50% of the patients. Elevated bilirubin (up to 6 mg/dL), transaminase (approximately 20 times than normal values), and serum bile acid levels (higher than 10 μmol/L) are the hallmark laboratory findings. However, the most sensitive diagnostic biomarker is the elevation in the fasting serum bile acid level, which is used to classify the disease as mild, moderate, or severe (mild: 10–39 μmol/mL, moderate: 40–99 μmol/mL and severe: ≥100 μmol/mL) [7].

1.2.3 Obstetric Management

Obstetric management of IHCP might affect the outcomes of the mother and the baby [10–16]. Medical treatment of pruritis during the perinatal period includes ursodeoxycholic acid, which is an FDA class B drug during pregnancy. Delivery of the baby at the fetal maturity is planned. In mild cases, delivery can be performed at term. However, in moderate or severe cases, early delivery at 36 weeks gestation should be considered due to the increased risk of preterm labor and/or birth, meconium staining of amniotic fluid, fetal loss, and abnormal fetal heart rate changes [2–4, 7].

1.2.4 Anesthetic Management

Choice of anesthesia for delivery seems to be controversial in IHCP. Due to the physiologic decrease in gallbladder contractility resulting in cholestasis, pregnant women tend to have a malabsorption of vitamin K, which is a cofactor responsible for synthesis of coagulation factors II, VII, IX, and X [11–15]. Because of the theoretical concern, studies have been conducted to elucidate whether alterations in coagulation status might be problematic in parturients with IHCP for the anesthesiologists [10, 16].

In a retrospective study (n = 319), estimated blood loss and the incidence of coagulopathy in IHCP parturients with (n = 223) or without (n = 96) preoperative coagulation tests (PT, PTT and platelets) were compared. No significant differences in estimated blood loss were found between them and no neuraxial hematoma was observed in subjects who received neuraxial analgesia and anesthesia. The incidence of postpartum hemorrhage (PPH) was reported to be 2.4% and 6.3% after vaginal and cesarean delivery, respectively. Of note, no abnormal coagulation studies were encountered postpartum even in the presence of preoperative increased liver enzymes in 13 subjects [16]. These authors reported that the presence of coagulopathy in parturients with isolated IHCP was very low and they concluded that use of neuraxial analgesia and/or anesthesia may not necessarily be delayed. Although preoperative coagulation test is not routine for performing neuraxial analgesia and/or anesthesia in isolated IHCP, it is recommended particularly in case of coexisting preeclampsia with IHCP [16]. In a recent retrospective study, maternal, fetal, and neonatal outcomes of parturients according to the severity of IHCP who delivered in 1 year at Gazi University were documented. The incidence of IHCP in Gazi University was 2% [10].

Delivery modes and anesthesia types in studies with IHCP patients were comparatively presented in Table 1.2 [7, 10, 16]. Severity of IHCP especially bile acid levels higher than 40 µmol/L may affect pregnancy outcomes. Parturients with severe IHCP delivered were preterm, whereas mild and moderate groups delivered at term [7, 10]. The CS rates were 14%, 73%, and 65.5% [7, 10, 16].

The rates of mild, moderate, and severe IHCP in Gazi University were 65%, 21%, and 14%, respectively. Twenty-seven percent of the cases had normal spontaneous vaginal delivery whereas the rest of the parturients (73%) underwent cesarean section (CS), 18.5% being not elective. The rates of neuraxial and general anesthesia for CSs were 85% and 15%, respectively. The most common neuraxial anesthesia type was spinal anesthesia (96%) [10].

1.2.5 Prognosis

There is no increased risk in maternal death rate and maternal outcomes are good because the disease disappears rapidly after delivery and it rarely progresses to cirrhosis [3]. According to the latest records, coagulation tests including PT, PTT, INR, and platelet counts did not differ between the preoperative and postoperative periods. But increased preoperative transaminases and AP in parturients with IHCP significantly returned to almost normal clinical laboratory limits on the 3rd postoperative day [10].

1.2.6 Maternal, Fetal, and Neonatal Outcomes

Comparison of maternal, fetal, and neonatal outcomes in three studies was summarized in Table 1.2. In general, documented adverse fetal and neonatal outcomes were comparable among the studies [7, 10, 16].

1.3 HELLP Syndrome

1.3.1 Definition and Incidence

The acronym for HELLP comes from hemolysis, elevated liver enzymes, and low platelet count. HELLP syndrome, either alone or associated with severe preeclampsia was first described by Weinstein in 1982 [17]. HELLP has an incidence of 0.1–0.6% that develops usually in the third trimester (Table 1.1). The rate of HELLP patients with severe preeclampsia varies between 4% and 12%,

Table 1.2 Delivery modes, anesthesia types and maternal, fetal, and neonatal outcomes

	J Clin Anesth 2014 [16] (n = 319)		Am J Obstet Gynecol 2015 [7] (n = 215)			Türk J Med Sci 2017 [10] (n = 37)		
			Mild (n = 108)	Moderate (n = 86)	Severe (n = 21)	Mild (n = 24)	Moderate (n = 8)	Severe (n = 5)
Severity of IHCP (n)	Not documented clearly							
Gestational age (week)	37.2 (36.8–38.1)		Term	Term	Preterm	Term	Term	Preterm
Preoperative coagulation tests (PT, PTT, platelet count)	Yes (n = 96)	No (n = 223)	Not documented			Yes (n = 37)		
Postoperative coagulation tests (PT, PTT, platelet count)	Yes (n = 319)		Not documented			Yes (n = 37)		
Preoperative liver enzymes and bilirubin levels	Not documented clearly		Highest data throughout the pregnancy were documented (n = 215)			Documented (n = 37) Elevated transaminases and AP Normal GGT, LDH, and bilirubin		
Postoperative liver enzymes and bilirubin levels	Not documented clearly					Documented (n = 37) Transaminases, AP, GGT, LDH, and bilirubin are normal		
VD (n (percent))	111 (34.5%)		185 (86%)			0 (27%)		
CS (n (percent))	208 (65.5%)		30 (14%)			27 (73%)		
Neuraxial analgesia for labor (n)	Not documented clearly		Not documented clearly			CSE: 1		
Anesthesia type for CS (n)	Not documented clearly		Not documented clearly			Spinal: 22 General: 4 CSE:1		
Adverse fetal and neonatal outcome (n)	Not documented clearly		74 (preterm birth, perinatal death, meconium stained fluid, and asphyxia)			7 (preterm labor and birth, perinatal death, newborn hepatitis)		
Adverse maternal outcome (PPH)	Overall rate 3.4% (6.3% after CS)		Overall rate 7.4%			0%		

CS cesarean section, VD vaginal delivery, PPH postpartum hemorrhage while 70% of patients with HELLP syndrome present before delivery, 30% of them develop postpartum mostly in the first 48 h [1, 18–21].

1.3.2 Pathophysiology

Approximately 20% of preeclamptic women with severe features develop HELLP. Mechanism of preeclampsia might be explained because of failed remodeling of spiral arteries by the cytotrophoblasts leading to hypoperfusion and ischemia of the placenta. The fetal consequence is intrauterine growth retardation. On the maternal side ischemic placenta releases several factors that provoke a generalized endothelial dysfunction which in turn is responsible for maternal symptoms and complications. Pathophysiology of HELLP with or without preeclampsia includes endothelial injury with fibrin deposits that causes microangiopathic hemolytic anemia and platelet activation-consumption leading to thrombocytopenia [17–20].

1.3.3 Diagnosis and Classification

Accurate diagnosis is made mainly by laboratory tests. Low platelet count (<100,000/μL), increased AST or ALT (≥70 IU/L) and LDH levels (≥600 IU/L) are required for complete diagnosis but if only one or two of these abnormalities are present it becomes partial HELLP syndrome. However, 50% patients with HELLP syndrome might be free of all diagnostic criteria [20, 22].

The severity of HELLP syndrome is basically classified depending on the platelet count [22]. According to the Mississippi classification, elevated AST and LDH associated with platelet count ≤50,000/μL are in class 1, platelet count between 50,000–10,0000/μL in class 2, and platelet count between 100,000–150,000/μL in class 3. However, in Tennessee classification, diagnosis is either complete or partial (severe preeclampsia + one or more of the hallmark laboratory findings) [22].

In the guidelines of Antwerp University, anesthetic technique can be chosen according to the platelet count. If platelet count is >90,000/μL, any anesthetic technique (either regional or general) can be chosen, if platelet count is between 60,000 and 90,000/μL some prefer single shot spinal anesthesia and as for platelet count <60,000/μL commonly general anesthesia is performed [23].

1.3.4 Obstetric Management

HELLP syndrome often progresses and may eventually compromise maternal and fetal outcomes. Therefore, obstetric management includes delivery at ≥34 weeks' gestation. Vaginal delivery may be proceeded in active labor, if there is no fetal distress or risk of disseminated intravascular coagulopathy (DIC). However, in the presence of coexisting multi-organ dysfunction, renal failure, or abruption, immediate cesarean delivery should be performed and induction of labor is avoided [1, 15, 24].

1.3.5   Medical Treatment

Basically, three drug groups (corticosteroids, antihypertensives, and anticonvulsants) are used for perinatal and expectant management of HELLP. Benefit of using IV corticosteroids before 34 weeks' gestation is recommended for fetal lung maturation in standard dose (betamethasone 6 mg twice a day). High doses may be preferred in patients with extremely low platelets, high liver enzymes, and low urine output. As an antihypertensive medication, labetalol is one of the first line drugs used to lower high blood pressure and monitoring blood pressure at least postpartum 24 h is required. Even if the HELLP diagnosis is not complete, hypertension crisis should be controlled by either hydralazine or labetalol within the first 1 h urgently. Intravenous magnesium sulphate 4–6 gram (g) of loading dose in 20 min followed by 1–2 g/h infusion should be administered for seizure prophylaxis in mild or severe preeclampsia complicated with HELLP and for treatment of ongoing seizures during labor until postpartum 24 h at least. Recommended therapeutic magnesium concentration is kept between 4–7 mg/dL by checking serum magnesium levels every 4 h along with monitoring urine output, respiratory rate, SpO_2, and patellar reflexes [24].

1.3.6   Preoperative Transfusion

Platelet transfusion is generally required in patients with HELLP when preoperative platelet count is <20,000/µL or <50,000/µL and cesarean delivery is mandatory. It is advisable to keep platelet count above 50,000/µL to avoid risk of bleeding. Of note, there is no need to transfuse platelet more than once, since thrombocytopenia improves usually 24 h after delivery [25]. Plasmapheresis might be a supportive therapeutic option in refractory patients [24].

1.3.7   Choice of Anesthesia

General anesthesia for CS has been the safest and most commonly preferred technique in HELLP syndrome. However, high rate of use of regional anesthesia for CS has been documented in 102 cases with preterm HELLP syndrome (antepartum $n = 95$, postpartum $n = 7$). Mean gestational age was 30.6 ± 2.7 weeks. Most of the parturients underwent regional anesthesia ($n = 65$). Cases having mean preoperative platelet count of 113,000/µL ($n = 53$) underwent CS under CSE, while patients ($n = 12$) with mean preoperative platelet count of 95,000/µL underwent spinal anesthesia. Interestingly, two patients with platelet count <50,000/µL underwent CS with CSE. Only one of them received platelet transfusion immediately before CSE. No epidural hematoma has been reported in that retrospective study [23].

1.3.8 Prognosis

HELLP syndrome is associated with increased risk of maternal and fetal morbidity and mortality. Rate of maternal death is approximately 1%. According to the latest revision in Mississippi classification related to composite major maternal morbidity (CMMM), patients with class 1 HELLP have higher CMMM [26]. Noteworthy maternal complications include pulmonary edema, acute renal failure, DIC, abruptio placenta, liver hemorrhage or failure, ARDS, retinal detachment, stroke, adverse events due to blood transfusion and neuraxial hematoma. The rate of perinatal death varies between 7.4% and 20.4%, depending on the gestational age and concurrent factors related to the pregnancy. The highest morbidity and mortality rates are observed <28 weeks' gestation. Most perinatal morbidity is due to prematurity that may cause respiratory distress syndrome, bronchopulmonary dysplasia, intracerebral hemorrhage, or necrotizing enterocolitis [1, 27–29].

1.3.9 Complications

A subarachnoid hematoma after CS under spinal anesthesia in a 39-year-old severe preeclamptic parturient associated with HELLP syndrome was reported. Complete recovery of motor block occurred 5 h after spinal block. Although preoperative platelet count was 91,000/μL, it declined progressively to 30,000/μL on the second postoperative day and patient started to suffer from sensory and motor deficit in the lower extremity, urinary retention, and flaccid paraparesis. Magnetic resonance imaging (MRI) revealed spinal subarachnoid hematoma compressing cauda equina. Three months after conservative medical treatment (Vit B12, PG E1, oral neostigmine + bladder exercise, flurbiprofen and rehabilitation), complete recovery with hematoma regression on the MRI was observed [29]. Another severe complication is massive hepatic infarction requiring surgical intervention 24 h after emergency CS which has been reported in a severe preeclamptic parturient with HELLP [30].

1.3.10 Follow-Up

Despite careful perioperative fluid therapy, patients should be monitored to avoid pulmonary edema for at least 48 h postpartum. Laboratory abnormalities usually regress 24 h postpartum and complete recovery occurs 48 h postpartum [1].

1.4 Acute Fatty Liver of Pregnancy

1.4.1 Definition and Incidence

Acute fatty liver of pregnancy was described as yellow atrophy of the liver in early 1950s. AFLP is an idiopathic fatal disease with a 10–85% mortality rate. The incidence is between 1/7000–1/16000 or 1:10,000–15,000 pregnancies. It often develops between 27 and 40 weeks' gestation, but may be undiagnosed until the postpartum period [1, 31].

1.4.2 Risk Factors

Advanced maternal age, primiparity, multiple pregnancies, preeclampsia, male fetus, being underweight, the use of non-steroidal anti-inflammatory drugs and previous AFLP are considered to be some of the risk factors [1, 32].

1.4.3 Pathophysiology

The incidence of AFLP is high in women with a genetic mutation. Basically, mitochondrial fatty acid oxidation pathway is affected. Fetus has a long-chain 3-hydroxyacyl-coenzyme A dehydrogenase deficiency [31].

1.4.4 Clinical Features and Laboratory Findings

Patient is presented with fatigue, vomiting, headache, hypoglycemia, lactic acidosis. Prolonged prothrombin time, depressed antithrombin III, elevated liver enzymes, persistent DIC, elevated direct bilirubin, creatinine, AP and leukocytosis are observed in almost all cases. Profound hypoglycemia might occur due to impaired glycogenolysis [33, 34].

1.4.5 Prognosis

Decision to make immediate delivery is extremely important because of high maternal (23%) and fetal (18%) mortality rate. If early diagnosis is made and properly treated, AFLP is a reversible peripartum liver failure. Most of the patients recover within 48–72 h after delivery with improved aminotransferase levels [35].

1.4.6 Diagnosis

Currently, there are no uniform diagnostic criteria for AFLP [36–39]. However, markedly elevated levels of serum transaminases (>200 U/L) and direct bilirubin

(60 μmol/L) should be considered in the accurate diagnosis because perinatal death was linked to elevated levels of direct bilirubin [38].

1.4.7 Obstetric Management

Early diagnosis, prompt delivery, and intensive supportive treatment by close monitoring are essential, since recovery before delivery is not possible. For severe cases, plasmapheresis and liver transplantation may be considered [33–35, 40].

1.4.8 Anesthetic Management

General anesthesia is usually required in patients with coagulopathy because of the concern for regional anesthesia related hematoma risk. Perioperative anesthesia care includes establishing adequate intravenous accesses readily available for cross matched blood and blood products against increased risk of PPH [1, 11].

1.4.9 Postoperative Care

Patients with coagulopathy, encephalopathy, or hypoglycemia may require admission to intensive care unit [33–38, 40].

Remarkable clinical and laboratory findings, anesthesia types, maternal, fetal, and neonatal outcomes from retrospective AFLP studies were summarized in Table 1.3 [36–39].

1.5 Hyperemesis Gravidarum

HG is characterized by severe and persistent form of nausea and vomiting resulting in dehydration, malnutrition, and weight loss [3]. It is always managed by the obstetricians, since planned anesthetic support is not needed for the disease during early pregnancy. Sometimes differential diagnosis may be required to rule out any gastrointestinal pathology (e.g., Helicobacter pylori infection) in serious cases refractory to treatment. Such a particular case was referred to outpatient anesthesia clinic after first unsuccessful awake endoscopy attempt without sedation. For the 2nd endoscopic procedure, propofol, which is a safe intravenous anesthetic agent in liver disease, was used under monitored anesthesia care [41]. Dose adjustment is made due to 10% decrease in propofol requirement in the first trimester [5].

Table 1.3 Anesthesia types and outcomes as potential predictors

Retrospective AFLP studies	Anesthesia types and outcomes
Zhou et al. [36] Retrospective analysis of AFLP 28 cases from Shanghai Public Health Center over 5 years. Gynecol Obstet Invest 2013	2 maternal deaths (7.1%) without fetal deaths CS under neuraxial ($n = 16$) and general anesthesia with RSI ($n = 12$)
Cheng et al. [37] AFLP: A retrospective study of 32 cases in South China J Matern Fetal Neonatal Med 2014	18 parturients recovered due to rapid diagnosis, early termination of pregnancy and supportive treatments Newborn male sex and vaginal delivery were risk factors of fetal outcome
Zang et al. [38] A retrospective analysis of 56 cases Chinese Med J 2016	PT/INR are risk factors for fatal complications – Perinatal mortality is linked to FDP
Qu Y et al. [39] Retrospective analysis of anesthetic and perioperative management in patients of AFLP in Peking University Zhonghua Yi Xue Za Zhi. 2017	12 cases were identified (91.7% primigravid, 50% twin pregnancies and 1 with concomitant preeclampsia) CS under neuraxial ($n = 1$) and general anesthesia with RSI ($n = 9$) 1 patient admitted after delivery died postpartum 6 out of the 18 fetuses were transferred to the pediatric department due to preterm, low birth weight, intrauterine restriction or asphyxia and they all survived

RSI rapid sequence induction

1.6   General Considerations for Anesthesia Management

1.6.1   Anesthesia Technique

During liver dysfunction and/or failure, metabolism of general anesthetic drugs is delayed. Therefore, regional anesthesia, either a neuraxial or peripheral block, is considered in the absence of coagulopathy whenever possible. Regional anesthesia is superior to general anesthesia in patients with particularly advanced liver disease because of the less systemic effects of the neuraxial and locally administered drugs. Additionally, regional anesthesia blunts hemodynamic effects of stress hormones in the circulation better than general anesthesia [1, 11, 15].

1.6.2   Local Anesthetics

Anesthetists must consider the altered pharmacokinetics in liver disease. Total drug dose used for a peripheral block should be cautiously calculated and possible side effects should be closely monitored. Regarding local anesthetic drugs, lidocaine has the longest $t_{1/2elim}$. Meanwhile, increased volume of distribution (Vd) of lidocaine may offer some protection against it. Toxicity is mostly dependent on the free fraction of the local anesthetic drug. Fortunately, $\alpha 1$ acid glycoprotein (GP), which is the main plasma protein that binds local anesthetics, is synthesized even in end stage liver disease. Noteworthy, clearance of ropivacaine is less in the end stage liver disease than normal. For metabolism of ester type local anesthetic drugs, though pseudocholinesterase enzyme production in the liver may decrease in disease state, overall clearance of chloroprocaine is unclear [15].

1.6.3 Intravenous and Inhalation Anesthetics

The elimination half-life of propofol is unaffected although its clearance may be higher. As for thiopental, the elimination half-life is 2.5 times longer than normal, which is explained by the marked increase in Vd despite increased clearance [5]. Considering inhalation anesthetics, when sevoflurane or desflurane was compared with isoflurane, sevoflurane seems to be advantageous without significant differences. Nitrous oxide is no more commonly preferred to provide perioperative analgesia [1, 15]. However, liver cell injury with xenon anesthesia has been shown to be impossible which might be a promising alternative agent if available [42, 43].

Since minimum alveolar concentration (MAC) of volatile anesthetics is decreased up to 40% in pregnancy, despite bispectral index (BIS) monitorization is not a standard tool it might be helpful in adjusting inhaled anesthetic requirements [3, 5].

1.6.4 Muscle Relaxants

Either atracurium or cisatracurium is a reasonable option due to its independent liver metabolism. Despite reduced pseudocholinesterase activity, suxamethonium is used for rapid sequence induction (RSI) since it does not result in clinically relevant prolongation in liver dysfunction and during pregnancy [1, 3, 5]. Although aminosteroid type muscle relaxants have enhanced sensitivity in liver disease, rocuronium induced prolonged neuromuscular block could be completely antagonized by sugammadex. Therefore, muscle relaxants are used by neuromuscular block monitoring [15, 44].

1.6.5 Practice of General Anesthesia

General anesthesia induction and maintenance are provided with possibly safe IV and inhalation anesthetic drugs under standard monitorization including heart rate, ECG, non-invasive blood pressure, peripheral oxygen saturation, and end tidal carbon dioxide pressure measurement. Among intravenous anesthetic agents for induction of anesthesia, propofol is the most favorable because of its rapid metabolism even in cirrhosis. Isoflurane, desflurane, or sevoflurane with or without small doses of fentanyl seems to be reasonable for maintenance of anesthesia. Fentanyl, if used in relatively moderate doses, is a good choice without affecting oxygen supply. Long acting narcotics and benzodiazepines should be avoided in cirrhotic patients [1, 3, 5, 15]. Total intravenous anesthesia (TIVA) with RSI using target controlled infusion (TCI) of propofol and remifentanil was reported. Rocuronium 1.2 mg/kg was used to facilitate endotracheal intubation. For induction of anesthesia, TCI propofol (4 ng/mL) and remifentanil (3 ng/mL) were used and maintenance of anesthesia was provided with 3 ng/mL of propofol and remifentanil. Recently, an emergency CS was performed with total intravenous anesthesia in a severe preeclamptic parturient associated with HELLP and renal insufficiency [45]. In another case report using TIVA, anesthesia induction with remifentanil and propofol with RSI using succinylcholine followed by propofol and remifentanil infusion [46].

Fetal heart rate monitoring is mandatory by a qualified obstetrician during expectant management of the parturient when necessary. However, invasive monitoring (intraarterial or central venous pressure) is not a must for anesthesia practice. Continuous invasive monitoring of intraarterial blood pressure is indicated only in patients with poorly controlled high blood pressure, rapid need for lowering blood pressure and frequent use of blood gases. Central venous pressure monitoring is only indicated in case of assessment of renal oliguria and response to fluid administration. Thus, careful fluid administration is required because of the increased risk of pulmonary edema particularly with which is one of the leading causes of morbidity in preeclamptic HELLP patients. According to the most recent meta-analysis investigating the incidence of pulmonary edema associated with colloid versus crystalloid administration in preeclampsia, no significant differences were found between them. The authors recommended an individually tailored fluid management with the aid of non-invasive modalities of hemodynamic measurement such as lung ultrasound, transthoracic echocardiography, or pulse waveform monitors if available [47].

1.6.6 Postoperative Care

Even though delayed clearance is a concern in severe liver disease, intravenous or neuraxial opioids can be administered to provide postoperative analgesia. Since advanced liver disease has an increased risk of hepatic encephalopathy, residual effects of anesthetics or analgesics may result in neurologic deterioration in the postoperative period. Therefore, neurologic and liver function monitoring is essential [1, 3, 15, 23].

Conclusion

Recent evidences about the anesthetic management in parturients with pregnancy induced liver diseases are not clear regarding the best approach. General anesthesia technique with RSI is the preferred choice in case of coagulopathy. Regardless of the selection of any anesthesia technique, hepatic blood flow and oxygenation should be maintained and hemodynamic alterations and sympathetic stimulation should be avoided at all times. Management of anesthesia in this particular group needs special attention and care with rational choice of available local and general anesthetic drugs that provide greater stability both for general and regional anesthesia under continuous careful monitoring.

Key Learning Points
- Isolated IHCP may be managed in the same manner like a healthy parturi-ent. Coagulopathy should be excluded or corrected before regional anes-thesia if possible. Since presence of coagulopathy in parturients with isolated IHCP is very low, neuraxial analgesia and/or anesthesia may not necessarily be delayed. Preoperative coagulation tests are recommended in case of coexisting preeclampsia with IHCP.
- General anesthesia with RSI is the safest choice in class I and II HELLP patients scheduled to undergo CS. Total intravenous anesthesia with pro-pofol and remifentanil was reported in a severe preeclamptic parturient associated with HELLP and renal insufficiency for emergency CS. Spinal anesthesia may be selected if there is no progressive thrombocytopenia. Close patient monitoring is a must against hemorrhagic complications, DIC or eclampsia at all times.
- Anesthesia selection should be individualized in patients with AFLP. General anesthesia with RSI is recommended in case of severe coagulopathy. Perioperative anesthetic care includes establishing adequate IV access with readily available cross matched blood and blood products against anticipated PPH.
- Despite its rarity, when anesthesia support is needed in a patient with severe HG, anesthesia is provided with safe IV drugs under monitored anesthesia care.

References

1. Gunaydin B, Tas Tuna A. Anesthetic considerations for liver diseases unique to pregnancy. World J Anaesthesiol. 2016;5:54–61.
2. Hepburn IS, Schade RR. Pregnancy-associated liver disorders. Dig Dis Sci. 2008;53:2334–58.
3. Wax DB, Beilin Y, Frolich M. Liver disease. In: Chestnut DH, Wong CA, Tsen LC, Ngan Kee WD, Beilin Y, Mhyre JM, editors. Chestnut's obstetric anesthesia principles and practice. 5th ed. Philadelphia: Elsevier; 2014. p. 1068–80.
4. Lee NM, Brady CW. Liver disease in pregnancy. World J Gastroenterol. 2009;15:897–906.
5. Gaiser R. Physiologic changes of pregnancy. In: Chestnut DH, Wong CA, Tsen LC, Ngan Kee WD, Beilin Y, Mhyre JM, editors. Chestnut's obstetric anesthesia principles and practice. 5th ed. Philadelphia: Elsevier; 2014. p. 15–38.
6. Than NN, Neuberger J. Liver abnormalities in pregnancy. Best Pract Res Clin Gastroenterol. 2013;27:565–75.
7. Brouwers L, Koster MP, Page-Christiaens GC, Kemperman H, Boon J, Evers IM, et al. Intrahepatic cholestasis of pregnancy: maternal and fetal outcomes associated with elevated bile acid levels. Am J Obstet Gynecol. 2015;212:100.e1–7.

8. Knox TA, Olans LB. Liver disease in pregnancy. N Engl J Med. 1996;335:569–76.
9. Reyes H. Sex hormones and bile acids in intrahepatic cholestasis of pregnancy. Hepatology. 2008;47:376–9.
10. Gunaydin B, Bayram M, Altug M, Cevher S, Bozkurt N. Retrospective analysis of maternal, fetal and neonatal outcomes of intrahepatic cholestasis of pregnancy at Gazi University. Turk J Med Sci. 2017;47:583–6.
11. Kamimura K, Abe H, Kawai H, Kamimura H, Kobayashi Y, Nomoto M, et al. Advances in understanding and treating liver diseases during pregnancy: a review. World J Gastroenterol. 2015;21:5183–90.
12. Bacq Y. Liver diseases unique to pregnancy: a 2010 update. Clin Res Hepatol Gastroenterol. 2011;35:182–93.
13. Ahmed KT, Almashhrawi AA, Rahman RN, Hammoud GM, Ibdah JA. Liver diseases in pregnancy: diseases unique to pregnancy. World J Gastroenterol. 2013;19:7639–46.
14. Goel A, Jamwal KD, Ramalingam A, Balasubramanian KA, Eapen CE. Pregnancy-related liver disorders. J Clin Exp Hepatol. 2014;4:151–62.
15. Rahimzadeh P, Safari S, Faiz SH, Alavian SM. Anesthesia for patients with liver disease. Hepat Mon. 2014;14:e19881.
16. DeLeon A, De Oliveira GS, Kalayil M, Narang S, McCarthy RJ, Wong CA. The incidence of coagulopathy in pregnant patients with intrahepatic cholestasis: should we delay or avoid neuraxial analgesia? J Clin Anesth. 2014;26:623–7.
17. Weinstein L. Syndrome of hemolysis, elevated liver enyzmes and low platelet count: a severe consequence of hypertension in pregnancy. Am J Obstet Gynecol. 1982;142:159–67.
18. Mihu D, Costin N, Mihu CM, Seicean A, Ciortea R. HELLP syndrome – a multisystemic disorder. J Gastrointest Liver Dis. 2007;16:419–24.
19. Fitzpatrick KE, Hinshaw K, Kurinczuk JJ, Knight M. Risk factors, management, and outcomes of hemolysis, elevated liver enzymes, and low platelets syndrome and elevated liver enzymes, low platelets syndrome. Obstet Gynecol. 2014;123:618–27.
20. Audibert F, Friedman SA, Frangieh AY, Sibai BM. Clinical utility of strict diagnostic criteria for the HELLP (hemolysis, elevated liver enzymes, and low platelets) syndrome. Am J Obstet Gynecol. 1996;175:460–4.
21. Martin JN, Blake PG, Lowry SL, Perry KG, Files JC, Morrison JC. Pregnancy complicated by preeclampsia-eclampsia with the syndrome of hemolysis, elevated liver enzymes, and low platelet count: how rapid is postpartum recovery? Obstet Gynecol. 1990;6:737–41.
22. Rahman H. Pinning down HELLP: a review. Biomed J Sci Tech Res. 2017;1:1–5.
23. Palit S, Palit G, Vercauteren M, Jacquemyn Y. Regional anaesthesia for primary caesarean section in patients with preterm HELLP syndrome: a review of 102 cases. Clin Exp Obstet Gynecol. 2009;36:230–4.
24. Del-Rio-Vellosillo M, Garcia-Medina JJ. Anesthetic considerations in HELLP syndrome. Acta Anaesthesiol Scand. 2016;60:144–57.
25. Padden MO. HELLP syndrome: recognition and perinatal management. Am Fam Physician. 1999;60:829–36.
26. Martin JN Jr, Brewer JM, Wallace K, Sunesara I, Canizaro A, Blake PG, et al. HELLP syndrome and composite major maternal morbidity (CMMM): importance of Mississipi classification. Patients with class 1HELLP have higher CMMM. J Matern Fetal Neonatal Med. 2013;26:1201–6.
27. Geary M. The HELLP syndrome. Br J Obstet Gynaecol. 1997;104:887–91.
28. Habli M, Eftekhari N, Wiebracht E, Bombrys A, Khabbaz M, How H, et al. Long-term maternal and subsequent pregnancy outcomes 5 years after hemolysis, elevated liver enzymes, and low platelets (HELLP) syndrome. Am J Obstet Gynecol. 2009;201:385.e1–5.
29. Koyama S, Tomimatsu T, Kanagawa T, Sawada K, Tsutsui T, Kimura T, et al. Spinal subarachnoid hematoma following spinal anesthesia in a patient with HELLP syndrome. Int J Obstet Anesth. 2010;19:87–91.
30. Mikolajczyk AE, Renz J, Diaz G, Alpert L, Hart J, Te HS. Massive hepatic infarction caused by HELLP syndrome. ACG Case Rep J. 2017;4:1–4.

31. Watson WJ, Seeds JW. Acute fatty liver of pregnancy. Obstet Gynecol Surv. 1990;45:585–91.
32. Ibdah JA. Acute fatty liver of pregnancy: an update on pathogenesis and clinical implications. World J Gastroenterol. 2006;12:7397–404.
33. Ko H, Yoshida EM. Acute fatty liver of pregnancy. Can J Gastroenterol. 2006;20:25–30.
34. Knight M, Nelson-Piercy C, Kurinczuk JJ, Spark P, Brocklehurst P. A prospective national study of acute fatty liver of pregnancy in the UK. Gut. 2008;57:951–6.
35. Nelson DB, Yost NP, Cunningham FG. Acute fatty liver of pregnancy: clinical outcomes and expected duration of recovery. Am J Obstet Gynecol. 2013;209:456.e1–7.
36. Zhou G, Zhang X, Ge S. Retrospective analysis of acute fatty liver of pregnancy: twenty-eight cases and discussion of anesthesia. Gynecol Obstet Invest. 2013;76:83–9.
37. Cheng N, Xiang T, Wu X, Li M, Xie Y, Zhang L. AFLP: a retrospective study of 32 cases in South China. J Matern Fetal Neonatal Med. 2014;27:1693–7.
38. Zang YP, Kong WQ, Zhou SP, Gong YH, Zhou R. Acute fatty liver of pregnancy: a retrospective analysis of 56 cases. Chin Med J (Engl). 2016;20(129):1208–14.
39. Qu YY, Zeng H, Guo XY, Li M. Retrospective analysis of anesthetic and perioperative management in patients of acute fatty liver of pregnancy. Zhonghua Yi Xue Za Zhi. 2017;27(97):1878–82.
40. Browning MF, Levy HL, Wilkins-Haug LE, Larson C, Shih VE. Fetal fatty acid oxidation defects and maternal liver disease in pregnancy. Obstet Gynecol. 2006;107:115–20.
41. Gunaydin B, Özek A, Özterlemez NT, Tuna A. Unique liver disease of pregnancy requiring anaesthesia support: a case with severe hyperemesis gravidarum. Turk J Anaesthesiol Reanim. 2017;45:234–6.
42. Bovill JG. Inhalation anaesthesia: from diethyl ether to xenon. Handb Exp Pharmacol. 2008;82:121–42.
43. Dabbagh A, Rajaei S. Xenon: a solution for anesthesia in liver disease. Hepat Mon. 2012;12:e8437.
44. Nonaka T, Fujimoto M, Nishi M, Yamamoto T. The effect of rocuronium and sugammadex in hepatic tumor patients without preoperative hepatic impairment. Masui. 2013;62:304–8.
45. Zuccolotto EB, Neto EP, Nogueira CG, Nociti JR. Anesthesia in pregnant women with HELLP syndrome: case report. Rev Bras Anestesiol. 2016;66:657–60.
46. Wang J, Wang N, Han Z. Anesthetic management of a parturient with hemolysis, elevated liver enzyme levels, and low platelet syndrome complicated by renal insufficiency and coagulopathy. Anesth Essays Res. 2017;11:1126–8.
47. Pretorius T, Van Rensburg G, Dyer RA, Biccard BM. The influence of fluid management on outcomes in preeclampsia: a systematic review and meta-analysis. Int J Obstet Anesth. 2018;34:85–95.

Anesthetic Management of Pregnant Patients with Hypertensive Disorders

2

Samina Ismail

2.1 Introduction

Hypertensive disorders of pregnancy are significant cause of both maternal and fetal morbidity and mortality [1]. It poses a global health threat in both developed and developing countries [2, 3]. However, the impact of the disease is more in the developing countries due to the late presentation of the disease making medical interventions less effective [4, 5]. Anesthesiologists being part of the multidisciplinary team are involved in the initial management for provision of analgesia/anesthesia and for subsequent management in the postpartum period. Therefore, this chapter will outline the role of anesthesiologist as a member of the multidisciplinary team in the anesthetic management of pregnant patients with hypertensive disorders. Since preeclampsia is a multisystem disease unique to human pregnancy, this chapter will focus mainly on this particular disorder.

2.2 Classification of Hypertensive Disorders of Pregnancy

The National High Blood Pressure Education Program (NHBPEP) Working Group on high blood pressure in pregnancy published a classification scheme in 2000 that achieved international acceptance [6]. They classified hypertensive disorders of pregnancy into (1) gestational hypertension, (2) preeclampsia, (3) chronic hypertension, and (4) chronic hypertension with superimposed preeclampsia:

1. *Gestational hypertension:* It is the most common hypertensive disorder of pregnancy with less severe outcomes almost similar to that of a normotensive parturient [7, 8]. Women are labeled as having gestational hypertension when they

S. Ismail
Department of Anaesthesiology, Aga Khan University, Karachi, Pakistan
e-mail: samina.ismail@aku.edu

© Springer International Publishing AG, part of Springer Nature 2018
B. Gunaydin, S. Ismail (eds.), *Obstetric Anesthesia for Co-morbid Conditions*,
https://doi.org/10.1007/978-3-319-93163-0_2

17

present with hypertension after the 20th week of pregnancy with no previous history of hypertension or signs and symptoms of preeclampsia. Hypertension resolves after 12 weeks postpartum [8].

2. *Preeclampsia:* The diagnosis of preeclampsia is made when hypertension is diagnosed for the first time after the 20th week of gestation and there is involvement of either one or more than one organ systems. The disease processes involving the organ system show resolution by 3 months in the postpartum period. Depending upon its severity, it is further classified into mild or severe. It can progress to *eclampsia* when the central nervous system involvement leads to seizures [9].

3. *Chronic hypertension:* Diagnosed as having hypertension prepregnancy or when hypertension fails to resolve after 12 weeks postpartum.

4. *Chronic hypertension with superimposed preeclampsia:* When a parturient with a prepregnancy diagnosis of chronic hypertension develops sudden new onset of proteinuria or sudden increase in the levels of blood pressure or when the symptoms of severe preeclampsia develop. The outcomes are worse with increased morbidity as compared to patient with preeclampsia alone [10].

2.3 Pathophysiology

The current widely accepted explanation is failure of placenta to embed adequately leading to hypoxia due to poor placental perfusion [11]. This in turn leads to vasospasm and activation of coagulation cascade with microthrombi formation and end-organ damage [12]. The resultant endothelial damage is responsible for the maternal syndrome of preeclampsia, manifesting as hypertension and proteinuria with or without systemic manifestation [13]. The fetal syndrome of preeclampsia includes fetal growth retardation, oligohydramnios, and abnormal oxygenation [6]. The pathophysiology of eclampsia is due to the presence of placenta and not because of the fetus as it can occur with woman having molar pregnancy.

2.4 Diagnostic Challenges of Preeclampsia

In order to establish the diagnoses of preeclampsia, there has to be a sustained increase in blood pressure on repeated measurement usually done at 4 hourly interval with disease process involving either one or more than one organ systems. The abnormalities of organ systems can either be of central nervous system, cardiovascular system, gastrointestinal system, hematological system, renal system, or uteroplacental systems [14].

Preeclampsia presenting before 20 weeks of gestation occurs in parturient having hydatidiform mole, fetal or placental abnormalities, multiple pregnancy, antiphospholipid syndrome, or severe renal disease [14].

Other causes of hypertension during pregnancy include renal disease, pheochromocytoma, coarctation of aorta, subclavian artery stenosis, aortic dissection, and vasculitis [15]. These conditions are caused by different pathologies, which need to be differentiated from preeclampsia as treatment options are entirely different.

In addition, severe hepatic dysfunctions due to causes other than preeclampsia need to be identified. This includes development of the acute fatty liver in pregnancy, which is not associated with hypertension [16].

One type of severe preeclampsia is HELLP syndrome characterized by hemolysis, elevated liver enzymes, and low platelet count. There is fragmentation of red blood cells and appearance of schistocytes on a blood film, rise in lactate dehydrogenase and total bilirubin levels often combined with declining hematocrit, and evidence of a bleeding diathesis [15].

Conditions like hemolytic uremic syndrome and thrombotic thrombocytopenic purpura, which have features like thrombocytopenia, hemolytic anemia associated with microangiopathies, and abnormalities of the central nervous system and renal system, need to be differentiated from HELLP syndrome, as treatment and/or interventions are entirely different [15].

2.5 Severity of Preeclampsia

This term is used when preeclampsia progresses in severity with rise in blood pressure to a level of systolic blood pressure equal or higher than 160 mmHg and diastolic blood pressure to a level equal or higher than 110 mmHg with severe decline in organ functions of involved body systems. The central nervous system involvement may progress to severe headache, visual disturbances, impaired consciousness, and seizures (eclampsia). Renal function impairment is observed by increase in the excretion of urinary protein to >5 gram (g). Severe preeclampsia also presents itself as HELLP syndrome.

2.6 Anesthetic Management

Early involvement of anesthesiologist is important as woman with mild preeclampsia can progress rapidly to severe category requiring anesthesia management and stabilization before delivery [17]. The importance of experienced multidisciplinary teamwork has been highlighted in literature [18–20].

Preanesthetic assessment and preparation should focus on airway examination, reduction of blood pressure, hemodynamic monitoring, fluid balance, and prevention and treatment of seizures. Routine investigations including coagulation profile are required to determine the possible need of any replacement therapy.

2.6.1 Airway

Airway changes in hypertensive parturient are due to soft tissue edema owing to fluid retention, increased cell permeability, and low plasma oncotic pressure [21]. Therefore, anesthesiologists need to anticipate the possibility of difficult airway and be prepared for it.

2.6.2 Control of Rising Blood Pressure

Parturients are labeled as having *non-severe hypertension* when systolic and diastolic blood pressures rise to a range of 140–159 mmHg and 90–109 mmHg, respectively. Agents considered safe for use in these patients include methyldopa, low-dose diazoxide, nifedipine, and some beta adrenoceptor blockers including labetalol, metoprolol, or pindolol [22]. Atenolol is avoided as it causes fetal growth restriction. Other agents that are contraindicated in parturient include angiotensin-converting enzyme inhibitors and angiotensin type-2 receptor blockers [23, 24]. When systolic pressure rises to more than 160 mmHg and diastolic pressure to more than 110 mmHg, the condition is termed as severe hypertension. Systolic blood pressure rising to more than 180 mmHg is labeled as a hypertensive crisis [18]. This condition is associated with high incidence of intracerebral hemorrhage if immediate medical intervention is not provided [19]. In order to prevent hemorrhagic stroke, various guidelines recommend using oral labetalol as the drug of choice to maintain systolic blood pressure below 150 mmHg and a diastolic blood pressure below 100 mmHg [25]. It is advisable to avoid sudden fall in blood pressure which may lead to adverse maternal and fetal complications. Blood pressure should be lowered at a rate of 10–20 mmHg every 10–20 min to levels of systolic blood pressure between 140 and 150 mmHg and diastolic pressures between 80 and 100 mmHg. Fetal heart rate monitoring should be monitored continuously until the blood pressure is stable [26].

Drugs that are considered to be safe for lowering of blood pressure include labetalol, hydralazine, and nifedipine. However, there is paucity of good randomized controlled trial comparing hydralazine with intravenous labetalol or oral nifedipine [25]. Intravenous hydralazine is usually administered by intermittent bolus of 5 mg or by continuous infusion in the dose of 0.5–10.0 mg/h for more refractory cases. Sodium nitroprusside is known to be associated with adverse maternal side effects of hypotension and paradoxical bradycardia and fetal cyanide toxicity in fetus; therefore it is rarely used in pregnancy [4].

Glyceryl trinitrate is the drug of choice in preeclamptic patients who develop acute pulmonary edema. It is given in an infusion of 5 μg/min increasing every 3–5 min to a maximum dose of 100 μg/min [4].

2.6.3 Hemodynamic Monitoring

Fluctuations in blood pressure are expected in patients with severe preeclampsia as a result of progression of disease and in response to administration of antihypertensive agents. Since patients with preeclampsia are volume contracted and fluid depleted, clinical assessment of intravascular volume can become difficult necessitating the use of invasive monitoring.

Continuous monitoring of blood pressure is indicated in case of poorly controlled maternal blood pressure or a rapid need to lower blood pressure using sodium nitroprusside or glyceryl trinitrate, frequent use of blood gases, or when general anesthesia is required in patients with severe preeclampsia.

Central venous pressure monitoring is advisable in assessment of oliguria and its response to fluid administration [9]. However, there is no indication of central hemodynamic monitoring that is specific to preeclampsia, as it is a disease of peripheral circulation and not of central circulation. Therefore, the indication for invasive central monitoring is the same for any multisystem disorders including severe sepsis, pulmonary edema, and cardiomyopathy [9].

2.6.4 Prevention and Treatment of Seizures

Patients with preeclampsia are at risk of developing seizures. Magnesium sulfate has shown to be the first-line drug treatment for both ongoing seizures (eclampsia) and for prevention of recurrent seizures [27, 28]. When compared to drugs like phenytoin, diazepam, or lytic cocktail (combination of chlorpromazine, promethazine, and pethidine), the use of magnesium sulfate has shown to decrease the incidence of maternal death, seizure recurrence, pneumonia, need for ventilation, or admission to an intensive care unit [27–29]. Magnesium sulfate can be used effectively by parenteral route. Collaborative Eclampsia Trial recommends the use of $MgSO_4$ in the dose of 4–5 g intravenously over 5 min, followed by an infusion of 1 g/h for 24 h. An additional 2 g intravenous $MgSO_4$ should be administered in case of recurrent seizures [30].

The use of magnesium sulfate for prevention of seizures is established in severe preeclampsia, but its use in mild disease is controversial. The investigators have found that the number needed to treat to prevent one woman having seizure was approximately 100 in mild disease as compared to 50 in patients with severe disease [31]. However, selective administration of magnesium sulfate to women with severe preeclampsia resulted in increased number of women developing eclampsia who required general anesthesia with adverse neonatal outcomes [32].

Magnesium sulfate is not recommended as an antihypertensive agent, and its clinical use does not reverse or prevent the progression of the disease [24, 26]. Proper guidelines need to be in place in health-care centers for the safe use of magnesium sulfate. This includes monitoring by clinical parameters like measuring urinary output, respiratory rate, oxygen saturation, and patellar reflexes. If any of the clinical parameter is indicated toward magnesium toxicity, it is mandatory to check serum magnesium levels. Magnesium toxicity is often apparent when the serum magnesium levels are above 3.5 mmol/L. Patients having any additional systemic manifestation like renal insufficiency are more likely to develop magnesium toxicity. The drug used for treatment of magnesium sulfate toxicity is 10% calcium gluconate given in the dose of 1 g over 10 min [15].

2.6.5 Fluid Balance

Careful fluid management is an important aspect in the management of patient with preeclampsia. Pulmonary edema is one of the leading causes of morbidity in preeclampsia leading to intensive care admission and death [33]. Evidence suggests that intravenous fluids should not be administered in preeclampsia for the purpose of volume expansion or for the treatment of oliguria when renal functions and serum creatinine concentration are within normal range [34].

2.6.6 Laboratory Investigations Including the Coagulation Status

As there is a marked variation in the normal values during pregnancy at different gestational periods, pregnancy-specific range is accepted for blood tests.
  (a) Useful blood tests in preeclampsia include [35]:
    • Full blood count with special emphasis on platelet count.
    • Clotting screen is needed if platelets are $<100 \times 10^{-9}$/L, liver function test (LFT) is abnormal, or unexplained bleeding or bruising is present. A blood film is required if HELLP syndrome is suspected.
    • Serum urea, electrolytes, creatinine, and urate levels.
    • Liver function tests including serum transaminase (AST) and alanine aminotransferase (ALT) are sent to detect liver disorders and liver damage.
  (b) Glucose needs to be checked in cases of acute fatty liver of pregnancy and diabetes or if patient's ALT is more than 150 IU/L.
  (c) Urine tests in preeclampsia include:
    • Urine dipstick.
    • Urinary protein/creatinine ratio (PCR) from a random sample (<30 mg/mmol excludes significant proteinuria; >30 mg/mmol does not reliably confirm or quantify proteinuria).
    • 24-h urine collection for proteinuria ($\geq$300 mg/24 h both confirm and quantify proteinuria).
    • Midstream specimen of urine to exclude infection.
    • Urine output must be accurately monitored and recorded.
Further investigations are warranted according to clinical presentation.

2.7 Neuraxial Blockade in Preeclamptic Parturient

Neuraxial blockade is the preferred method for both anesthesia and analgesia in parturient diagnosed with preeclampsia [25, 36, 37]. However, coagulopathy needs to be ruled out before institution of neuraxial block. Common reasons for coagulopathy in preeclampsia include thrombocytopenia and less commonly disseminated intravascular coagulation [15]. Studies using thromboelastography to determine safe levels of platelet count in preeclampsia have recommended that counts less than 100×10^9/L were associated with coagulation abnormality in severe preeclampsia requiring additional investigation of coagulation status [15].

Regarding the lower limit of the platelet count, there is no definitive evidence; however, indirect conclusions from current standard of practice and thromboelastography studies have shown that in the absence of other coagulation abnormalities, the risk of hematoma associated with neuraxial anesthesia with platelet counts >75 × 10⁹/L is very low [15].

2.7.1 Neuraxial Technique and Its Associated Complications in Preeclamptic Patients

The estimated incidence of major complications after neuraxial techniques in pregnant women in general is approximately 1/20,000–30,000 for spinal anesthesia and 1/25,000 for epidural analgesia [38]. The risk of epidural hematomas increases in preeclampsia as thrombocytopenia is shown to be present in 30–50% of parturient having severe preeclampsia [39]. In addition the presence of engorged epidural venous plexus combined with low platelet count further increases the risk.

Therefore, neuraxial anesthetic techniques may be avoided in pregnancy-induced hypertension if there is concomitant thrombocytopenia and coagulopathy. It is recommended to follow the trend and get a coagulation profile if there is a declining trend.

2.7.2 Neuraxial Labor Analgesia for Labor and Delivery

Currently neuraxial technique for labor analgesia is considered as a gold standard technique for number of reasons. The advantages of neuraxial blocks include improved intervillous blood flow due to sympathetic blockade causing decrease in uteroplacental resistance [40]. In addition it causes reduction in pain-mediated hypertensive responses by causing reduction in serum catecholamine levels. Investigators have shown better neonatal acid-base status and Apgar score at 1 and 5 min with labor epidural analgesia compared to no analgesia and systemic opioids [41]. In addition the presence of a functioning epidural catheter enables the use of the epidural catheter for cesarean delivery.

Epidural labor analgesia is maintained by either continuous infusion, intermittent boluses, or patient-controlled epidural analgesia (PCEA) using a combination of local anesthetics and preservative-free opioids. The PCEA has the advantage over other techniques as parturients are able to self-administer prefixed doses of epidural medication whenever needed and a lock out time interval provides a safety from over dosage of local anesthetics [42]. However, the choice of delivery mostly depends on the availability of equipment.

2.8 Anesthesia for Cesarean Delivery

2.8.1 Technique of Anesthesia

Availability of time, maternal or fetal status, and communication with the obstetrical team have a vital role to play in the decision of the anesthetic technique for cesarean delivery. When there is no maternal and fetal compromise with no time constraint, spinal anesthesia or epidural top-up of a pre-existing epidural catheter is the technique of choice. On the other hand, when there is a maternal and fetal compromise, coagulation abnormality, or a parturient with ongoing seizures, general anesthesia may be considered over regional anesthetic technique.

Neuraxial anesthesia is preferred over general anesthesia as an anesthetic technique for cesarean delivery as the risk of aspiration, possibility of encountering difficult or failed intubations, and sympathetic response to laryngoscopy and intubation associated with general anesthetic can be avoided [15]. A population-based study with a sample size of total 303,862 women who had undergone cesarean delivery showed an increased risk of maternal stroke in preeclamptic women receiving general anesthesia for cesarean delivery [43].

Neuraxial techniques that have been used effectively include single-shot spinal, combined spinal-epidural, and epidural anesthesia. However, no evidence has suggested advantage of one technique over the other. Spinal anesthesia is the most commonly used technique as it has a rapid onset, dense block and can provide an effective postoperative analgesia when long-acting intrathecal opioids are used [44]. Studies have shown two times lower incidence of spinal-induced hypotension and vasopressor requirement in preeclamptic parturient when compared with normal parturient undergoing cesarean delivery [45]. Vasoactive drugs including 3–5 mg bolus of intravenous ephedrine or 50–100 µg bolus of intravenous phenylephrine are used in titrated doses to successfully manage episodes of hypotension [37, 46]. It is best to avoid adrenaline-containing local anesthetic in preeclampsia for the anticipated risk of hypertensive crisis due to absorbed adrenaline [15].

Hypertensive response to intubation during general anesthesia has been identified as a cause of direct maternal mortality [18, 19]. Numbers of drugs have been used to attenuate this response, which includes short-acting narcotics like fentanyl, alfentanil, and remifentanil. In addition $MgSO_4$ lidocaine and esmolol have been used for this purpose. Choice of the drug depends on its availability and physicians' familiarity with the drug [47]. Special attention needs to be paid to complications like aspiration, hypertensive response, and acute pulmonary edema that are commonly encountered at the time of emergence from anesthesia.

2.8.2 Recommended Monitoring for Cesarean Delivery

Continuous intra-arterial blood pressure monitoring is recommended for cesarean delivery in parturient with severe hypertension [25]. In addition to beat-to-beat arterial pressure recording, it is useful for frequent blood sampling required for the assessment of electrolytes, acid-base balance, and abnormalities of respiratory, hematological, and hepatic systems [15].

Other invasive monitoring like central venous pressure and pulmonary artery pressure are used very occasionally [34]. Transthoracic echocardiography is considered a better option as it has the advantage of providing information related to cardiac structural and functional performance and responses to interventions [48].

2.9 Postpartum Management

Patients with severe preeclampsia should be monitored in the postpartum period by trained staff in an appropriately monitored setting [19]. Important consideration in the postpartum period is for analgesia, thromboprophylaxis, decision to discontinue magnesium sulfate, and identification and management of postpartum complications.

2.9.1 Analgesia

Although analgesic modalities like the use of intravenous opioids, paracetamol, local anesthetic, and neuraxial techniques have been used frequently in the postpartum management, enough literature is not available for preeclampsia [49]. Nonsteroidal anti-inflammatory agents have well-documented adverse effects and are contraindicated in women with preeclampsia [50].

2.9.2 Thromboprophylaxis

It should be considered for all women with preeclampsia, and neuraxial technique should be timed accordingly.

2.9.3 Discontinuation of Intravenous Magnesium Sulfate

There has been recommendation to continue it for 12–24 h [51]. However, it has been suggested to use improvement in clinical parameters rather than time to make a decision to discontinue $MgSO_4$. Clinical improvement includes normalization of blood pressure to less than 150/100 mmHg without the need of antihypertensive medications and urine output of more than 100 mL/h for at least in the last couple of hours and with no headache, pain in the epigastrium, or vision abnormality [52].

2.9.4 Identification and Management of Postpartum Complications

Some of the common postpartum complications observed in the postpartum period among preeclamptic parturient include severe hypertension, acute pulmonary edema, and decrease in urine output and acute renal decompensation.

Postpartum hypertension is a cause of postpartum morbidity and mortality, and medications commonly employed for treatment include hydralazine, methyldopa, furosemide, and nifedipine [53].

Incidence of pulmonary edema in preeclampsia is 2.9% with 70% occurring in the postpartum period [54]. Treatment options are similar to those used in the non-obstetric population.

Oliguria in the postpartum period can be due to a number of causes, and no treatment is required including the use of furosemide or low-dose dopamine if renal and respiratory functions are normal [55].

2.10   Recent Advances

2.10.1 Echocardiography

Is emerging as an extremely useful tool to enable more informed decisions in the management of women with preeclampsia especially pertaining to fluid therapy and choice of antihypertensive agents [56]. In addition it can provide a more definitive evaluation of cardiac function in the hypertensive pregnant patient.

2.10.2 Placental Growth Factor

Placenta produces an angiogenic factor called placental growth factor (PlGF) which shows a peak in concentrations between 26 and 30 weeks of gestation. Women with preeclampsia have shown to have reduced levels of PlGF with the lowest levels corresponding to earlier onset and increased severity of the disease. The importance of this biomarker lies in its ability to diagnose preeclampsia before the onset of hypertension and proteinuria, thus allowing earlier treatment and multidisciplinary planning for delivery. As the levels of PlGF naturally decline during the third trimester, therefore the test becomes less reliable after 35 weeks [57]. There is a need for randomized controlled trials to assess whether diagnosing preeclampsia with PlGF rather than current methods can improve maternal and/or fetal outcomes.

Conclusion

Hypertensive disorders of pregnancy especially preeclampsia will continue to remain a significant cause of maternal and fetal morbidity in both developed and developing countries. Anesthesiologists, as part of the multidisciplinary team, play a vital role in the provision of safe anesthesia/analgesia, resuscitation, and critical care management in the postpartum period. Therefore, it is imperative for the anesthesiologists to have a thorough understanding of this disease which is unique to pregnancy. The skill, knowledge, and awareness of potential intra- and postoperative problems and the ability to respond quickly in emergency situation are the key factors for successful management of these patients.

Key Learning Points

- Hypertensive disorders of pregnancy are significant cause of both maternal and fetal morbidity and mortality.
- The National High Blood Pressure Education Program (NHBPEP) Working Group on high blood pressure in pregnancy classified hypertensive disorders of pregnancy into (1) gestational hypertension, (2) preeclampsia, (3) chronic hypertension, and (4) chronic hypertension with superimposed preeclampsia.
- The diagnosis of preeclampsia is made when there is a new onset of hypertension after the 20th week of gestation with one or more organ system involvement and resolution of the disease by 3 months postpartum.
- The current widely accepted explanation is failure of placenta to embed adequately leading to hypoxia due to poor placental perfusion. This in turn leads to vasospasm and activation of coagulation cascade with microthrombi formation leading to endothelial damage with organ damage responsible for systemic manifestation.
- Severe preeclampsia is defined as progression in severity with blood pressure showing a substantial increase of systolic >160 mmHg and diastolic >110 mmHg with marked derangements of organ functions.
- Preanesthetic assessment and preparation should focus on airway examination, reduction of blood pressure, hemodynamic monitoring, prevention and treatment of seizures, fluid balance, and investigations including the coagulation status and need for replacement therapies if needed.
- Antihypertensive drugs that are considered safe in these patients include labetalol, hydralazine, and nifedipine.
- Continuous arterial blood pressure monitoring is indicated in cases of poorly controlled maternal blood pressure, frequent use of blood gases especially in the setting of patient with pulmonary edema, rapid need to lower blood pressure using sodium nitroprusside or glyceryl trinitrate, and when using general anesthesia in patients with severe preeclampsia.
- As preeclampsia is a disease of peripheral circulation and not the central circulation, there is no indication of central hemodynamic monitoring that is specific to preeclampsia.
- Neuraxial anesthesia is preferred over general anesthesia as an anesthetic technique for cesarean delivery as the risk of aspiration, possibility of encountering difficult or failed intubations, and sympathetic response to laryngoscopy and intubation associated with general anesthetic can be avoided. However coagulopathy needs to be ruled out before institution of neuraxial block.
- Hypertensive response to intubation has been identified as a cause of direct maternal mortality. Therfore, particular attention needs to be paid to attenuate this response when general anesthesia is used as technique of anesthesia.

- Important consideration in the postpartum period is for analgesia, thromboprophylaxis, and decision to discontinue magnesium sulfate.
- In addition there is a need for identification and management of postpartum complications.
- Some of the common postpartum complications observed in preeclampsia include severe hypertension, acute pulmonary edema, oliguria, and acute renal decompensation.

References

1. Mammaro A, Carrara S, Cavaliere A, Ermito S, Dinatale A, Pappalardo EM, et al. Hypertensive disorders of pregnancy. J Prenat Med. 2009;3:1.
2. National Institute for Health and Care Excellence (NICE). Hypertension in pregnancy: the management of hypertensive disorders during pregnancy. In: NICE CG 107. Manchester: National Institute for Health and Clinical Excellence; 2010. Available from http://www.nice.org.uk/guidance/cg107/resources/guidance-hypertension-in-pregnancy-pdf. Accessed 5 Jan 2018.
3. Bujold E, Morency AM, Roberge S, Lacasse Y, Forest JC, Giguere Y. Acetylsalicylic acid for the prevention or preeclampsia and intra-uterine growth restriction in women with abnormal uterine artery Doppler: a systematic review and meta-analysis. J Obstet Gynaecol Can. 2009;31:818–26.
4. Regitz-Zagrosek V, Lundqvist CB, Borghi C, Cifkova R, Ferreira R, Foidart JM, et al. European Society of Cardiology Guidelines on the management of cardiovascular diseases during pregnancy: the Task Force on the Management of Cardiovascular Diseases during Pregnancy of the European Society of Cardiology (ESC). Eur Heart J. 2011;32:3147–97.
5. Fitzpatrick K, Hinshaw K, Kurinczuk J, Knight M. Risk factors, management, and outcomes of hemolysis, elevated liver enzymes, and low platelets syndrome and elevated liver enzymes, low platelets syndrome. Obstet Gynecol. 2014;123:618–27.
6. Gifford RW. Report of the national high blood pressure education program working group on high blood pressure in pregnancy. Am J Obstet Gynecol. 2000;183:1–22.
7. Hauth JC, Ewell MG, Levine RJ, Esterlitz JR, Sibai B, Calcium for Preeclampsia Prevention Study Group, et al. Pregnancy outcomes in healthy nulliparas who developed hypertension. Obstet Gynecol. 2000;95(1):24–8.
8. Barton JR, O'Brien JM, Bergauer NK, Jacques DL, Sibai BM. Mild gestational hypertension remote from term: progression and outcome. Am J Obstet Gynecol. 2001;184(5):979–83.
9. Polly LS. Hypertension disorders. In: Chestnut DH, Tsen LC, Polly LS, Wong CA, editors. Chesnut's obstetric anesthesia: principles and practice. 4th ed. Philadelphia: Mosby Elsevier; 2004. p. 975–1008.
10. Giannubilo SR, Dell'Uomo B, Tranquilli AL. Perinatal outcomes, blood pressure patterns and risk assessment of superimposed preeclampsia in mild chronic hypertensive pregnancy. Eur J Obstet Gynecol Reprod Biol. 2006;126:63–7.
11. Uzan J, Carbonnel M, Piconne O, Asmar R, Ayoubi JM. Preeclampsia: pathophysiology, diagnosis, management. Vasc Health Risk Manag. 2011;7:467–74.
12. Bell MJ. A historical overview of preeclampsia-eclampsia. J Obstet Gynecol Neonatal Nurs. 2010;39:510–8.
13. Alladin AA, Harrison M. Preeclampsia: systemic endothelial damage leading to increased activation of the blood coagulation cascade. J Biotech Res. 2012;4:26–43.
14. Pickering TG, Hall JE, Appel LJ, Falkner BE, Graves J, Hill MN, et al. Recommendations for blood pressure measurement in humans and experimental animals: part 1: blood pressure

measurement in humans: a statement for professionals from the Subcommittee of Professional and Public Education of the American Heart Association Council on High Blood Pressure Research. Hypertension. 2005;45:142–61.

15. Dennis AT. Management of pre-eclampsia: issues for anaesthetists. Anaesthesia. 2012;67:1009–20.

16. Bacq Y. Liver diseases unique to pregnancy: a 2010 update. Clin Res Hepatol Gastroenterol. 2011;35:182–93.

17. Healthcare Improvement Scotland. Scottish confidential audit of severe maternal morbidity, 7th annual report. Edinburgh; 2011. http://www.healthcareimprovementscotland.org/pro-grammes/reproductive_maternal_child/programme_resources/scasmm.aspx. Accessed 3 Nov 2017.

18. Cantwell R, Clutton-Brock T, Cooper G, Dawson A, Drife J, Garrod D, et al. Saving mothers' lives: reviewing maternal deaths to make motherhood safer: 2006–2008. The eighth report of the confidential enquiries into maternal deaths in the United Kingdom. BJOG. 2011;118:1–203.

19. Lewis G, editor. The confidential enquiry into maternal and child health (CEMACH). Saving mothers' lives: reviewing maternal deaths to make motherhood safer – 2003–2005. The sev-enth report on confidential enquiries into maternal deaths in the United Kingdom. London: CEMACH; 2007.

20. Dyer RA, Piercy JL, Reed AR. The role of the anaesthetist in the management of the pre-eclamptic patient. Curr Opin Anaesthesiol. 2007;20:168–74.

21. Izci B, Riha RL, Martin SE, Vennelle M, Liston WA, Dundas KC, et al. The upper airway in pregnancy and preeclampsia. Am J Respir Crit Care Med. 2003;167:137–40.

22. Hennessy A, Thornton CE, Makris A, Ogle RF, Henderson-Smart DJ, Gillin AG, et al. A ran-domized comparison of hydralazine and mini-bolus diazoxide for hypertensive emergencies in pregnancy: the PIVOT trial. Aust N Z J Obstet Gynaecol. 2007;47:279–85.

23. Abalos E, Duley L, Steyn DW, Henderson-Smart DJ. Antihypertensive drug therapy for mild to moderate hypertension during pregnancy. Cochrane Database Syst Rev. 2007;1:CD002252.

24. Podymow T, August P. Update on the use of antihypertensive drugs in pregnancy. Hypertension. 2008;51:960–9.

25. National Collaborating Centre for Women's and Children's Health. Hypertension in pregnancy. The management of hypertensive disorders during pregnancy. National Institute for Health and Clinical Excellence Guideline 107. August 2010 revised reprint January 2011 ed. London: RCOG; 2011. http://www.nice.org.uk/nicemedia/live/13098/50475/50475.pdf. Accessed 30 Dec 2011.

26. Rowe T. Diagnosis, evaluation, and management of the hypertensive disorders of pregnancy. J Obstet Gynaecol Can. 2008;30:1–48.

27. Duley L, Gülmezoglu AM, Chou D. Magnesium sulphate versus lytic cocktail for eclampsia. Cochrane Database Syst Rev. 2010;9:CD002960.

28. Duley L, Henderson-Smart DJ, Walker GJA, Chou D. Magnesium sulphate versus diazepam for eclampsia. Cochrane Database Syst Rev. 2010;12:CD000127.

29. Duley L, Henderson-Smart DJ, Chou D. Magnesium sulphate versus phenytoin for eclampsia. Cochrane Database Syst Rev. 2010;10:CD000128.

30. The Collaborative Eclampsia Trial Group. Which anticonvulsant for women with eclampsia? Evidence from the Collaborative Eclampsia Trial. Lancet. 1995;345:1455–63.

31. Duley L, Gülmezoglu AM, Henderson-Smart DJ, Chou D. Magnesium sulphate and other anti-convulsants for women with preeclampsia. Cochrane Database Syst Rev. 2010;11:CD000025.

32. Alexander JM, McIntire DD, Leveno KJ, Cunningham FG. Selective magnesium sulfate prophylaxis for the prevention of eclampsia in women with gestational hypertension. Obstet Gynecol. 2006;108:826–32.

33. Ganzevoort W, Rep A, Bonsel GJ, Fetter WP, van Sonderen L, De Vries JI, et al. A randomised controlled trial comparing two temporising management strategies, one with and one without plasma volume expansion, for severe and early onset pre-eclampsia. BJOG. 2005;112:1358–68.

34. Duley L, Williams J, Henderson-Smart DJ. Plasma volume expansion for treatment of pre-eclampsia. Cochrane Database Syst Rev. 1999;4:CD001805.

35. Krishnachetty B, Plaat F. Management of hypertensive disorders of pregnancy. ATOTW Weekly. 2014;304:1–13.

36. Lucas MJ, Sharma SK, McIntire DD, Wiley J, Sidawi JE, Ramin SM, et al. A randomized trial of labor analgesia in women with pregnancy-induced hypertension. Am J Obstet Gynecol. 2001;185:970–5.
37. Visalyaputra S, Rodanant O, Somboonviboon W, Tantivitayatan K, Thienthong S, Saengchote W. Spinal versus epidural anesthesia for cesarean delivery in severe preeclampsia: a prospective randomized, multicenter study. Anesth Analg. 2005;101:862–8.
38. Moen V, Dahlgren N, Irestedt L. Severe neurological complications after central neuraxial blockades in Sweden 1990–1999. Anesthesiology. 2004;101:950–9.
39. Valera MC, Parant O, Vayssiere C, Arnal JF, Payrastre B. Physiologic and pathologic changes of platelets in pregnancy. Platelets. 2010;21:587–95.
40. Ginosar Y, Nadjari M, Hoffman A, Firman N, Davidson EM, Weiniger CF, et al. Antepartum continuous epidural ropivacaine therapy reduces uterine artery vascular resistance in pre-eclampsia: a randomized, dose-ranging, placebo-controlled study. Br J Anaesth. 2009;102:369–78.
41. Reynolds F. Labour analgesia and the baby: good news is no news. Int J Obstet Anesth. 2011;20:38–50.
42. Fettes PD, Moore CS, Whiteside JB, McLeod GA, Wildsmith JA. Intermittent vs. continuous administration of epidural ropivacaine with fentanyl for analgesia during labour. Br J Anaesth. 2006;97:359–64.
43. Huang CJ, Fan YC, Tsai PS. Differential impacts of modes of anaesthesia on the risk of stroke among preeclamptic women who undergo caesarean delivery: a population-based study. Br J Anaesth. 2010;105:818–26.
44. Sia AT, Fun WL, Tan TU. The ongoing challenges of regional and general anaesthesia in obstetrics. Best Pract Res Clin Obstet Gynaecol. 2010;24:303–12.
45. Aya AG, Vialles N, Tanoubi I, Mangin R, Ferrer JM, Robert C, et al. Spinal anesthesia-induced hypotension: a risk comparison between patients with severe preeclampsia and healthy women undergoing preterm cesarean delivery. Anesth Analg. 2005;101:869–75.
46. Berends N, Teunkens A, Vandermeersch E, Van de Velde M. A randomized trial comparing low-dose combined spinal-epidural anesthesia and conventional epidural anesthesia for cesarean section in severe preeclampsia. Acta Anaesthesiol Belg. 2005;56:155–62.
47. Dyer RA, Els I, Farbas J, Torr GJ, Schoeman LK, James MF. Prospective, randomized trial comparing general with spinal anesthesia for cesarean delivery in preeclamptic patients with a nonreassuring fetal heart trace. Anesthesiology. 2003;99:561. Discussion 5A-6A.
48. Dennis AT. Transthoracic echocardiography in obstetric anaesthesia and obstetric critical illness. Int J Obstet Anesth. 2011;20:160–8.
49. Macintyre PE, Schug SA, Scott DA, Visser EJ, Walker SM, Acute Pain Management: Scientific Evidence Working Group of the Australian and New Zealand College of Anaesthetists and Faculty of Pain Medicine. Acute pain management: scientific evidence. 3rd ed. Melbourne: Australian and New Zealand College of Anaesthetists and the Faculty of Pain Medicine; 2010.
50. Makris A, Thornton C, Hennessy A. Postpartum hypertension and nonsteroidal analgesia. Am J Obstet Gynecol. 2004;190:577–8.
51. Ehrenberg HM, Mercer BM. Abbreviated postpartum magnesium sulfate therapy for women with mild preeclampsia: a randomized controlled trial. Obstet Gynecol. 2006;108:833–8.
52. Isler CM, Barrilleaux PS, Rinehart BK, Magann EF, Martin JN Jr. Postpartum seizure prophylaxis: using maternal clinical parameters to guide therapy. Obstet Gynecol. 2003;101:66–9.
53. Magee L, Sadeghi S, von Dadelszen P. Prevention and treatment of postpartum hypertension. Cochrane Database Syst Rev. 2005;1:CD004351.
54. Norwitz ER, Hsu CD, Repke JT. Acute complications of preeclampsia. Clin Obstet Gynecol. 2002;45:308–29.
55. Steyn DW, Steyn P. Low-dose dopamine for women with severe pre-eclampsia. Cochrane Database Syst Rev. 2007;1:CD003515.
56. Dennis A, Castro J. Transthoracic echocardiography in women with treated severe preeclampsia. Anaesthesia. 2014;69:436–44.
57. Chappell L, Duckworth S, Seed P, Griffin M, Myers J, Mackillop L, et al. Diagnostic accuracy of placental growth factor in women with suspected preeclampsia. Circulation. 2013;128:2121–31.

Anesthesia for the Pregnant Diabetic Patient

3

Emine Aysu Salviz

3.1 Introduction

3.1.1 Diabetes Mellitus Definition, Epidemiology, and Classification

Diabetes mellitus (DM) is a group of metabolic disorders characterized by hyperglycemia. Type 1 DM (juvenile or insulin-dependent autoimmune disorder) is an immunologic destruction of the pancreas, causing deficiency in insulin secretion. Type 2 DM (adult-onset or noninsulin-dependent disorder) results from the combination of an inadequate insulin secretion, an increased resistance of the pancreatic cells to insulin action, and an excessive or inappropriate glucagon secretion. It accounts for 90–95% of all diabetic patients, and it has a prevalence of 6.8–8.2% in the general adult population in the USA. Its incidence has been increasing steadily, mostly because of continuing epidemic of obesity [1–5]. This has led to more Type 2 DM in women of childbearing age, with an increase in the number of parturients without previous diagnosis [6].

For a long time, gestational diabetes mellitus (GDM) was defined as any degree of carbohydrate intolerance that had first been diagnosed during pregnancy, regardless of whether the condition may have begun before the pregnancy or persisted after the pregnancy [7]. However, parturients diagnosed with DM in the first trimester should be classified as having pre-existing Type 2 DM or, rarely, Type 1 DM. Currently, parturients, who are unable to produce enough insulin to compensate insulin resistance at the receptor and postreceptor levels, are diagnosed with GDM. GDM is explained as DM that is first diagnosed in the second or third trimester of pregnancy which is not clearly either pre-existing Type 1 or Type 2 DM [1, 4].

E. A. Salviz
Istanbul University, Istanbul Faculty of Medicine, Department of Anesthesiology and Intensive Care, Istanbul, Turkey

© Springer International Publishing AG, part of Springer Nature 2018
B. Gunaydin, S. Ismail (eds.), *Obstetric Anesthesia for Co-morbid Conditions*,
https://doi.org/10.1007/978-3-319-93163-0_3

Table 3.1 White's classification system of diabetes mellitus during pregnancy class definition [8, 9]

A_1	GDM that is diet controlled
A_2	GDM that requires insulin
B	Pre-existing DM with onset >age 20 and duration <10 years without complications
C	Pre-existing DM with onset between ages 10 and 19 or duration of ages 10–19 without complications
D	Pre-existing DM with onset age <10 or duration >20 years. Without complications
F	Pre-existing DM complicated by nephropathy
R	Pre-existing DM complicated by proliferative retinopathy
T	Pre-existing DM and status/post kidney transplant
H	Pre-existing DM complicated by ischemic heart disease

GDM gestational diabetes mellitus, *DM* diabetes mellitus

The GDM prevalence varies from 1.4% to 14% (usually between 2% and 5%) in the USA, and the amount varies in direct proportion to the prevalence of Type 2 DM [5].

A classification system was proposed for DM in pregnancy, to emphasize the relationship between the duration of DM, complications of DM, and poor fetal outcome, in 1949 (Table 3.1) [8]. In the 1950s, fetal survival rates were determined as 100% for class A, 67% for class B, 48% for class C, 32% for class D, and 3% class F [9].

3.2 Pathophysiology

The women are carbohydrate-intolerant during pregnancy. Glucose fasting levels are decreased, and serum levels following a meal or glucose load are increased compared to the nonpregnant state. In all pregnancies, circulating concentrations of insulin antagonists such as cortisol, prolactin, human placental lactogen (HPL) and leptin rise and insulin resistance increases as the pregnancy advances. This resistance results in increased insulin demand in pregnant women with pre-existing DM or predisposes some parturients to develop GDM. All these changes affect fetal placental unit growth and rapidly become reversed after delivery. This "facilitated anabolism" reveals appropriate changes in carbohydrate, amino acid, and lipid metabolism and ensures adequate nutrients for the developing fetus [1, 4].

Deficient β-cell reserve, as in any type of DM, would result in the abnormal carbohydrate, protein, and fat metabolism adaptation. Insulin is required to compensate increasing caloric needs, increasing adiposity, decreasing exercise, and increasing anti-insulin hormones in Type 1 DM. The required insulin dose to maintain normoglycemia and prevent maternal ketosis may increase up to threefold during pregnancy in Type 1 DM. Parturients with Type 2 DM may also need insulin treatment at high doses, because of physical inactivity and obesity [10, 11].

3.3 Clinical Presentation and Diagnosis of Gestational Diabetes Mellitus

Advanced maternal age; obesity (especially central obesity, dyslipidemia with high triglycerides, and/or low HDL cholesterol); glycosuria; family history of Type 2 DM, GDM, and polycystic ovarian syndrome; and/or history of fetal malformation or macrosomia, prior stillbirth, and neonatal death are the factors leading up to GDM. On the other hand, clinical presentation of DM and GDM can be associated with acute (diabetic ketoacidosis, hyperglycemic nonketotic state, and hypoglycemia) and chronic (macrovascular atherosclerosis, coronary, cerebrovascular, and peripheral vascular; microvascular, retinopathy and nephropathy; neuropathy, autonomic and somatic) complications [12].

Inadequate insulin therapy and infection are the most common triggering factors for both diabetic ketoacidosis (DKA) and hyperglycemic nonketotic state (HNS) [13]. DKA usually occurs in patients with Type 1 DM and may sometimes be the first clinical sign of it during pregnancy [14, 15]. The incidence of DKA is 1–2% in parturients with DM [16, 17]. DKA results from decreased uptake of glucose by tissues and greater use of free fatty acids instead and is associated with metabolic acidosis, hyperglycemia, and dehydration secondary to osmotic diuresis. Signs and symptoms such as nausea and vomiting, weakness, tachypnea, hypotension, tachycardia, stupor, and acetone on the breath frequently occur, and its diagnosis depends on the laboratory findings of hyperglycemia, ketosis, and acidosis [13, 18]. The HNS usually occurs in patients with Type 2 DM. Laboratory findings are hyperglycemia (blood glucose >600 mg/dL), hyperosmolarity (>320 mOsm/kg), and moderate azotemia (blood urea nitrogen >60 mg/dL), without ketonemia or significant acidosis.

Hypoglycemia results from an imbalance between DM medical therapy and available metabolic fuels. It is a continuing health threat for patients with both Type 1 DM and Type 2 DM [13]. The risk of hypoglycemia in parturients with Type 1 DM increases with tight glucose control [19–21]. Its rate is 3–15 times higher than the nonpregnant patients with Type 1 DM, and 80–84% of severe hypoglycemia episodes occur before 20 weeks of gestation [19, 20, 22, 23]. In contrast, it was demonstrated in a study that parturients with pre-existing Type 2 DM or GDM requiring insulin therapy experienced no episodes of severe hypoglycemia [22]. Hypoglycemia has three levels of classification, and the International Hypoglycaemia Study Group reported their related recommendations regarding severity of hypoglycemia:

Level 1: glucose level ≥ 70 mg/dL (3.9 mmol/L), often related to symptomatic hypoglycemia and important for dose adjustment of glucose-lowering drugs
Level 2: glucose level < 54 mg/dL (3.0 mmol/L), clinically significant
Level 3: severe, no specific glucose threshold, and may be associated with severe cognitive impairment requiring assistance [24, 25]

The prevalence of complications generally increases with the obesity, hypertension, and duration of DM [26–30]. The evidence of obesity management is strong and consistent that it can delay the progression from prediabetes to Type 2 DM and may be also beneficial in the treatment of Type 2 DM [26, 27, 31–34]. The Diabetes Control and Complications Trial including patients with Type 1 DM demonstrated a positive relationship between tight glucose control and a lowered incidence or rate of progression of diabetic chronic complications (retinopathy, nephropathy, neuropathy, coronary atherosclerosis, cardiomyopathy) [35, 36]. Another study including patients with Type 2 DM—the UK Prospective Diabetes Study (UKPDS)—showed that the tight glucose control reduced the incidence of microvascular complications but not macrovascular complications or patient mortality. In parturients with pre-existing Type 1 DM, systolic and diastolic blood pressures are higher, and these have three times more gestational hypertension risk than nondiabetic patients [37, 38]. In addition, the risk of preeclampsia is also directly proportional to the severity of DM [39]. In patients with Type 2 DM and hypertension, antihypertensive therapy lowered the incidence of both macrovascular complications and mortality [28].

The Hyperglycemia and Adverse Pregnancy Outcome (HAPO) study, which is a multicentral trial including more than 23,000 parturients, demonstrated that adverse maternal, fetal, and neonatal risks were continuously increased as a function of maternal glycemia at 24–28 weeks, even within ranges previously considered normal for pregnancy [40]. Although not all adverse outcomes are of equal clinical importance, these results showed that GDM carries risks for both the mother and the neonate and deserve careful reconsideration of the risk assessment, screening, and diagnostic criteria for GDM.

The American Diabetes Association recommended an approach for screening and diagnosis of GDM in 2008, which divides parturients into three GDM risk categories on the basis of history: (1) low risk, (2) very high risk, and (3) higher than low risk. As low-risk patients do not require any testing, very high-risk patients undergo standard nonpregnant testing (Table 3.2), and higher-than-low-risk category parturients undergo one of the two different screening and diagnosis approaches (one- or two-step strategies) at 24–28 weeks of gestation (Table 3.3) [1, 29, 41].

One-Step Strategy Based on a recommendation of the International Association of Diabetes and Pregnancy Study Groups (IADPSG), in the 2011 Standards of Care, the ADA recommended that all parturients not known to have prior DM undergo a 75 g oral glucose tolerance test (OGTT) at 24–28 weeks of gestation (Table 3.3) [1, 42, 43]. This one-step strategy was anticipated to significantly increase the incidence of GDM (from 5–6% to 15–20%), primarily because only one abnormal value became enough to make the diagnosis. Although the ADA recognized that the anticipated increase in the incidence of GDM would have the potential to "medicalize" pregnancies previously categorized as "normal", they still recommended these diagnostic criteria changes with the intent of optimizing gestational outcomes, because these were the only ones based on pregnancy outcomes.

Table 3.2 Risk assessment at the first prenatal visit for gestational diabetes mellitus [1, 29, 41]

Low-risk
The parturients at low-risk status must meet all of the following criteria and do not require screening
Criteria for low-risk status:
• Age < 25 years
• Weight normal before pregnancy
• Member of an ethnic group with a low prevalence of DM
• No known DM in first-degree relatives
• No history of abnormal glucose tolerance
• No history of poor obstetric outcome
Very high-risk
The parturients at very high-risk status should be screened with *standard DM diagnostic testing* as soon as pregnancy is confirmed
Criteria for very-high-risk status:
• Severe obesity
• Prior history of GDM or delivery of large-for-gestational-age infant
• Presence of glycosuria
• Diagnosis of polycystic ovarian syndrome
• Strong family history of type 2 DM
Standard DM diagnostic testing:
• Fasting plasma glucose (FPG) ≥126 mg/dL (7.0 mmol/L) Fasting is defined as no caloric intake for at least 8 h[a]
OR
• 2-h plasma glucose (PG) ≥200 mg/dL (11.1 mmol/L) during an OGTT The test should be performed by using a glucose load containing the equivalent of 75 g anhydrous glucose dissolved in water[a]
OR
• HbA1c ≥ 6.5% (48 mmol/mol) (normal range is 4.1–5.9%) The test should be performed in a laboratory (using a method that is NGSP certified and standardized to the DCCT assay)[a]
OR
• A random plasma glucose ≥200 mg/dL (11.1 mmol/L) in a patient with classic symptoms of hyperglycemia or hyperglycemic crisis

DM diabetes mellitus, *GDM* gestational diabetes mellitus
[a]In the absence of unequivocal hyperglycemia, results should be confirmed by repeat testing

Two-Step Strategy The National Institutes of Health (NIH) including representatives from obstetrics/gynecology, maternal-fetal medicine, pediatrics, diabetes research, biostatistics, and other related fields convened a consensus development conference to consider diagnostic criteria of GDM. The panel recommended a two-step strategy for screening that used a 1-h 50 g glucose load test (GLT) followed by a 3-h 100 g OGTT for the ones screened positive (Table 3.3) [1, 44].

Data comparing one-step versus two-step strategies have been conflicting to date [45, 46]. The American College of Obstetricians and Gynecologists (ACOG)

Table 3.3 Screening and diagnosis for gestational diabetes mellitus [1, 47–49]

One-step strategy		
Plasma glucose level measurements at 24–28 weeks of gestation in women, not previously diagnosed with overt DM		
Perform a 75 g OGTT in the morning after an overnight fasting of at least 8 h.		
GDM is diagnosed when any of the following plasma glucose values are met or exceeded:		
Fasting	92 mg/dL (5.1 mmol/L)	
1-h	180 mg/dL (10.0 mmol/L)	
2-h	153 mg/dL (8.5 mmol/L)	

Two-step strategy		
Step 1: Plasma glucose level measurements at 24–28 weeks of gestation in women, not previously diagnosed with overt DM.		
Perform a 50 g GLT (nonfasting), with plasma glucose measurement at 1 h		
If the plasma glucose level measured 1 h after the load is ≥130 mg/dL (7.2 mmol/L), 135 mg/dL (7.5 mmol/L) or 140 mg/dLᵃ (7.8 mmol/L), proceed to a 100 g OGTT		

Step 2: The 100 g OGTT should be performed when the patient is fasting
GDM is diagnosed if at least two of the following four plasma glucose levels are met or exceeded:

	Carpenter/Coustan (48)	NDDG §(49)
Fasting	95 mg/dL (5.3 mmol/L)	105 mg/dL (5.8 mmol/L)
1-h	180 mg/dL (10.0 mmol/L)	190 mg/dL (10.6 mmol/L)
2-h	155 mg/dL (8.6 mmol/L)	165 mg/dL (9.2 mmol/L)
3-h	140 mg/dL (7.8 mmol/L)	145 mg/dL (8.0 mmol/L)

GDM: gestational diabetes mellitus
DM: diabetes mellitus
OGTT: oral glucose tolerance test
GLT: glucose load test
*The American College of Obstetricians and Gynecologists (ACOG) (47) recommends either 135 mg/dL (7.5 mmol/L) or 140 mg/dL (7.8 mmol/L). §NDDG, National Diabetes Data Group.

updated its guidelines supporting the two-step approach in 2013 and recommended either of two sets of diagnostic thresholds for the 3-h 100 g OGTT [47–49]. GDM-diagnosed pregnancies per the IADPSG criteria, but not recognized as such, have comparable outcomes to GDM-diagnosed pregnancies by the more rigid two-step criteria [50, 51]. As the one-step strategy has been adopted internationally and pregnancy outcomes were improved with cost savings, one-step strategy seems to become the preferred approach [52].

3.4 Interaction of Diabetes Mellitus with Pregnancy

3.4.1 The Effect of Pregnancy on Diabetes Mellitus [4, 12]

1. Insulin antagonist hormones such as HPL, placental growth hormone (GH), cortisol, and progesterone rise and cause progressive resistance to insulin.
2. Pancreatic islet cell mass and glucose sensitivity increase secondary to progesterone and lactogenic hormone stimuli in the endocrine pancreas [53, 54].

3. Maternal adipokines play a role in insulin resistance and facilitate the supply of maternal fuels for the fetus.
4. In parturients with GDM, peripheral insulin resistance cannot be sufficiently compensated. GDM can be seen as a preclinical state of glucose intolerance in some patients, which is not detectable before pregnancy.
5. In parturients with pre-existing DM, insulin requirements generally increase progressively during pregnancy [55]. However, maternal overnight insulin requirements decrease near term, because the growing fetus gets maternal fuels [56].
6. In parturients without DM, endogenous insulin secretion can be affected by several factors, and only one of them is plasma glucose concentration. During painful labor of these patients, glucose production and utilization are higher; however, plasma insulin concentrations increase briefly during the third stage of labor and immediately postpartum. This finding shows that glucose use during labor is largely independent of insulin whether the patient is with or without analgesia [57, 58].
7. In parturients with Type 1 DM, insulin requirements decrease with the onset of the first stage and increase during the second stage of labor. The use of epidural analgesia or oxytocin does not affect exogenous insulin requirements during the first two stages of labor [59, 60]. Insulin requirements decrease markedly after delivery for at least several days and then gradually return to prepregnancy levels within several weeks of delivery [56, 61, 62].

Several complications including both the mother and the fetus occur in these patients during pregnancy and delivery, and even after delivery. This should be kept in mind that both Type 1 and Type 2 DM confer significantly greater maternal and fetal risk than GDM [4, 63].

3.4.2 The Effect of Diabetes Mellitus on Parturient [4, 12]

1. The parturients with GDM are at increased risk for Type 2 DM later in life.
2. The parturients with pre-existing DM require more insulin during pregnancy.
3. The parturients with Type 1 DM are at significant risk for hypoglycemia development, especially during early pregnancy, despite increased insulin requirements.
4. The relative insulin resistance in parturients with Type 1 DM is associated with enhanced lipolysis and ketogenesis; and DKA can occur at significantly lower glucose levels (200–250 mg/dL) than is typically associated with DKA in nonpregnant patients. It most commonly occurs in the second and third trimesters and may be triggered by the infection and the administration of β-adrenergic drugs for tocolysis and glucocorticoids for fetal lung maturation.
5. The incidence of preeclampsia is increased in parturients with any type of DM.
6. Polyhydramnios is more common in parturients with DM.

3.4.3   The Effect of Diabetes Mellitus on Fetus [4, 12]

1. DM in pregnancy may increase the risk of obesity and Type 2 DM in offspring later in life.
2. Non-reassuring fetal heart rate patterns may also be associated with the presence of DKA. Fortunately, these patterns usually resolve once the maternal metabolic abnormalities have been corrected. Therefore, fetal intervention and/ or preterm delivery should be avoided, unless the heart rate abnormalities persist after DKA treatment.
3. An increased incidence of abnormal fetal heart rate patterns may lead to the reduction in uteroplacental perfusion.
4. Uteroplacental perfusion is decreased by 35–45% in patients with DM compared to patients without DM. Blood flow may also decrease in women with well-controlled GDM.
5. The intrauterine fetal death/spontaneous abortion incidence is increased in parturients with DM. Reduced uteroplacental perfusion is thought to be a significant contributing factor. Nevertheless, aggressive antenatal fetal surveillance in parturients with DM has been successful in decreasing the number of intrauterine fetal deaths.
6. The risk of congenital anomalies is increased in parturients with pre-existing DM and is now the leading cause of perinatal mortality in diabetic pregnancies [64]. The incidence of major malformations is 8.5–10%, which is a two- to sixfold increase compared to patients without DM. The most common complications are cardiovascular (transposition of great vessels, ventricular septal defect, situs inversus, single ventricle, hypoplastic left ventricle) and central nervous system (anencephaly, encephalocele, meningomyelocele, spina bifida, holoprosencephaly) malformations. Skeletal (caudal regression), renal (agenesis, multicystic dysplasia), gastrointestinal (anal or rectal atresia, small left colon), and pulmonary (hypoplasia) complications can also be seen. Although the etiology is usually multifactorial, the most important factor seems to be the poor glucose control during organogenesis. Therefore, initiation of tight glycemic control during the preconception period decreases the incidence of congenital anomalies.
7. Fetal macrosomia, large for gestational age, is also common in parturients with any type of DM. Pre-existing DM results in fetal macrosomia in 9–25% of parturients—a four- to sixfold higher rate than patients without DM. The risks of shoulder dystocia and birth injury are increased in these macrosomic fetuses during vaginal delivery. Therefore, Cesarean delivery is more likely performed.
8. Neonatal hypoglycemia occurs in 5–12% of parturients with pre-existing DM and GDM [65]. This is a 6- to 16-fold increase compared to infants of nondiabetic mothers. The fetal hyperinsulinemia that arises in response to maternal hyperglycemia is believed to be the reason.
9. DM was thought to be as one of the independent risk factors for fetal lung immaturity and infant respiratory distress syndrome (RDS), especially in

infants whose mothers had poor glycemic control during pregnancy. Then, it was understood that RDS is more common among newborns, who are delivered preterm or are surgically delivered. Later studies have not demonstrated a significant difference in the incidence of neonatal RSD between diabetic and non-diabetic pregnancies [65–67].

10. Intrauterine or neonatal death during pregnancy, neonatal hyperbilirubinemia, glucose intolerance, and cognitive impairment are also DM-related complications.

11. Offsprings of mothers with DM are at increased risk for development of DM because of a combination of genetic and intrauterine environmental factors. Studies of monozygotic human twins have demonstrated that genetic factors have a greater role in Type 2 DM than in Type 1 DM (100% vs 20–50% concordance, respectively) [68]. Moreover, fathers with Type 1 DM are five times more likely than mothers to have a child with Type 1 DM.

3.5 Obstetric Management

Optimal glycemic control is the major focus at each phase of obstetric care of parturients with DM, as it minimizes fetal structural malformations. In the preconception period, the women of childbearing age with DM should be counseled about the importance of tight glycemic control and prevention of complications and given appropriate treatment to avoid hyperglycemia. They should be informed that the elevations in HbA1c during the first 10 weeks of pregnancy are directly proportional to increased risk of diabetic embryopathy, anencephaly, microcephaly, congenital heart disease, and caudal regression. The optimal glycemic control prior to conception and during pregnancy (HbA1c < 6–6.5% (42–48 mmol/mol)) is associated with the lowest risk of congenital anomalies [69–74].

During early pregnancy, parturients with Type 1 DM are sensitive to insulin, and their glucose levels and insulin requirements are lower. Later on, during the second and third trimesters, this situation rapidly reverses as insulin resistance increases and insulin requirement progressively increases. In parturients with normal pancreatic function, insulin production is sufficient to meet the challenge of this insulin resistance and to maintain normal glucose levels. Nevertheless, in women with pre-existing DM and GDM, hyperglycemia occurs if treatment with diet, exercise, and insulin therapy is not appropriate [1]. Self-monitoring of glucose measurements with a reflectance meter and transdermal or subcutaneous glucose monitoring systems is performed several times each day during pregnancy. In order to maintain adequate glycemic control, insulin therapy is frequently changed with progressively increasing requirements throughout pregnancy. The treatment regimen may include three to four insulin injections per day or continuous subcutaneous insulin pump [4].

Fasting, preprandial and postprandial monitoring of blood glucose are recommended to achieve metabolic control in parturients with DM. Preprandial monitoring is recommended for patients with pre-existing DM using insulin pumps or basal bolus therapy, and postprandial monitoring is associated with better glycemic control and lower risk of preeclampsia [75–77].

The American College of Obstetricians and Gynecologists [47] and the ADA (1) recommended the similar following blood glucose target values for women with Type 1 DM, Type 2 DM, or GDM:

- Fasting ≤95 mg/dL (5.3 mmol/L)
- 1-h postprandial ≤140 mg/dL (7.8 mmol/L) or 2-h postprandial ≤120 mg/dL (6.7 mmol/L)

These are optimal control values if they can be achieved safely. If patients cannot achieve these targets without significant hypoglycemia, the ADA suggests less strict targets based on clinical experience and individualization of care [1].

Treatment of GDM begins with medical nutrition therapy, physical activity, and weight control. Studies recommend that 70–85% of women diagnosed with GDM can control their GDM with lifestyle modification alone, depending on the population [1]. Early initiation of pharmacologic treatment may be needed for the women with greater initial degrees of hyperglycemia, and it has been demonstrated to improve perinatal outcomes [78]. Insulin is the first-line agent recommended for treatment of GDM in the USA and is the preferred agent for management of both Type 1 and Type 2 DM in pregnancy. Previously, oral antidiabetic agents were not used extensively in pregnancy, because of concerns about potential teratogenicity and fetal hyperinsulinemia. In current practice, many women with GDM are treated with glyburide, glipizide, or metformin [79, 80]. The short-term safety and efficacy of metformin (lowers the risk of neonatal hypoglycemia and maternal weight gain and however may increase the risk of prematurity) and glyburide (associated with a higher rate of neonatal hypoglycemia and macrosomia) have also been shown. However, long-term safety data are not available [1, 81–84].

The complications of DM can also occur in parturients, and their management is usually similar to those for nonpregnant patients [4]:

1. DKA: Frequent arterial blood gas assessments, serum glucose, and electrolyte measurements are essential. Intensive intravenous hydration with normal saline is required because of volume depletion. Intravenous insulin treatment is administered to control glucose levels. An intravenous potassium infusion (10–20 mEq/h) should be initiated, if the serum potassium level is reduced. Bicarbonate is administered when the patients have severe acidosis (pH < 7.1).
2. Fetal heart rate abnormalities: Maneuvers to optimize the fetal status include left uterine displacement and supplemental oxygen. Fetal condition usually improves with suitable medical therapy of the mother without any intervention.
3. Intrauterine fetal death: Routine antenatal fetal surveillance is important during the third trimester. At 28–32 weeks of gestation, most obstetricians begin non-stress tests twice weekly [55, 85, 86]. A nonreactive test will lead to performance of a contraction stress test or a fetal biophysical profile to evaluate fetal status. If fetal testing is reassuring, delivery can be delayed until after 38 weeks of gestation [55, 85]. If fetal testing is abnormal and amniotic fluid analysis shows fetal pulmonary maturity, the fetus should be delivered as soon as possible. In the

abnormal fetal testing and immature fetal lungs confirmed by amniotic fluid analysis, timing of delivery decisions is more difficult. Both the timing and the route of delivery are of great importance in parturients with DM, because the goal of obstetricians is to deliver an infant with mature lungs while avoiding an intrauterine fetal death in pregnancy.

4. Fetal macrosomia: The decision of delivery method requires consideration of estimated fetal weight and condition, cervical dilation and effacement, and previous obstetric history. Some obstetricians choose elective induction of labor at 38–40 weeks of gestation for not only avoiding complication of late stillbirth but also the associated risks with fetal macrosomia including shoulder dystocia and birth injury. The others often prefer elective Cesarean delivery in diabetic parturients for similar reasons.

3.6   Anesthetic Management

There have been few studies regarding anesthetic management of parturients with DM. Clinical decisions of these patients are usually guided by logical extensions of the studies of nonpregnant patients with DM and parturients without DM.

The anesthesiologist should focus on the glycemic control in parturients with DM in addition to the usual preanesthetic evaluation including history and physical examination. In women with pre-existing disease, DM-related acute and chronic complications should be determined. Possible complications include cardiac, vascular, and renal involvements as well as autonomic neuropathy and dysfunction. Parturients with DM have additional risks associated with autonomic neuropathy such as hypertension, orthostatic hypotension, painless myocardial infarction, decreased heart rate variability, decreased response to some medications (atropine and propranolol), resting tachycardia, neurogenic atonic bladder, decreased cough reflex threshold, and increased incidence of obstructive sleep apnea and gastroparesis. In patients with long-standing DM, ischemic heart disease or autonomic dysfunction can be identified by an electrocardiogram (ECG). In the anesthetic management of these patients, major concerns include hypotension requiring aggressive hydration and vasopressors, and aspiration [4, 87, 88].

On the other hand, the women with Type 1 DM should be screened for evidence of the "stiff joint" syndrome by looking for the "prayer sign," despite its rarity. This syndrome may be associated with the limited movement of atlanto-occipital joint, which may lead to difficult direct laryngoscopy and intubation [4, 12].

3.6.1   Management and Analgesia for Labor and Vaginal Delivery

Epidural analgesia is beneficial for labor pain management in patients with DM. It provides excellent analgesia for labor itself, instrumentally assists delivery and episiotomy, attenuates the physiologic response to pain, and results in decreased maternal plasma catecholamine concentrations.

As uteroplacental blood flow is reduced in parturients with DM, the decrease in catecholamine levels associated with neuraxial analgesia would also lead to improved uteroplacental perfusion. Additionally, as catecholamines are insulin antagonist hormones that oppose insulin activity, the theory is that epidural labor analgesia improves glucose control during labor and delivery. This improvement indirectly increases placental blood flow and reduces the maternal lactic acid production and hence fetal acidosis.

Certain precautions should be taken into consideration when administering epidural analgesia to parturients with DM. Patients with pre-existing DM and autonomic neuropathy are especially prone to hypotension during the initiation of sympathetic blockade. Therefore, aggressive volume expansion with a non-dextrose-containing solution and slow dosing of the epidural catheter to accomplish a slower onset of sympathetic blockade during epidural analgesia should be emphasized. Otherwise, hypotension related to epidural analgesia may lead to fetal compromise because of the reduction in uteroplacental perfusion associated with DM. If hypotension occurs, it should be treated promptly and aggressively with ephedrine. Uteroplacental blood flow reduction by 35–45% in parturients with DM increases the risk for fetal distress during labor and necessitates an urgent Cesarean delivery. Hence, epidural analgesia is usually preferable to combined spinal-epidural (CSE) analgesia in many parturients with DM, especially in the ones with non-reassuring fetal heart rate tracings [4, 88].

3.6.2   Anesthesia for Cesarean Delivery

Cesarean delivery is more likely in patients with DM compared to the healthy ones, and regional anesthesia is generally preferred over general anesthesia throughout all parturients. Previously, an association was found between spinal-epidural anesthesia for Cesarean delivery and umbilical cord-neonatal acidosis in parturients with DM. However, later on, the reasons for the acidosis were determined to be the dextrose-containing fluids (5% dextrose), maternal hyperglycemia, and hypotension [4, 89, 90]. When providing epidural or spinal anesthesia in a parturient with DM, adequate hydration with a non-dextrose-containing solution should be accomplished, maternal glycemic control should be satisfactory, and hypotension should be treated promptly and aggressively with vasopressors to avoid neonatal acidosis [91, 92]. To date, the comparison of spinal and epidural anesthesia techniques for Cesarean delivery in parturients with DM has not been made in terms of the maternal or neonatal effects. However, when the Cesarean delivery is elective and there is adequate time to initiate epidural anesthesia, it may be preferable. Epidural anesthesia is also of choice when a parturient with DM has a chronic uteroplacental insufficiency. Its slower onset of sympathetic blockade could decrease the risk of anesthesia-induced hypotension/hemodynamic alterations, and the avoidance of hypotension is important to ensure fetal well-being in patients with DM. When the

Cesarean delivery is urgent and does not allow time for epidural block, spinal anesthesia is usually preferred over general anesthesia because of its safety profile, despite its hypotension risk. If hypotension occurs, it can quickly be treated with a vasopressor to avoid fetal compromise [4].

Although spinal and epidural anesthesia techniques are more commonly used, we should keep in mind that patients with DM are more vulnerable to neurologic injury for the reasons including susceptibility to infection, having vascular diseases and peripheral neuropathy. These patients are at increased risk for spontaneous or catheter-associated epidural abscess, anterior spinal artery syndrome, and worsening of neuropathy [93–97]. On the other hand, after epidural anesthesia for Cesarean delivery, an increased incidence of neonatal hypoglycemia was observed in patients with pre-existing DM. In this study, maternal glycemic control was fair (mean fasting plasma glucose (FPG) was 127 mg/dL), a non-dextrose-containing solution was used for hydration, and intravenous insulin therapy was adjusted on the basis of frequent blood glucose determinations. This illustrates the neonate's vulnerability to hypoglycemia despite meticulous anesthesia care at the time of delivery [92].

Parturients with DM undergo general anesthesia either because of urgent Cesarean delivery (especially if an epidural catheter has not been placed for labor analgesia) or contraindications that preclude neuraxial anesthesia. The same principles are valid to provide general anesthesia for any parturient when caring for women with DM. General anesthesia can sometimes be problematic because of limited atlanto-occipital joint extension, increased hemodynamic response to intubation, and impaired insulin antagonist hormone responses to hypoglycemia and gastroparesis [98, 99]. No published data has been published indicating the effects of DM on the pharmacokinetics and pharmacodynamics of anesthetic agents in parturients. However, in nonpregnant women, DM was found to be associated with delayed onset of muscle relaxation with tubocurarine and prolonged blockade with vecuronium [100, 101].

Some special considerations exist in patients with pre-existing DM, because these are at risk for autonomic neuropathy. The anesthesiologist should be prepared for more frequent and severe hypotension attacks in these parturients. Left uterine displacement and intravenous hydration are the methods used preoperatively and intraoperatively to prevent hypotension. If prompt hypotension occurs, aggressive therapy is necessary. It was shown that autonomic dysfunction was associated with increased vasopressor requirements during general anesthesia in nonpregnant patients with DM [87]. In addition, the increased risk of aspiration secondary to gastroparesis can also be minimized by the administration of metoclopramide.

Finally, the "prayer sign" occurs in patients with long-standing, pre-existing DM and is associated with nonfamilial short stature, joint contractures, tight skin, limited atlanto-occipital joint movement, and noncompliant epidural space [12, 93, 102]. Therefore, the anesthesiologist should carefully evaluate the parturients with DM for the risk of difficulty in direct laryngoscopy, intubation, and requirement for awake intubation [4, 12].

3.7   Postpartum Management

In the postpartum period, insulin requirements usually decrease significantly, and after labor and delivery, glycemic control does not need to be as tight as before. If an insulin infusion is utilized during labor, it should not be continued after delivery to avoid maternal hypoglycemia [4].

Most patients with GDM return to normal glucose tolerance after delivery but remain at increased risk for Type 2 DM and the recurrence of GDM later in life [103]. The prevalence of postpartum DM has been reported as 2.4% in the UK, and the recurrence rate for GDM is 35–70% [104, 105].

As GDM may represent pre-existing undiagnosed Type 1 or Type 2 DM, women with GDM should be tested for persistent DM or prediabetes at 4–12 weeks of postpartum with a 75 g OGTT using nonpregnancy criteria. The OGTT is recommended over HbA1c at that time point, because HbA1c may be persistently lowered by the increased red blood cell turnover related to pregnancy or blood loss at delivery. The OGTT is also more sensitive at detecting glucose intolerance, including both prediabetes and DM [1].

Women at reproductive age with prediabetes may develop Type 2 DM during their next pregnancy and will need evaluation. As GDM is associated with increased maternal risk for DM, although the 4–12 weeks of 75 g OGTT is normal, women should be tested every 1–3 years thereafter. The frequency of testing depends on other risk factors including family history, prepregnancy body mass index, and insulin- or oral glucose-lowering medication requirement during pregnancy. The evaluation may be continued with any recommended glycemic test including HbA1c, FPG, or 75 g OGTT using nonpregnant thresholds [1].

Key Learning Points
- Gestational DM (GDM) is described as DM that is first diagnosed in the second or third trimester of pregnancy, which is not clearly either pre-existing Type 1 or Type 2 DM.
- Clinical presentation of DM and GDM can be associated with acute (diabetic ketoacidosis, hyperglycemic nonketotic state, and hypoglycemia) and chronic (macrovascular atherosclerosis, coronary, cerebrovascular, and peripheral vascular; microvascular, retinopathy and nephropathy; neuropathy, autonomic and somatic) complications.
- Optimal glycemic control is the major focus at each phase of obstetric care of parturients with DM, as it minimizes fetal structural malformations. Treatment of GDM begins with medical nutrition therapy, physical activity, and weight control. Insulin, glyburide, glipizide, and metformin are the other possible medical therapy options.
- During preanesthetic evaluation, anesthesiologist should focus on the glycemic control in parturients with DM in addition to routine history and physical examination. In women with pre-existing disease, DM-related

acute and chronic complications including cardiac, vascular, and renal involvements as well as autonomic neuropathy and dysfunction should be determined. These patients may have additional risks associated with autonomic neuropathy such as hypertension, orthostatic hypotension, painless myocardial infarction, decreased heart rate variability, decreased response to some medications (atropine and propranolol), resting tachycardia, neurogenic atonic bladder, decreased cough reflex threshold, and increased incidence of obstructive sleep apnea and gastroparesis. The women with Type 1 DM may present with "stiff joint" syndrome, and this syndrome is associated with the limited movement of atlanto-occipital joint, which may lead to difficult direct laryngoscopy and intubation

- For labor pain management, epidural technique provides excellent analgesia in parturients with DM, especially if instrumentally assisted delivery and episiotomy are required. Additionally, the decrease in catecholamine levels associated with neuraxial analgesia leads to improved uteroplacental perfusion.

- Certain precautions should be taken into consideration when administering epidural analgesia to parturients with DM. Patients with pre-existing DM and autonomic neuropathy are especially prone to hypotension during the initiation of sympathetic blockade. Therefore, aggressive volume expansion with a non-dextrose-containing solution and slow dosing of the epidural catheter to accomplish a slower onset of sympathetic blockade should be emphasized.

- Cesarean delivery is more likely in patients with DM compared to the healthy ones, and regional anesthesia is generally preferred over general anesthesia throughout all parturients. During epidural or spinal anesthesia performance in a parturient with DM, adequate hydration with a non-dextrose-containing solution should be accomplished, maternal glycemic control should be satisfactory, and hypotension should be treated promptly and aggressively with vasopressors to avoid neonatal acidosis.

- When the Cesarean delivery is elective and there is adequate time, epidural anesthesia is a preferable option with its slower onset of sympathetic blockade. However, if the Cesarean delivery is urgent and does not allow time for epidural block, spinal anesthesia would usually be preferred over general anesthesia because of its safety profile, despite its hypotension risk.

- Parturients with DM undergo general anesthesia either because of urgent Cesarean delivery (especially if an epidural catheter has not been placed for labor analgesia) or contraindications that preclude neuraxial anesthesia. General anesthesia can sometimes be problematic because of limited atlanto-occipital joint extension, increased hemodynamic response to intubation, and impaired insulin antagonist hormone responses to hypoglycemia and gastroparesis.

References

1. American Diabetes Association. Standards of medical care in diabetes-2017. Diabetes Care. 2017;40(Suppl1):S1–135.
2. Ioannou GN, Bryson CL, Boyko EJ. Prevalence and trends of insulin resistance, impaired fasting glucose, and diabetes. J Diabetes Complicat. 2007;21(6):363–70.
3. Bays HE, Bazata DD, Clark NG, Gavin JR 3rd, Green AJ, Lewis SJ, et al. Prevalence of self-reported diagnosis of diabetes mellitus and associated risk factors in a national survey in the US population: SHIELD (study to help improve early evaluation and management of risk factors leading to diabetes). BMC Public Health. 2007;7:277.
4. Fragneto RY. The high-risk obstetric patient. In: Braveman F, editor. Obstetric and gynecologic anesthesia. The requisites in anesthesiology. 1st ed. Philadelphia: Elsevier; 2006. p. 79–113.
5. ACOG Practice Bulletin. Clinical management guidelines for obstetrician-gynecologists. Number 30. Obstet Gynecol. 2001;98(3):525–38.
6. Lawrence JM, Contreras R, Chen W, Sacks DA. Trends in the prevalence of preexisting diabetes and gestational diabetes mellitus among a racially/ethnically diverse population of pregnant women, 1999–2005. Diabetes Care. 2008;31(5):899–904.
7. Expert Committee on the Diagnosis and Classification of Diabetes Mellitus. Report of the expert committee on the diagnosis and classification of diabetes mellitus. Diabetes Care. 1997;20(7):1183–97.
8. White P. Pregnancy complicating diabetes. Am J Med. 1949;7(5):609–16.
9. White P. Classification of obstetric diabetes. Am J Obstet Gynecol. 1978;130(2):228–30.
10. Kapoor N, Sankaran S, Hyer S, Shehata H. Diabetes in pregnancy: a review of current evidence. Curr Opin Obstet Gynecol. 2007;19(6):586–90.
11. McCance DR. Diabetes in pregnancy. Best Pract Res Clin Obstet Gynaecol. 2015;29(5):685–99.
12. Wissler RN. Endocrine disorders. In: Chestnut DH, Polley LS, Tsen LC, Wong CA, editors. Chestnut's obstetric anesthesia. Principles and practice. 4th ed. Philadelphia: Elsevier; 2009. p. 913–41.
13. Kitabchi AE, Nyenwe EA. Hyperglycemic crises in diabetes mellitus: diabetic ketoacidosis and hyperglycemic hyperosmolar state. Endocrinol Metab Clin North Am. 2006;35(4):725–51, viii.
14. Montoro MN, Myers VP, Mestman JH, Xu Y, Anderson BG, Golde SH. Outcome of pregnancy in diabetic ketoacidosis. Am J Perinatol. 1993;10(1):17–20.
15. Robertson G, Wheatley T, Robinson RE. Ketoacidosis in pregnancy: an unusual presentation of diabetes mellitus: case reports. Br J Obstet Gynaecol. 1986;93(10):1088–90.
16. Cousins L. Pregnancy complications among diabetic women: review 1965-1985. Obstet Gynecol Surv. 1987;42(3):140–9.
17. Parker JA, Conway DL. Diabetic ketoacidosis in pregnancy. Obstet Gynecol Clin North Am. 2007;34(3):533–43, xii.
18. Wallace TM, Matthews DR. Recent advances in the monitoring and management of diabetic ketoacidosis. QJM. 2004;97(12):773–80.
19. ter Braak EW, Evers IM, Willem Erkelens D, Visser GH. Maternal hypoglycemia during pregnancy in type I diabetes: maternal and fetal consequences. Diabetes Metab Res Rev. 2002;18(2):96–105.
20. Kimmerle R, Heinemann L, Delecki A, Berger M. Severe hypoglycemia incidence and predisposing factors in 85 pregnancies of type I diabetic women. Diabetes Care. 1992;15(8):1034–7.
21. Rosenn BM, Miodovnik M, Holcberg G, Khoury JC, Siddiqi TA. Hypoglycemia: the price of intensive insulin therapy for pregnant women with insulin-dependent diabetes mellitus. Obstet Gynecol. 1995;85(3):417–22.
22. Lankford HV, Bartholomew SP. Severe hypoglycemia in diabetic pregnancy. Va Med Q. 1992;119(3):172–4.

23. Nielsen LR, Pedersen-Bjergaard U, Thorsteinsson B, Johansen M, Damm P, Mathiesen ER. Hypoglycemia in pregnant women with type 1 diabetes: predictors and role of metabolic control. Diabetes Care. 2008;31(1):9–14.
24. International Hypoglycaemia Study Group. Glucose concentrations of less than 3.0 mmol/L (54 mg/dL) should be reported in clinical trials: a joint position statement of the American Diabetes Association and the European Association for the Study of Diabetes. Diabetes Care. 2017;40(1):155–7.
25. Seaquist ER, Anderson J, Childs B, Cryer P, Dagogo-Jack S, Fish L, et al. Hypoglycemia and diabetes: a report of a workgroup of the American Diabetes Association and the Endocrine Society. Diabetes Care. 2013;36(5):1384–95.
26. Tuomilehto J. The emerging global epidemic of type 1 diabetes. Curr Diab Rep. 2013;13(6):795–804.
27. Knowler WC, Barrett-Connor E, Fowler SE, Hamman RF, Lachin JM, Diabetes Prevention Program Research Group, et al. Reduction in the incidence of type 2 diabetes with lifestyle intervention or metformin. N Engl J Med. 2002;346(6):393–403.
28. King P, Peacock I, Donnelly R. The UK prospective diabetes study (UKPDS): clinical and therapeutic implications for type 2 diabetes. Br J Clin Pharmacol. 1999;48(5):643–8.
29. American Diabetes Association. Standards of medical care in diabetes-2008. Diabetes Care. 2008;31(Suppl 1):S12–54.
30. Santiago JV. Overview of the complications of diabetes. Clin Chem. 1986;32(10 Suppl):B48–53.
31. Pastors JG, Warshaw H, Daly A, Franz M, Kulkarni K. The evidence for the effectiveness of medical nutrition therapy in diabetes management. Diabetes Care. 2002;25(3):608–13.
32. Lim EL, Hollingsworth KG, Aribisala BS, Chen MJ, Mathers JC, Taylor R. Reversal of type 2 diabetes: normalisation of beta cell function in association with decreased pancreas and liver triacylglycerol. Diabetologia. 2011;54(10):2506–14.
33. Jackness C, Karmally W, Febres G, Conwell IM, Ahmed L, Bessler M, et al. Very low-calorie diet mimics the early beneficial effect of Roux-en-Y gastric bypass on insulin sensitivity and b-cell function in type 2 diabetic patients. Diabetes. 2013;62(9):3027–32.
34. Rothberg AE, McEwen LN, Kraftson AT, Fowler CE, Herman WH. Very-low-energy diet for type 2 diabetes: an underutilized therapy? J Diabetes Complicat. 2014;28(4):506–10.
35. Diabetes Control and Complications Trial Research Group, Nathan DM, Genuth S, Lachin J, Cleary P, Crofford O, et al. The effect of intensive treatment of diabetes on the development and progression of long-term complications in insulin-dependent diabetes mellitus. N Engl J Med. 1993;329(14):977–86.
36. Amour J, Kersten JR. Diabetic cardiomyopathy and anesthesia: bench to bedside. Anesthesiology. 2008;108(3):524–30.
37. Peterson CM, Jovanovic-Peterson L, Mills JL, Conley MR, Knopp RH, Reed GF, et al. The diabetes in early pregnancy study: changes in cholesterol, triglycerides, body weight, and blood pressure. Am J Obstet Gynecol. 1992;166(2):513–8.
38. Siddiqi T, Rosenn B, Mimouni F, Khoury J, Miodovnik M. Hypertension during pregnancy in insulin-dependent diabetic women. Obstet Gynecol. 1991;77(4):514–9.
39. Sibai BM, Caritis S, Hauth J, Lindheimer M, Van Dorsten JP, Mac Pherson C, et al. Risks of preeclampsia and adverse neonatal outcomes among women with pregestational diabetes mellitus. Am J Obstet Gynecol. 2000;182(2):364–9.
40. HAPO Study Cooperative Research Group, Metzger BE, Lowe LP, Dyer AR, Trimble ER, Chaovarindr U, et al. Hyperglycemia and adverse pregnancy outcomes. N Engl J Med. 2008;358(19):1991–2002.
41. O'Kane MJ, Lynch PL, Moles KW, Magee SE. Determination of a diabetes control and complications trial-aligned HbA(1c) reference range in pregnancy. Clin Chim Acta. 2001;311(2):157–9.
42. International Association of Diabetes and Pregnancy Study Groups Consensus Panel, Metzger BE, Gabbe SG, Persson B, Buchanan TA, Catalano PA, et al. International Association of

Diabetes and Pregnancy Study Groups recommendations on the diagnosis and classification of hyperglycemia in pregnancy. Diabetes Care. 2010;33(3):676–82.

43. American Diabetes Association. Standards of medical care in diabetes 2011. Diabetes Care. 2011;34(Suppl. 1):S11–61.

44. Vandorsten JP, Dodson WC, Espeland MA, Grobman WA, Guise JM, Mercer BM, et al. NIH consensus development conference: diagnosing gestational diabetes mellitus. NIH Consens State Sci Statements. 2013;29(1):1–31.

45. Wei Y, Yang H, Zhu W, Yang H, Li H, Yan J, et al. International Association of Diabetes and Pregnancy Study Group criteria is suitable for gestational diabetes mellitus diagnosis: further evidence from China. Chin Med J. 2014;127(20):3553–6.

46. Feldman RK, Tieu RS, Yasumura L. Gestational diabetes screening: the International Association of the Diabetes and Pregnancy Study Groups compared with Carpenter-Coustan screening. Obstet Gynecol. 2016;127(1):10–7.

47. Committee on Practice Bulletins-Obstetrics. Practice Bulletin No. 137: gestational diabetes mellitus. Obstet Gynecol. 2013;122:406–46.

48. Carpenter MW, Coustan DR. Criteria for screening tests for gestational diabetes. Am J Obstet Gynecol. 1982;144(7):768–73.

49. National Diabetes Data Group. Classification and diagnosis of diabetes mellitus and other categories of glucose intolerance. Diabetes. 1979;28(12):1039–57.

50. Ethridge JK Jr, Catalano PM, Waters TP. Perinatal outcomes associated with the diagnosis of gestational diabetes made by the International Association of the Diabetes and Pregnancy Study Groups criteria. Obstet Gynecol. 2014;124(3):571–8.

51. Mayo K, Melamed N, Vandenberghe H, Berger H. The impact of adoption of the International Association of Diabetes in Pregnancy Study Group criteria for the screening and diagnosis of gestational diabetes. Am J Obstet Gynecol. 2015;212(2):224.e1–9.

52. Duran A, Saenz S, Torrejon MJ, Bordiu E, Del Valle L, Galindo M, et al. Introduction of IADPSG criteria for the screening and diagnosis of gestational diabetes mellitus results in improved pregnancy outcomes at a lower cost in a large cohort of pregnant women: the St. Carlos Gestational Diabetes Study. Diabetes Care. 2014;37(9):2442–50.

53. Sorenson RL, Brelje TC. Adaptation of islets of Langerhans to pregnancy: Beta-cell growth, enhanced insulin secretion and the role of lactogenic hormones. Horm Metab Res. 1997;29(6):301–7.

54. Picard F, Wanatabe M, Schoonjans K, Lydon J, O'Malley BW, Auwerx J. Progesterone receptor knockout mice have an improved glucose homeostasis secondary to beta-cell proliferation. Proc Natl Acad Sci U S A. 2002;99(24):15644–8.

55. Jovanovic-Peterson L, Peterson CM. Pregnancy in the diabetic woman: guidelines for a successful outcome. Endocrinol Metab Clin N Am. 1992;21(2):433–56.

56. Hare JW. Insulin management of type I and type II diabetes in pregnancy. Clin Obstet Gynecol. 1991;34(3):494–504.

57. Maheux PC, Bonin B, Dizazo A, Guimond P, Monier D, Bourque J, et al. Glucose homeostasis during spontaneous labor in normal human pregnancy. J Clin Endocrinol Metab. 1996;81(1):209–15.

58. Holst N, Jenssen TG, Burhol PG, Jorde R, Maltau JM. Plasma vasoactive intestinal peptide, insulin, gastric inhibitory polypeptide, and blood glucose in late pregnancy and during and after delivery. Am J Obstet Gynecol. 1986;155(1):126–31.

59. Jovanovic L, Peterson CM. Insulin and glucose requirements during the first stage of labor in insulin-dependent diabetic women. Am J Med. 1983;75(4):607–12.

60. Caplan RH, Pagliara AS, Beguin EA, Smiley CA, Bina-Frymark M, Goettl KA, et al. Constant intravenous insulin infusion during labor and delivery in diabetes mellitus. Diabetes Care. 1982;5(1):6–10.

61. Crombach G, Siebolds M, Mies R. Insulin use in pregnancy: clinical pharmacokinetic considerations. Clin Pharmacokinet. 1993;24(2):89–100.

62. Davies HA, Clark JD, Dalton KJ, Edwards OM. Insulin requirements of diabetic women who breast feed. BMJ. 1989;298(6684):1357–8.
63. Horvath K, Koch K, Jeitler K, Matyas E, Bender R, Bastian H, et al. Effects of treatment in women with gestational diabetes mellitus: systematic review and meta-analysis. BMJ. 2010;340:c1395.
64. Reece EA, Homko CJ. Prepregnancy care and the prevention of fetal malformations in the pregnancy complicated by diabetes. Clin Obstet Gynecol. 2007;50(4):990–7.
65. Jacobson JD, Cousins L. A population-based study of maternal and perinatal outcome in patients with gestational diabetes. Am J Obstet Gynecol. 1989;161(4):981–6.
66. Mimouni F, Miodovnik M, Whitsett JA, Holroyde JC, Siddiqi TA, Tsang RC. Respiratory distress syndrome in infants of diabetic mothers in the 1980s: no direct adverse effect of maternal diabetes with modern management. Obstet Gynecol. 1987;69(2):191–5.
67. Piper JM, Langer O. Does maternal diabetes delay fetal pulmonary maturity? Am J Obstet Gynecol. 1993;168(3 Pt 1):783–6.
68. Bo S, Menato G, Gallo ML, Bardelli C, Lezo A, Signorile A, et al. Mild gestational hyperglycemia, the metabolic syndrome and adverse neonatal outcomes. Acta Obstet Gynecol Scand. 2004;83(4):335–40.
69. Guerin A, Nisenbaum R, Ray JG. Use of maternal GHb concentration to estimate the risk of congenital anomalies in the offspring of women with prepregnancy diabetes. Diabetes Care. 2007;30(7):1920–5.
70. Jensen DM, Korsholm L, Ovesen P, Beck-Nielsen H, Moelsted-Pedersen L, Westergaard JG, et al. Peri-conceptional A1C and risk of serious adverse pregnancy outcome in 933 women with type 1 diabetes. Diabetes Care. 2009;32(6):1046–8.
71. Charron-Prochownik D, Downs J. Diabetes and reproductive health for girls. Alexandria: American Diabetes Association; 2016.
72. Nielsen GL, Møller M, Sørensen HT. HbA1c in early diabetic pregnancy and pregnancy outcomes: a Danish population-based cohort study of 573 pregnancies in women with type 1 diabetes. Diabetes Care. 2006;29(12):2612–6.
73. Suhonen L, Hiilesmaa V, Teramo K. Glycaemic control during early pregnancy and fetal malformations in women with type 1 diabetes mellitus. Diabetologia. 2000;43(1):79–82.
74. Maresh MJ, Holmes VA, Patterson CC, Young IS, Pearson DW, Diabetes and Pre-eclampsia Intervention Trial Study Group, et al. Glycemic targets in the second and third trimester of pregnancy for women with type 1 diabetes. Diabetes Care. 2015;38(1):34–42.
75. Manderson JG, Patterson CC, Hadden DR, Traub AI, Ennis C, McCance DR. Preprandial versus postprandial blood glucose monitoring in type 1 diabetic pregnancy: a randomized controlled clinical trial. Am J Obstet Gynecol. 2003;189(2):507–12.
76. de Veciana M, Major CA, Morgan MA, Asrat T, Toohey JS, Lien JM, et al. Postprandial versus preprandial blood glucose monitoring in women with gestational diabetes mellitus requiring insulin therapy. N Engl J Med. 1995;333(19):1237–41.
77. Jovanovic-Peterson L, Peterson CM, Reed GF, Metzger BE, Mills JL, Knopp RH, et al. Maternal postprandial glucose levels and infant birth weight: the Diabetes in Early Pregnancy Study. The National Institute of Child Health and Human Development – Diabetes in Early Pregnancy Study. Am J Obstet Gynecol. 1991;164(1 Pt 1):103–11.
78. Hartling L, Dryden DM, Guthrie A, Muise M, Vandermeer B, Donovan L. Benefits and harms of treating gestational diabetes mellitus: a systematic review and meta-analysis for the U.S. Preventive Services Task Force and the National Institutes of Health Office of Medical Applications of Research. Ann Intern Med. 2013;159(2):123–9.
79. Langer O. From educated guess to accepted practice: the use of oral antidiabetic agents in pregnancy. Clin Obstet Gynecol. 2007;50(4):959–71.
80. Feig DS, Briggs GG, Koren G. Oral antidiabetic agents in pregnancy and lactation: a paradigm shift? Ann Pharmacother. 2007;41(7):1174–80.

81. Rowan JA, Hague WM, Gao W, Battin MR, Moore MP, MiG Trial Investigators. Metformin versus insulin for the treatment of gestational diabetes. N Engl J Med. 2008;358(19): 2003–15.
82. Gui J, Liu Q, Feng L. Metformin vs insulin in the management of gestational diabetes: a meta-analysis. PLoS One. 2013;8(5):e64585.
83. Langer O, Conway DL, Berkus MD, Xenakis EM, Gonzales O. A comparison of glyburide and insulin in women with gestational diabetes mellitus. N Engl J Med. 2000;343(16):1134–8.
84. Coustan DR. Pharmacological management of gestational diabetes: an overview. Diabetes Care. 2007;30(Suppl. 2):S206–8.
85. Landon MB, Gabbe SG, Sachs L. Management of diabetes mellitus and pregnancy: a survey of obstetricians and maternal-fetal specialists. Obstet Gynecol. 1990;75(4):635–40.
86. American College of Obstetricians and Gynecologists. Pregestational diabetes mellitus. ACOG Practice Bulletin No. 60. Washington DC, March 2005. Obstet Gynecol. 2005;105:675–84.
87. Burgos LG, Ebert TJ, Asiddao C, Turner LA, Pattison CZ, Wang-Cheng R, et al. Increased intraoperative cardiovascular morbidity in diabetics with autonomic neuropathy. Anesthesiology. 1989;70(4):591–7.
88. Pani N, Mishra SB, Rath SK. Diabetic parturient-anaesthetic implications. Indian J Anaesth. 2010;54(5):387–93.
89. Datta S, Brown WU Jr. Acid-base status in diabetic mothers and their infants following general or spinal anesthesia for cesarean section. Anesthesiology. 1977;47(3):272–6.
90. Datta S, Brown WU Jr, Ostheimer GW, Weiss JB, Alper MH. Epidural anesthesia for cesarean section in diabetic parturients: maternal and neonatal acid-base status and bupivacaine concentration. Anesth Analg. 1981;60(8):574–8.
91. Datta S, Kitzmiller JL, Naulty JS, Ostheimer GW, Weiss JB. Acid-base status of diabetic mothers and their infants following spinal anesthesia for cesarean section. Anesth Analg. 1982;61(8):662–5.
92. Ramanathan S, Khoo P, Arismendy J. Perioperative maternal and neonatal acid-base status and glucose metabolism in patients with insulin-dependent diabetes mellitus. Anesth Analg. 1991;73(2):105–11.
93. Eastwood DW. Anterior spinal artery syndrome after epidural anesthesia in a pregnant diabetic patient with scleredema. Anesth Analg. 1991;73(1):90–1.
94. Rodrigo N, Perera KN, Ranwala R, Jayasinghe S, Warnakulasuriya A, Hapuarachchi S. Aspergillus meningitis following spinal anaesthesia for caesarean section in Colombo, Sri Lanka. Int J Obstet Anesth. 2007;16(3):256–60.
95. Moen V, Dahlgren N, Irestedt L. Severe neurological complications after central neuraxial blockades in Sweden, 1990-1999. Anesthesiology. 2004;101(4):950–9.
96. Wang LP, Hauerberg J, Schmidt JF. Incidence of spinal epidural abscess after epidural analgesia: a national 1-year survey. Anesthesiology. 1999;91(6):1928–36.
97. Hebl JR, Kopp SL, Schroeder DR, Horlocker TT. Neurologic complications after neuraxial anesthesia or analgesia in patients with preexisting peripheral sensorimotor neuropathy or diabetic polyneuropathy. Anesth Analg. 2006;103(5):1294–9.
98. Vohra A, Kumar S, Charlton AJ, Olukoga AO, Boulton AJ, McLeod D. Effect of diabetes mellitus on the cardiovascular responses to induction of anesthesia and tracheal intubation. Br J Anaesth. 1993;71(2):258–61.
99. Lev-Ran A. Sharp temporary drop in insulin requirement after caesarean section in diabetic patients. Am J Obstet Gynecol. 1974;120(7):905–8.
100. Attallah MM, Daif AA, Saied MMA, Sonbul ZM. Neuromuscular blocking activity of tubocurarine in patients with diabetes mellitus. Br J Anaesth. 1992;68(6):567–9.
101. Saitoh Y, Kaneda K, Hattori H, Nakajima H, Murakawa M. Monitoring of neuromuscular block after administration of vecuronium in patients with diabetes mellitus. Br J Anaesth. 2003;90(4):480–6.

102. Rosenbloom AL. Skeletal and joint manifestations of childhood diabetes. Pediatr Clin North Am. 1984;31(3):569–89.
103. Metzger BE. Long-term outcomes in mothers diagnosed with gestational diabetes mellitus and their offspring. Clin Obstet Gynecol. 2007;50(4):972–9.
104. Holt RI, Goddard JR, Clarke P, Coleman MA. A postnatal fasting plasma glucose is useful in determining which women with gestational diabetes should undergo a postnatal oral glucose tolerance test. Diabet Med. 2003;20(7):594–8.
105. Bottalico JN. Recurrent gestational diabetes: risk factors, diagnosis, management, and implications. Semin Perinatol. 2007;31(3):176–84.

Anesthesia for the Morbidly Obese Pregnant Patient

4

Holly Ende and Bhavani Kodali

4.1 Introduction

4.1.1 Epidemiology

Rates of obesity have been increasing exponentially for the past several decades, with an estimated 1.46 billion overweight and 602 million obese adults worldwide [1]. In the United States, approximately 36% of adults are overweight or obese, and this prevalence is higher among women [2]. Depending on the population studied, there is an approximately 20% incidence of obesity in pregnancy [3]. The management of morbidly obese women during pregnancy presents a challenge to obstetric and anesthesia providers alike. This is mainly due to frequently comorbid disease states including hypertension, diabetes, cardiovascular, and thromboembolic disease. However, obesity itself can have negative effects on pregnancy course and outcomes, including increased rates of pregnancy-induced hypertension, gestational diabetes, cesarean delivery, hemorrhage, fetal macrosomia, preterm birth, and stillbirth [4].

Studies evaluating morbidity and mortality associated with a diagnosis of obesity in pregnancy are confounded by variability in widely accepted definitions. The World Health Organization classifies obesity according to body mass index (BMI) which is defined as weight in kilograms divided by the square of height in meters. Overweight is defined as BMI greater than or equal to 25, with obesity further categorized into three categories—class 1 (BMI 30–34.9 kg/m^2), class 2 (BMI 35–39.9 kg/m^2), and class 3 (BMI > 40 kg/m^2).

H. Ende (✉)
Vanderbilt University Medical Center, Department of Anesthesiology, Nashville, TN, USA
e-mail: holly.ende@vanderbilt.edu

B. Kodali
Brigham and Women's Hospital, Department of Anesthesiology, Perioperative, and Pain Medicine, Boston, MA, USA

© Springer International Publishing AG, part of Springer Nature 2018
B. Gunaydin, S. Ismail (eds.), *Obstetric Anesthesia for Co-morbid Conditions*,
https://doi.org/10.1007/978-3-319-93163-0_4

4.2 Physiologic Changes of Obesity and Pregnancy

4.2.1 Cardiovascular Changes

Both obesity and pregnancy increase the amount of tissue requiring perfusion as well as oxygen demand; and therefore, both increase overall demand on the cardiovascular system. Heart rate, stroke volume, cardiac output, and blood volume increase with both obesity and pregnancy. Cardiac output (CO) is increased 30–50 ml/min for each additional 100 g of adipose tissue. Pregnancy further increases CO up to 50%. Endothelial dysfunction which accompanies obesity as a result of higher levels of leptin, insulin, and other inflammatory mediators predisposes obese patients to hypertension as a result of increased systemic vascular resistance (SVR). Pregnancy, on the other hand, tends to decrease SVR, and these changes may offset. Pulmonary vascular resistance (PVR) and pulmonary artery pressure (PAP) are also increased as a result of obesity due to potential left ventricular hypertrophy and dysfunction, increased pulmonary blood flow, and sleep apnea with resulting chronic hypoxia. While pregnancy itself does not affect systolic or diastolic function, obesity can impair both, leading to heart failure and other sequelae. The physiologic effects seen in obesity and pregnancy as well as the anticipated combined effects are summarized in Table 4.1.

4.2.2 Respiratory Changes

The respiratory system is considerably affected by both obesity and pregnancy. The most clinically significant ventilatory effects include decreases in functional residual capacity (FRC), residual volume (RV), and expiratory reserve volume (ERV) as a result of cephalad diaphragm movement due to the gravid uterus in pregnancy and abdominal and chest wall adiposity seen in obesity. These changes combined with increased oxygen consumption also seen in both pregnancy and obesity lead to rapid desaturation during apneic episodes. Tidal volume and minute ventilation increase during pregnancy as a result of progesterone's effects on the medullary respiratory centers. Overall, both pregnancy and obesity result in restrictive-type

Table 4.1 Physiologic changes of the cardiovascular system associated with pregnancy and obesity [5]

	Pregnancy	Obesity	Combined
Heart rate	↑	↑↑	↑↑
Stroke volume	↑↑	↑	↑
Cardiac output	↑↑	↑↑	↑↑↑
Systemic vascular resistance	↓↓	↑	↔ or ↓
Mean arterial pressure	↑	↑↑	↑↑
Systolic function	↔	↔ or ↓	↔ or ↓
Diastolic function	↔	↓	↓
Central venous pressure	↔	↑	↑↑
Pulmonary wedge pressure	↔	↑↑	↑↑

ventilatory patterns. Oxygenation can be impaired by both obesity and pregnancy if the FRC falls below the closing capacity (CC), resulting in shunting and ventilation/perfusion mismatching. Both pregnant and obese patients also tend to have lower baseline arterial oxygen partial pressures (P_aO_2), with this change amplified in morbidly obese parturients. Finally, both pregnancy and obesity can be associated with difficult airways as a result of capillary engorgement with mucosal edema or soft tissue adiposity, respectively. These airway changes can lead to the development of obstructive sleep apnea in both populations. For a full list of the physiology effects of obesity and pregnancy on the respiratory system, see Table 4.2.

4.2.3 Gastrointestinal Changes

Both obesity and pregnancy result in increased intra-abdominal pressure, decreased gastrointestinal motility, and decreased lower esophageal sphincter tone, putting morbidly obese parturients at greater risk of pulmonary aspiration of gastric contents. Changes in gastric volume and gastric pH associated with obesity and pregnancy are less clear, with some studies showing higher volumes of more acidic fluid, while others show no difference [6, 7]. Comorbid diabetes is frequently diagnosed in this patient population, which is also associated with delayed gastric emptying.

4.2.4 Endocrine Changes

Diabetes mellitus and gestational diabetes are both more common among obese parturients compared to those of normal weight. This most likely results from increased levels of inflammatory mediators which results in insulin resistance and hyperglycemia.

4.2.5 Hematologic Changes

Both pregnancy and obesity are independently associated with hypercoagulability, venous stasis, and endothelial injury, and together they combine to dramatically

Table 4.2 Physiologic changes of the respiratory system associated with pregnancy and obesity [5]

	Pregnancy	Obesity	Combined
Tidal volume	↑	↓	↑
Respiratory rate	↑	↔ or ↑	↑
Minute volume	↑	↓ or ↔	↑
Expiratory reserve volume	↓	↓↓	↓
Residual volume	↓	↓ or ↔	↓
Functional residual capacity	↓↓	↓↓↓	↓↓
Total lung capacity	↓	↓↓	↓
Compliance	↔	↓↓	↓
V/Q mismatch	↑	↑	↑↑

increase risk of venous thromboembolic events. Obesity increases the levels of plas-minogen activator inhibitor-1 which prevents fibrinolysis, leptin which encourages platelet aggregation, interleukin-6 which increases the production of coagulation factors by the liver, and C-reactive protein which activates platelets [8]. Venous stasis results from increased intra-abdominal pressure caused by both the gravid uterus and abdominal adiposity.

4.3 Morbidity and Mortality

4.3.1 Maternal Comorbidities Associated with Obesity and Pregnancy

Obesity is associated with a number of comorbidities which can complicate the care of the parturient. The relative risk of diabetes mellitus type II in obese women is 12 times that of controls of normal BMI and waist circumference. Obesity is addition-ally associated with increased incidence of hypertension, coronary artery disease, congestive heart failure, stroke, pulmonary embolism, asthma, gallbladder disease, chronic back pain, depression, and gastroesophageal reflux disease [9]. A comor-bidity with particular influence on anesthetic management is obstructive sleep apnea (OSA). OSA is more common in obese patients in general; however the definition of OSA in pregnancy is not widely agreed upon, and so the exact prevalence is unknown. Changes associated with pregnancy and labor have varying effects on the physiology of OSA, with weight gain and airway swelling potentially worsening symptoms, while increased minute ventilation and side sleeping may be protective [10].

4.3.2 Maternal Morbidity

Obese women also have a higher incidence of developing pregnancy-related com-plications, specifically hypertensive disorders of pregnancy, gestational diabetes, thromboembolic disease, and need for operative delivery. A prospective multicenter study found the odds ratio (OR) of developing gestation hypertension to be 2.5 and 3.2 for obesity and morbid obesity, respectively, while preeclampsia was also increased, with OR of 1.6 in obese and 3.3 in morbidly obese versus control patients of normal BMI (11). In addition to the higher likelihood of preexisting type II dia-betes, morbidly obese parturients are also four times as likely to develop gestational diabetes, most likely secondary to insufficient insulin production to offset the insu-lin resistance conferred by pregnancy. The implications of this are far-reaching, with higher chance of fetal malformations, macrosomia, and coexisting maternal cardiovascular and renal disease. Morbidly obese pregnant patients also carry a higher risk of thromboembolic complications, both during pregnancy and after delivery, with a relative risk of 3.5 for pulmonary embolism compared to lean con-trols [9]. Finally, the risk of operative delivery is increased in obesity, with OR of

1.7 and 3.0 for operative vaginal delivery and cesarean delivery, respectively, in the morbidly obese population [11]. There are many potential explanations for these increases, including higher rates of dysfunctional labor patterns, fetal macrosomia, abnormal fetal presentation, and induction of labor secondary to maternal medical conditions.

4.3.3 Maternal Mortality

In addition to the significantly increased morbidity associated with obesity in pregnancy, mortality rates are also higher in this cohort. A report published by the Centre for Maternal and Child Enquiries in the United Kingdom showed that half of all women with pregnancy-related deaths were overweight or obese. This percentage was even higher when evaluating women who died of thromboembolic or cardiac disease. Anesthesia-related maternal deaths are also more common in obese women [12]. These findings led to subsequent recommendations by the American Congress of Obstetricians and Gynecologists (ACOG) that all obese women should undergo antepartum consultation with an anesthesiologists and that multidisciplinary care is required to decrease morbidity and mortality in this population [13].

4.3.4 Fetal Morbidity and Mortality

Maternal obesity further has implications for fetal morbidity and mortality. Fetuses born to morbidly obese mothers have higher odds of fetal macrosomia, with ORs 1.9 and 2.4 for birth weight greater than 4000 g and 4500 g, respectively [11]. This higher incidence of fetal macrosomia also increases the risk of shoulder dystocia in the delivery of these infants. Furthermore, the odds of poor obstetric outcomes for the fetus are greater, including higher incidence of large for gestational age, fetal distress, meconium aspiration, intrauterine fetal demise, and early neonatal death [14]. Congenital malformations such as neural tube defects and cardiac anomalies are also more frequent in these infants [15].

4.4 Labor and Vaginal Delivery

4.4.1 Impact on Labor Progress

The progress of normal labor seems to be related to a patient's BMI. Morbidly obese parturients experience slower centimeter by centimeter labor progress with resultant longer latent and active phases of labor as well as higher chance of cesarean delivery performed for abnormal labor. A large multicenter trial conducted in the United States showed that morbidly obese nulliparous women took more than 2 h longer to progress from 4 cm to 10 cm dilation, while multiparous women took approximately 1 h longer. These same results of slower labor progress were demonstrated for both spontaneous and induced labor [16]. This may be due to higher incidence of fetal macrosomia in obese mothers, higher rates of induction, and/or dysfunctional uterine contractility or poor myometrial response to oxytocin. Zhang et al. [17] showed that the myometrium of obese parturients at the time of cesarean delivery contracted with less force and frequency and demonstrated less calcium flux when compared to control women of normal BMI. Thus obese parturients have a significantly increased risk of cesarean delivery, driven primarily by failed or obstructed labor. In an attempt to quantify this increased risk of cesarean delivery among overweight and obese women, Chu et al. conducted a meta-analysis of 33 studies in which they found unadjusted OR of cesarean delivery of 1.46 (1.34–1.60), 2.05 (1.86–2.27), and 2.89 (2.28–3.79) among overweight, obese, and morbidly obese patients, respectively [18]. Another study looking at greater than 16,000 patients found that the rate of cesarean delivery in obese nulliparous women was 47.4% versus 20.7% in those with a BMI less than 30. The odds ratio of having an operative vaginal delivery was also higher among morbidly obese patients compared to controls, with an OR of 1.7 (1.2–2.2) [11].

4.4.2 Anesthetic Management

Neuraxial analgesia represents the most effective option for pain control and is of particular benefit in obese patients given the higher rates of macrosomia, shoulder dystocia, operative vaginal delivery, and cesarean delivery (which may be emergent). A positive correlation between BMI and the severity of labor pain has also been demonstrated [19]. Technical challenges associated with neuraxial placement in this population, however, are numerous. These challenges include adipose tissue obscuring palpation of spinous processes and intervertebral spaces, greater depth of the epidural space which exaggerates needle inaccuracies, and presence of fat pockets which may cause false loss of resistance [20, 21]. Useful techniques to help mitigate these challenges may include the use of visible anatomic landmarks including the seventh cervical vertebrae and gluteal cleft, elicitation of patient feedback on perceived needle position, as well as ultrasound imaging prior to neuraxial placement. While ultrasound imaging in the obese population may not be able to identify depth to the epidural space because of lack of ultrasound penetration, the midline can often be identified which can provide some useful information. The sitting position is preferred by many practitioners for neuraxial placement in obese women because of improved identification of midline and shorter distance from skin to epidural space in this position [22]. After successful placement of an epidural, patients should subsequently be repositioned in the lateral position before securing the catheter. This is because redistribution of subcutaneous adipose tissue in the back may lead to an increased distance from the skin to epidural space and thus dislodgement of the catheter from the epidural space (Fig. 4.1) [23]. If unsecured at the skin, the catheter can instead be drawn in from the outside, preserving the depth residing within the epidural space.

Because of these many anatomical and positioning challenges associated with maternal obesity, epidural catheter placements on average require more attempts, take more time, are less likely to result in adequate analgesia for delivery, and are more likely to fail outright and require replacement [24, 25]. Although data is conflicting, inadvertent dural puncture may be more common in obese patients as a result of these technical difficulties [26]. Whether or not adjustments should be made to epidural dosing in morbidly obese patients remains unclear; although, data suggests that higher weight and BMI are likely associated with greater cephalad extent of neuroblockade [27, 28]. Finally, the decision of whether to utilize standard epidural or combined spinal-epidural (CSE) technique for labor analgesia in obese parturients is practitioner-dependent. The primary goals of neuraxial anesthesia in morbidly obese parturients are to provide patient comfort but also to ensure a properly functioning catheter in the high likelihood (compared to lean patients) that operative vaginal and cesarean delivery are necessary. Avoidance of general anesthesia in this patient population is of utmost importance because of the higher chance of encountering a difficult airway. Both the epidural and CSE techniques offer advantages and disadvantages in this respect. The CSE technique indirectly confirms correct positioning of the epidural needle and may be associated with higher initial success rates and decreased need for catheter replacement [29, 30]. On the other hand, the epidural catheter inserted with a CSE technique is unable to be

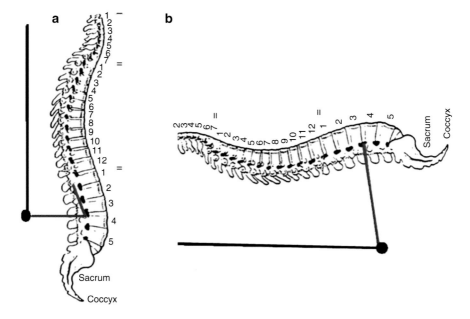

Fig. 4.1 Depth to the epidural space can increase with transition from sitting (**a**) to supine (**b**) position secondary to redistribution of subcutaneous adipose tissue. When this occurs, the catheter previously in the epidural space (blue line) can be dislodged leading to subsequent catheter failure

Fig. 4.2 Despite identifying the epidural space, the tip of the epidural needle may be off-midline. Confirmation with dural puncture (as with a CSE technique) confirms midline placement with flow of CSF

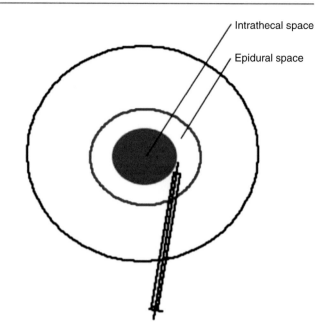

Intrathecal space

Epidural space

tested for reliability until the spinal anesthetic wears off. For this reason, some practitioners prefer standard epidural technique so that a solid and bilateral epidural anesthetic level can be confirmed from the outset. As previously mentioned, this standard epidural technique may be associated with higher catheter failure rate, potentially due to identification of the epidural space laterally as opposed to midline (Fig. 4.2).

4.5   Cesarean Delivery

4.5.1   Operative Variables

Many operative variables can be affected by a parturient's BMI including operative time, blood loss, and the need for uterotonics. Hood et al. [24] showed that cesarean delivery operative times for morbidly obese patients, which they defined as those weighing greater than 300 lbs., and controls were 76.7 ± 31.2 and 47.1 ± 14.4 min, respectively. Similarly increased operative times were demonstrated by Perlow et al. who reported that 48.8% of morbidly obese women had an operative time >60 min, compared to 9.3% of controls [31]. In this same study, 34.9% of morbidly obese women had an estimated blood loss of >1000 ml during their cesarean delivery, while only 9.3% of controls surpassed this cutoff. In a related finding, morbidly obese women are also more likely to require administration of uterotonics following delivery [31].

4.5.2 Anesthetic Management

4.5.2.1 Regional Anesthesia

In the obese parturient, regional anesthesia is preferred over general anesthesia for cesarean delivery. If a labor epidural is in situ, the catheter can be used for conversion to surgical anesthesia. If cesarean delivery is elective, or if a parturient has no epidural or a poorly functioning catheter, both spinal anesthesia and CSE are options in the morbidly obese population. CSE, however, may be advantageous for multiple reasons. Depending on the distribution of adipose tissue and specifically the degree of adiposity at the site of neuraxial placement, longer needles may be required. Spinal placement using a longer needle is certainly possible, but identifying the epidural space with a larger-gauge epidural needle may be technically easier, which can be followed with a needle-through-needle technique for intrathecal (IT) injection. Also, CSE offers the advantage of extending the timeframe of anesthesia should the duration of surgery be prolonged, which is commonly the case with morbidly obese parturients. The ability to prolong blockade can help to avoid the need to convert to general anesthesia and manipulate the airway, which as stated previously is more likely to pose difficulty with intubation. In patients with super-morbid obesity (BMI > 50 kg/m^2), occasionally a supra-umbilical vertical midline incision is required due to the large abdominal pannus. In these cases, a double neuraxial catheter technique has been described in which a lumbar spinal catheter and thoracic epidural catheter are placed for intraoperative and postoperative anesthesia, respectively [32]. The spinal catheter offers the advantage of reliable re-dosing compared to the epidural placed as part of a CSE technique, which remains untested until intraoperatively.

Deciding on the dose of local anesthetic for IT or epidural administration in the morbidly obese parturient can be challenging. On one hand, there is data to suggest that morbidly obese patients have decreased CSF volume, which is associated with greater cephalad extent of neural blockade for any given IT dose [33, 34]. On the other hand, erring too low on the local anesthetic dose may increase the risk of inadequate block and need for conversion to general anesthesia if a single-shot technique is used. Furthermore, despite the proven concept of CSF volume effecting cephalad spread, dose-finding studies in the obstetric population have failed to demonstrate differences in ED50 or ED95 of local anesthetics for cesarean delivery in morbidly obese versus nonobese patients [35, 36]. Data regarding the extent of cephalad blockade with epidural dosing is also conflicting; however, this is less of an issue as epidural local anesthetic can be titrated to effect.

Neuraxial morphine with or without the addition of a lipid-soluble opioid (e.g., fentanyl) is typically administered in addition to the local anesthetic for cesarean delivery. Dosing regimens are usually not adjusted for BMI; however, careful postoperative monitoring for respiratory depression is particularly important in the morbidly obese patient (see Sect. 4.5.3).

4.5.2.2 General Anesthesia

When general anesthesia is required, a thorough airway assessment is of utmost importance, as the incidence of difficult laryngoscopy in the obstetric population has been reported to be greater than 8%, with a reported incidence of 1 in 390 for failed intubations [37, 38]. Multiple aspects of obesity and pregnancy, including airway edema, enlarged breasts, greater anteroposterior chest diameter, and larger neck circumference, make difficult airway more likely, and difficult intubation is significantly associated with greater BMI [39]. One study reported an incidence for difficult intubation as high as 33% in women weighing greater than 300 lbs. [24]. Predictors of difficult intubation which have been evaluated in obstetric populations include modified Mallampati score (MMT), upper lip bite test, thyromental distance, ratio of height to thyromental distance (RHTMD), sternomental distance, mandible protrusion, neck circumference, and ratio of neck circumference to thyromental distance (NC/TMD). Savva et al. found that the MMT alone was neither sensitive nor specific in predicting difficult intubation [40]. Honarmand et al. subsequently found RHTMD to have the highest sensitivity, positive predictive value, and negative predictive value compared to other variables tested [37]. In obese parturients, however, NC/TMD may have the best combined sensitivity and specificity for identifying difficult laryngoscopy [39]. Positioning on the operating room table can be utilized to optimize laryngoscopic view, with a ramped position providing best alignment of the oral, pharyngeal, and tracheal axes. While retraction of a large panniculus may be necessary for surgical exposure, placement of these retractors should be used with caution, especially prior to intubation, as cephalad retraction of adiposity may hinder laryngoscopy and can also be associated with hypotension, ventilation difficulties, and fetal compromise.

Airway manipulation for cesarean delivery is further complicated by higher risk of aspiration in the obstetric and obese populations. Aspiration prophylaxis is recommended to mitigate this risk. Both nonparticulate antacids and H2 receptor blockers have been shown to increase gastric pH, while metoclopramide significantly decreases both nausea and vomiting when compared to placebo [41–43]. However, due to the extremely low incidence of aspiration events, none of these medications have data to support improved patient outcomes. Risk of aspiration exists during both induction and emergence of general anesthesia, necessitating rapid sequence induction (unless difficult airway is anticipated) and careful emergence and extubation at the end of the procedure.

Induction of general anesthesia should be preceded by adequate denitrogenation ("preoxygenation") as both pregnancy and obesity predispose to rapid oxygen desaturation and hypoxemia. There is evidence to suggest that both eight deep breaths over 1 min (8DB) and tidal volume breathing for 3 min are equally effective in achieving $ETO_2 > 90\%$, with the 8DM method having the advantage of the ability to perform more quickly in emergent situations [44]. Unless difficult intubation is anticipated, rapid sequence induction is indicated in pregnant patients undergoing cesarean delivery. A combination of hypnotic and neuromuscular blocker is typically administered for induction. Dosing of propofol (2–2.5 mg/kg) or thiopental (4–5 mg/kg) should be based on lean body weight (difference between total body weight and fat mass) [45]. Succinylcholine (1–1.5 mg/kg) is the neuromuscular blocker of choice in obese parturients, with dosing based on total body weight [45]. If rocuronium (1.2 mg/kg) is chosen for rapid sequence intubation, the dose should be based on ideal body weight, and sugammadex (16 mg/kg) should be immediately available to reverse the NMB should unanticipated difficult airway arise [45]. Specifically in the case of the morbidly obese parturient, additional airway equipment, including video laryngoscope, fiber-optic scope, various endotracheal tube sizes, and supraglottic airway devices, should be available in case of emergency.

Maintenance of anesthesia is usually accomplished with volatile agent or propofol infusion with or without nitrous oxide. While pregnancy is associated with decreased minimum alveolar concentration (MAC), obesity does not affect MAC any further. Desflurane or sevoflurane may be the preferred volatile agents in obesity as they are less lipid-soluble and therefore are associated with quicker times to extubation at the end of the case. Functional residual capacity (FRC) is decreased by both pregnancy and obesity, and these patients may require higher positive end-expiratory pressure and frequent recruitment maneuvers to prevent atelectasis and hypoxemia. At the end of the procedure, complete neuromuscular blockade reversal should be confirmed, and the patient should be fully awake prior to extubation. Obese parturients are at greater risk of airway obstruction following extubation, and careful monitoring of oxygen saturations should be continued into the postoperative period.

4.5.3 Postoperative Care

Women who undergo cesarean delivery under regional anesthesia typically receive neuraxial morphine as part of their anesthetic. Although there is some data to suggest that respiratory depression following IT morphine administration occurs more commonly in morbidly obese patients, the incidence is still remarkably low [46]. In women who receive general anesthesia, parenteral opioids are commonly required postoperatively and are usually administered via patient-controlled analgesia (PCA). Minimizing opioids in order to mitigate the risk of respiratory depression can typically be achieved by the use of multimodal analgesic regimens, which can include nonsteroidal anti-inflammatory drugs, acetaminophen, gabapentin, local wound infiltration, and transversus abdominis plane (TAP) blocks. In the general obstetric population, TAP blocks are not effective at reducing pain scores or opioid consumption when combined with IT morphine; however, they may be beneficial in patients who did not receive neuraxial opioids [47]. The performance of TAP blocks may be challenging or impossible in patients with excess abdominal adiposity.

4.6 Postpartum Complications

4.6.1 Respiratory Insufficiency

Obesity has been identified as a significant risk factor for airway obstruction and hypoventilation postoperatively. If a morbidly obese parturient has a diagnosis of obstructive sleep apnea, requires general anesthesia for cesarean delivery, and/or receives opioids for pain control, the American Society of Anesthesiologists recommends continuous pulse oximetry and close monitoring be continued after discharge from the PACU [48]. Supplemental oxygen may also be required until the parturient is able to maintain baseline oxygen saturation on room air.

4.6.2 Infection

Infectious morbidity is also increased in the obese and morbidly obese obstetric populations. In a study evaluating infectious morbidity in patients undergoing cesarean delivery, Myles et al. [49] reported that following elective and nonelective CD, respectively, 89.5% and 81.8% of those who developed postoperative infection were obese. Overall, endomyometritis was the most common infection reported, with 15.9% of obese patients diagnosed compared to 5.0% in normal BMI controls. Although not statistically significant, they also reported that 75% of wound infections occurred in the obese group [49]. In another case-control study of 43 "massively obese" (>300 pound) women who underwent cesarean delivery, 32.6% developed postoperative endometritis, while only 4.9% of controls developed this infectious complication [31].

4.6.3 Length of Stay

Length of stay (LOS) is another postoperative variable which is frequently assessed, both because it has financial implications for the patient and health system and also because it often represents a surrogate for ongoing medical morbidity. Obese patients have been shown to have significantly greater incidence of prolonged LOS, with 34.9% of morbidly obese patients requiring LOS > 4 days following cesarean delivery, compared to 2.3% in normal BMI controls [31]. In another study, morbidly obese patients stayed in the hospital on average 3.8 and 7.3 days following vaginal and cesarean delivery, respectively, while control patients stayed 2.9 and 5.4 days [24].

4.6.4 Venous Thromboembolism

Obesity is a significant risk factor for the development of thromboembolic complications both during and immediately after pregnancy. During pregnancy obesity is associated with venous thromboembolism (VTE) with an overall adjusted OR of 5.3, and this risk is even higher when evaluating patients who develop VTE prior to delivery (adjusted OR 9.7). Obesity is more strongly associated with risk of PE (adjusted OR 14.9) compared to deep vein thrombosis (adjusted OR 4.4) [50].

4.6.5 Postpartum Hemorrhage

Finally, excessive blood loss or postpartum hemorrhage (PPH) is more common in obese patients following both vaginal and cesarean delivery. As stated previously,

Perlow et al. showed that 34.9% of morbidly obese women had an estimated blood loss of >1000 ml, which is a commonly utilized definition for PPH. In this study, only 9.3% of controls experienced a PPH [31]. Another study also found that obese women have an increased incidence of excessive blood loss, defined as >600 ml, following spontaneous vaginal delivery, with an OR of 2.13 (1.18–3.84) compared to normal-weight women [17].

Key Learning Points
- Rates of obesity are increasing exponentially in both the general and obstetric populations.
- Physiologic changes in both the cardiovascular and pulmonary systems during pregnancy are exacerbated by obesity.
- Morbidly obese pregnant patients have higher pregnancy-related mortality compared to normal weight controls.
- Fetal morbidity and mortality are higher in the offspring of morbidly obese parturients.
- There are many implications for anesthetic management of obese parturients for both labor and cesarean delivery.
- Morbidly obese pregnant patients experience higher rates of postpartum complications, including infection, thromboembolism, and hemorrhage.

References

1. Finucane MM, Stevens GA, Cowan MJ, Danaei G, Lin JK, Paciorek CJ, et al. National, regional, and global trends in body-mass index since 1980: systematic analysis of health examination surveys and epidemiological studies with 960 country-years and 9.1 million participants. Lancet. 2011;377(9765):557–67.
2. Ogden CL, Carroll MD, Fryar CD, Flegal KM. Prevalence of obesity among adults and youth: United States, 2011-2014. NCHS Data Brief. 2015;219:1–8.
3. Kanagalingam MG, Forouhi NG, Greer IA, Sattar N. Changes in booking body mass index over a decade: retrospective analysis from a Glasgow Maternity Hospital. BJOG. 2005;112(10):1431–3.
4. Scott-Pillai R, Spence D, Cardwell CR, Hunter A, Holmes VA. The impact of body mass index on maternal and neonatal outcomes: a retrospective study in a UK obstetric population, 2004-2011. BJOG. 2013;120(8):932–9.
5. Saravanakumar K, Rao SG, Cooper GM. Obesity and obstetric anaesthesia. Anaesthesia. 2006;61(1):36–48.
6. Wisen O, Hellstrom PM. Gastrointestinal motility in obesity. J Intern Med. 1995;237(4):411–8.
7. Wong CA, McCarthy RJ, Fitzgerald PC, Raikoff K, Avram MJ. Gastric emptying of water in obese pregnant women at term. Anesth Analg. 2007;105(3):751–5.
8. Mertens I, Van Gaal LF. Obesity, haemostasis and the fibrinolytic system. Obes Rev. 2002;3(2):85–101.
9. Guh DP, Zhang W, Bansback N, Amarsi Z, Birmingham CL, Anis AH. The incidence of co-morbidities related to obesity and overweight: a systematic review and meta-analysis. BMC Public Health. 2009;9:88.
10. Maasilta P, Bachour A, Teramo K, Polo O, Laitinen LA. Sleep-related disordered breathing during pregnancy in obese women. Chest. 2001;120(5):1448–54.

11. Weiss JL, Malone FD, Emig D, Ball RH, Nyberg DA, Comstock CH, et al. Obesity, obstetric complications and cesarean delivery rate – a population-based screening study. Am J Obstet Gynecol. 2004;190(4):1091–7.
12. Cantwell R, Clutton-Brock T, Cooper G, Dawson A, Drife J, Garrod D, et al. Saving mothers' lives: reviewing maternal deaths to make motherhood safer: 2006-2008. The eighth report of the confidential enquiries into maternal deaths in the United Kingdom. BJOG. 2011;118(Suppl 1):1–203.
13. American College of Obstetricians, Gynecologists. ACOG Committee opinion number 315, September 2005. Obesity in pregnancy. Obstet Gynecol. 2005;106(3):671–5.
14. Cedergren MI. Maternal morbid obesity and the risk of adverse pregnancy outcome. Obstet Gynecol. 2004;103(2):219–24.
15. Cedergren MI, Kallen BA. Maternal obesity and infant heart defects. Obes Res. 2003;11(9):1065–71.
16. Kominiarek MA, Zhang J, Vanveldhuisen P, Troendle J, Beaver J, Hibbard JU. Contemporary labor patterns: the impact of maternal body mass index. Am J Obstet Gynecol. 2011;205(3):244 e1–8.
17. Zhang J, Bricker L, Wray S, Quenby S. Poor uterine contractility in obese women. BJOG. 2007;114(3):343–8.
18. Chu SY, Kim SY, Schmid CH, Dietz PM, Callaghan WM, Lau J, et al. Maternal obesity and risk of cesarean delivery: a meta-analysis. Obes Rev. 2007;8(5):385–94.
19. Melzack R, Kinch R, Dobkin P, Lebrun M, Taenzer P. Severity of labour pain: influence of physical as well as psychologic variables. Can Med Assoc J. 1984;130(5):579–84.
20. Ellinas EH, Eastwood DC, Patel SN, Maitra-D'Cruze AM, Ebert TJ. The effect of obesity on neuraxial technique difficulty in pregnant patients: a prospective, observational study. Anesth Analg. 2009;109(4):1225–31.
21. Clinkscales CP, Greenfield ML, Vanarase M, Polley LS. An observational study of the relationship between lumbar epidural space depth and body mass index in Michigan parturients. Int J Obstet Anesth. 2007;16(4):323–7.
22. Hamza J, Smida M, Benhamou D, Cohen SE. Parturient's posture during epidural puncture affects the distance from skin to epidural space. J Clin Anesth. 1995;7(1):1–4.
23. Hamilton CL, Riley ET, Cohen SE. Changes in the position of epidural catheters associated with patient movement. Anesthesiology. 1997;86(4):778–84. Discussion 29A.
24. Hood DD, Dewan DM. Anesthetic and obstetric outcome in morbidly obese parturients. Anesthesiology. 1993;79(6):1210–8.
25. Dresner M, Brocklesby J, Bamber J. Audit of the influence of body mass index on the performance of epidural analgesia in labour and the subsequent mode of delivery. BJOG. 2006;113(10):1178–81.
26. Faure E, Moreno R, Thisted R. Incidence of postdural puncture headache in morbidly obese parturients. Reg Anesth. 1994;19(5):361–3.
27. Hodgkinson R, Husain FJ. Obesity and the cephalad spread of analgesia following epidural administration of bupivacaine for cesarean section. Anesth Analg. 1980;59(2):89–92.
28. Panni MK, Columb MO. Obese parturients have lower epidural local anaesthetic requirements for analgesia in labour. Br J Anaesth. 2006;96(1):106–10.
29. Pan PH, Bogard TD, Owen MD. Incidence and characteristics of failures in obstetric neuraxial analgesia and anesthesia: a retrospective analysis of 19,259 deliveries. Int J Obstet Anesth. 2004;13(4):227–33.
30. Lee S, Lew E, Lim Y, Sia AT. Failure of augmentation of labor epidural analgesia for intrapartum cesarean delivery: a retrospective review. Anesth Analg. 2009;108(1):252–4.
31. Perlow JH, Morgan MA. Massive maternal obesity and perioperative cesarean morbidity. Am J Obstet Gynecol. 1994;170(2):560–5.
32. Polin CM, Hale B, Mauritz AA, Habib AS, Jones CA, Strouch ZY, et al. Anesthetic management of super-morbidly obese parturients for cesarean delivery with a double neuraxial catheter technique: a case series. Int J Obstet Anesth. 2015;24(3):276–80.

33. Hogan QH, Prost R, Kulier A, Taylor ML, Liu S, Mark L. Magnetic resonance imaging of cerebrospinal fluid volume and the influence of body habitus and abdominal pressure. Anesthesiology. 1996;84(6):1341–9.
34. Carpenter RL, Hogan QH, Liu SS, Crane B, Moore J. Lumbosacral cerebrospinal fluid volume is the primary determinant of sensory block extent and duration during spinal anesthesia. Anesthesiology. 1998;89(1):24–9.
35. Lee Y, Balki M, Parkes R, Carvalho JC. Dose requirement of intrathecal bupivacaine for cesarean delivery is similar in obese and normal weight women. Rev Bras Anestesiol. 2009;59(6):674–83.
36. Carvalho B, Collins J, Drover DR, Atkinson Ralls L, Riley ET. ED(50) and ED(95) of intrathecal bupivacaine in morbidly obese patients undergoing cesarean delivery. Anesthesiology. 2011;114(3):529–35.
37. Honarmand A, Safavi MR. Prediction of difficult laryngoscopy in obstetric patients scheduled for caesarean delivery. Eur J Anaesthesiol. 2008;25(9):714–20.
38. Kinsella SM, Winton AL, Mushambi MC, Ramaswamy K, Swales H, Quinn AC, et al. Failed tracheal intubation during obstetric general anaesthesia: a literature review. Int J Obstet Anesth. 2015;24(4):356–74.
39. Hirmanpour A, Safavi M, Honarmand A, Jabalameli M, Banisadr G. The predictive value of the ratio of neck circumference to thyromental distance in comparison with four predictive tests for difficult laryngoscopy in obstetric patients scheduled for caesarean delivery. Adv Biomed Res. 2014;3:200.
40. Savva D. Prediction of difficult tracheal intubation. Br J Anaesth. 1994;73(2):149–53.
41. Jasson J, Lefevre G, Tallet F, Talafre ML, Legagneux F, Conseiller C. Oral administration of sodium citrate before general anesthesia in elective cesarean section. Effect on pH and gastric volume. Ann Fr Anesth Reanim. 1989;8(1):12–8.
42. Lin CJ, Huang CL, Hsu HW, Chen TL. Prophylaxis against acid aspiration in regional anesthesia for elective cesarean section: a comparison between oral single-dose ranitidine, famotidine and omeprazole assessed with fiberoptic gastric aspiration. Acta Anaesthesiol Sin. 1996;34(4):179–84.
43. Pan PH, Moore CH. Comparing the efficacy of prophylactic metoclopramide, ondansetron, and placebo in cesarean section patients given epidural anesthesia. J Clin Anesth. 2001;13(6):430–5.
44. Chiron B, Laffon M, Ferrandiere M, Pittet JF, Marret H, Mercier C. Standard preoxygenation technique versus two rapid techniques in pregnant patients. Int J Obstet Anesth. 2004;13(1):11–4.
45. Ingrande J, Lemmens HJ. Dose adjustment of anaesthetics in the morbidly obese. Br J Anaesth. 2010;105(Suppl 1):i16–23.
46. Abouleish E, Rawal N, Rashad MN. The addition of 0.2 mg subarachnoid morphine to hyperbaric bupivacaine for cesarean delivery: a prospective study of 856 cases. Reg Anesth. 1991;16(3):137–40.
47. Mishriky BM, George RB, Habib AS. Transversus abdominis plane block for analgesia after Cesarean delivery: a systematic review and meta-analysis. Can J Anaesth. 2012;59(8):766–78.
48. American Society of Anesthesiologists Task Force on Perioperative Management of patients with obstructive sleep apnea. Practice guidelines for the perioperative management of patients with obstructive sleep apnea: an updated report by the American Society of Anesthesiologists Task Force on perioperative management of patients with obstructive sleep apnea. Anesthesiology. 2014;120(2):268–86.
49. Myles TD, Gooch J, Santolaya J. Obesity as an independent risk factor for infectious morbidity in patients who undergo cesarean delivery. Obstet Gynecol. 2002;100(5 Pt 1):959–64.
50. Larsen TB, Sorensen HT, Gislum M, Johnsen SP. Maternal smoking, obesity, and risk of venous thromboembolism during pregnancy and the puerperium: a population-based nested case-control study. Thromb Res. 2007;120(4):505–9.

Anesthesia for the Pregnant Patient with Asthma

5

Mukadder Orhan Sungur

5.1 Epidemiology and Effect of Asthma on Maternal and Fetal Outcomes

Asthma remains to be the most common respiratory problem in pregnant patients despite new developments in assessment and pharmacological and non-pharmacological interventions [1–3]. Asthma prevalence in pregnant patients is estimated between 3.2% and 8.4% in the United States [4]; however reported incidence may vary geographically [5]. Moreover, this prevalence is shown to increase in recent years, similar to asthma prevalence in general which translates to an important health burden [6].

The sole effect of the disease on outcomes is difficult to determine as several other comorbidities are associated with maternal asthma such as obesity, higher smoking, and alcohol consumption as well as increased incidence of other chronic diseases [6, 7]. Possible effects of therapy on outcomes further complicate the issue.

When studies or systematic reviews controlling for these confounding factors are considered, the effect of asthma on maternal and fetal adverse events can be summarized in Table 5.1. Of note, these outcome studies are largely retrospective analysis of databases so that increased observation frequency (i.e., increased doctor visits) and hence increased possibility of detecting adverse outcomes compared to non-asthmatic counterparts should be taken into account. Additionally, although studies conclude higher incidence of adverse outcomes in uncontrolled maternal asthma, not all studies could report an association between asthma control level and outcomes [8]. These underline the need for large, prospective studies.

Even though not demonstrated in Table 5.1, respiratory viral infections are more frequently encountered in asthmatic pregnant patients compared to non-asthmatics which can deteriorate maternal health, cause asthma exacerbations, increase

M. Orhan Sungur
Istanbul University, Istanbul Faculty of Medicine, Department of Anesthesiology and Intensive Care, Istanbul, Turkey

© Springer International Publishing AG, part of Springer Nature 2018
B. Gunaydin, S. Ismail (eds.), *Obstetric Anesthesia for Co-morbid Conditions*,
https://doi.org/10.1007/978-3-319-93163-0_5

Table 5.1 Maternal asthma-related adverse outcomes

Maternal	Peripartum	Fetal
Spontaneous abortion specifically in pregnant women with uncontrolled asthma	Pulmonary embolism	Low birth weight
	Maternal ICU admission	Small for gestational age
	Antepartum and postpartum hemorrhage due to placenta previa and placental abruption	Hyperbilirubinemia
Gestational hypertension, preeclampsia, eclampsia		Respiratory distress syndrome, transient tachypnea of newborn or asphyxia
Gestational diabetes mellitus	Premature contractions, preterm delivery	Intracerebral hemorrhage in term infants
Breech presentation		Anemia for term infants
		Congenital malformations
Cesarean section		Cleft lip with or without cleft palate
		Neonatal hospitalization, ICU admission
		Neonatal death

ICU intensive care unit

hospitalization, and increase risk of preeclampsia [9]. Respiratory viral infections can also increase asthma and subsequently wheezing risk in the offspring [10]. Influenza A pandemic in 2009 (H1N1) has clearly demonstrated that pregnant patients are at higher risk of morbidity and mortality during influenza infections and risk is further increased with maternal asthma [11].

5.2 Pathophysiology and Effect of Pregnancy on Maternal Asthma

Asthma is a chronic disease of bronchial hyperreactivity and inflammation. Combined effects of muscle spasm, airway inflammation, and mucus plugging result in edema, airway flow limitation, and remodeling of the tissues [12]. Different underlying etiologies have been proposed for this disease such as innate immunity imbalance between T-helper cells Th1, Th2, and Th17 (mainly due to Th2 inflammation [13], genetics, environmental factors, and exaggerated cholinergic activity). Pathological changes lead to clinical symptoms of partially/completely reversible bronchoconstriction [14].

Pregnancy has a complex effect on asthmatic patients. In terms of hormones, progesterone increases minute ventilation and causes bronchodilation via cyclic adenosine monophosphate (cAMP) pathway with resultant amelioration of asthmatic symptoms [15]. Yet, progesterone is also held responsible for changes in beta (ß)-2 adrenoreceptor responsiveness and airway inflammation [16].

Regarding immunological changes, pregnancy is a state of so-called physiological immunosuppression. This immunosuppression is vital for fetus to control maternal immune response against its expressed paternal antigens [13]. Immunosuppression of pregnancy is characterized by abundance of Th2 cells and regulatory T cells (Treg) that inhibit natural killer (NK) cells. NK cells offer protection against viral diseases. Increase of Treg cells in healthy pregnancy may explain viral infection susceptibility of the pregnant patients. Interestingly, there are conflicting immunological changes in asthmatic pregnant patients. There are findings of blunted lymphocyte activation (particularly CD4 and CD8 cells) in well-controlled asthmatic pregnant patients compared to nonpregnant asthmatics or healthy pregnant patients [17]. Contrary to this blunted response, there is an increase peripheral interferon (IFN)-γ-producing cells and interleukin (ILN)-4 levels [18]. Serum levels of inflammatory heat shock protein (Hsp)-70 [19] and lower levels of Treg cells in maternal asthma compared to healthy pregnant counterparts are also noted [20]. All these complex changes are speculated to be involved in maternal and fetal adverse outcomes of asthma such as preeclampsia and intrauterine growth retardation [21].

A study by Schatz et al. reviewing prospectively maintained asthma diaries and monthly spirometry showed that asthma clinic worsened in 35%, improved in 28%, and remained the same in 33% of pregnant asthma patients [22]. This study was the base of "one-third" rule stating that asthma progress can increase, decrease, or be left unchanged in one-third of pregnant patients. In this study, patients with progressed symptoms were particularly affected between 25 and 32 weeks of gestation. Luckily, asthma attack incidence and severity was decreased in the last month of pregnancy, and exacerbations were rare during labor [22].

5.3   Diagnosis

Characteristic symptoms of asthma (i.e., wheezing, cough, shortness of breath, and feeling of tightness in chest) can demonstrate intensity differences over time (symptoms usually worse at night or early in the morning) and can be triggered by a variety of causes (Table 5.2). On auscultation, wheezing can be heard, but its absence does not exclude diagnosis. For definitive diagnosis, at least a partially reversible airway obstruction should be demonstrated such as an increase greater than 12% (or 200 mL) in forced expiratory volume in 1 s (FEV_1) with bronchodilator short-acting ß-2 agonist (SABA) administration [12].

Pregnancy affects spirometry so that functional residual capacity (FRC, decreased by 17–20%), residual volume (RV, decreased by 20–25%), tidal volume (TV, increased by 30–50%), and expiratory reserve volume (ERV, decreased by 5–15%) are changed with resultant increased minute volume (MV) by 30–50%. Yet, FEV_1 and peak expiratory flow rate (PEFR) are unchanged in healthy pregnant women making these two measurements distinctive for asthma diagnosis and management [14]. There is also very modest increase in forced vital capacity (FVC) in healthy pregnant women, so that FEV_1/FVC ratio remains the same throughout pregnancy [14].

Spirometry, not handheld peak flow meters, should be performed for diagnosis though latter measurements can effectively monitor asthma progress. Peak expiratory flow rate (PEFR) is roughly 380–550 L/min in an otherwise healthy parturient.

Table 5.2 Asthma triggers and comorbidities

Trigger/comorbidity	Suggestion
Viral respiratory infections	Consider prevention by annual inactive influenza vaccination Consider antiviral medications during influenza pandemics for postexposure prophylaxis and treatment of infected individuals
Obesity	Counsel for weight control
Smoking	Patients should be questioned for smoking and advised and assisted to quit. Regular follow-up of smoking status should commence in doctor visits. In heavy-smoker pregnant asthmatic patients (>10 cigarettes/day), transdermal nicotine patches should be considered [24]
Indoor (e.g., mold, house dust mite, cockroach, animal dander, or secretory products) or outdoor (e.g., pollen) environmental triggers	Avoid triggers such as animal dander, house dust mites, cockroaches, pollens, and indoor mold. For indoor allergens mattress and pillow encasement in allergen-impermeable cover, washing bedding weekly in hot water, reduction of indoor humidity to <50%, and removal of carpeting and pets can offer protection
Irritants (e.g., tobacco smoke, strong odors, air pollutants, occupational chemicals, dusts and particulates, vapors, gases, and aerosols)	Avoid triggers. Starting immunotherapy (IT) for allergens not recommended for pregnant patients due to risk of anaphylaxis [23]
Emotions (e.g., fear, anger, frustration, hard crying, or laughing) and stress, depression	Depression can increase likelihood of uncontrolled asthma [1] and should be treated
Drugs (e.g., aspirin; and other nonsteroidal anti-inflammatory drugs, ß-blockers including eye drops, others)	Avoid triggers
Food, food additives, and preservatives (e.g., sulfites)	
Changes in weather, exposure to cold air	
Comorbid conditions (e.g., sinusitis, rhinitis, gastroesophageal reflux disease (GERD))	Discussed in diagnosis section

Asthma triggers and comorbidities should be identified, and patients should be educated for avoidance or treatment

Patients can self-monitor daily progress comparing measurements with their "personal best values" acquired in doctor visits as suggested by National Asthma Education and Prevention Program (NAEPP) of National Heart, Lung, and Blood Institute [12] and American College of Obstetricians and Gynecologists (ACOG) [23]. Severity of asthma is classified based on the occurrence of symptoms and these measurements as listed in Table 5.3.

In spite of the fact that bronchoprovocation with methacholine, histamine, or exercise challenge is used in suspicion of asthma for individuals with normal

Table 5.3 Asthma severity classification as advised by NAEPP [12] and ACOG [23]

Severity	Symptom	Nighttime awakening	Interference with normal activity (limitation of daily activity)	FEV$_1$ or peak flow (predicted % of personal best)	ACT score
Intermittent (well controlled)	≤2 days/week	≤Twice/month	None	>80%	≥20
Mild persistent (not well controlled)	>2 days/week but not daily	>Twice/month	Minor	>80%	16–19
Moderate persistent (not well controlled)	Daily	>Once/week	Some	60–80%	16–19
Severe persistent (very poorly controlled)	Throughout the day	≥4 times/week	Extreme	<60%	<15

This table can be used for both assessing severity in asthmatic patients who are not receiving long-term medications and controlling management to step up or down in patients with long-term medications. FEV$_1$ is forced expiratory volume in 1 s. ACT is Asthma Control Questionnaire [30]

spirometry, it is not recommended for pregnant patients [24]. Rather, a trial of therapy is advised in patients whom asthma suspicion could not be verified by spirometry. Similarly, skin testing for allergens is not recommended due to possibility of systemic anaphylaxis. If and when deemed necessary, immunoglobulin E antibodies for allergens can be tested in blood [25].

Differential diagnosis includes all causes of dyspnea in pregnancy including dyspnea of pregnancy (physiological dyspnea), gastroesophageal reflux, allergic rhinitis with postnasal drip, bronchitis, pneumonia, congestive heart failure, cardiomyopathy, pulmonary edema, amniotic fluid embolism, pulmonary embolism, and airway obstruction [25]. Of these, dyspnea of pregnancy is the most commonly seen in early pregnancy in 70% of the women [26], yet in this situation wheezing, cough, productive sputum, or chest tightness is not encountered.

Gastroesophageal reflux and non-allergic rhinitis due to hormonal changes in pregnancy can further exacerbate maternal asthma and should be treated accordingly [1]. For patients with allergic rhinitis, several recommendations such as avoiding triggers, intranasal hypertonic saline lavage, and intranasal corticosteroids are effective, but corticosteroids are shown to have no benefit in pregnancy-related non-allergic rhinitis. Other medications such as leukotriene receptor antagonist montelukast, intranasal or oral antihistamines, or local vasoconstrictor oxymetazoline have been used successfully in treatment of rhinitis. Oral decongestants with pseudoephedrine or phenylephrine should not be given specifically in early pregnancy as systemic vasoconstriction is linked with teratogenicity. For gastroesophageal reflux, lifestyle modifications coupled with antacids such as sucralfate or histamine (H)$_2$ receptor antagonists such as ranitidine can be used. Lifestyle modifications can be summarized as avoidance of triggering foods (e.g., coffee) or feeding within 3 h of bedtime, eating in smaller portions, and elevation of the head of the bed while sleeping [23].

In the recent years, use of exhaled nitric oxide (NO) has been suggested for diagnosis and management of asthma. Respiratory epithelium is the origin for exhaled NO via inducible NO synthase (iNOS). In asthmatic patients, expression of iNOS and subsequently fractional exhaled NO (FeNO) is increased due to Th2 cytokines [27]. Unfortunately, smoking can interfere with FeNO results, and its effectiveness needs further testing in pregnant population [28].

5.4 Medical Management

5.4.1 Components of Medical Management

Experts in NAEPP and Global Initiative for Asthma (GINA) [29] emphasize four important components of medical management as listed below:

1. Objective monitoring and assessment: Asthma severity and progress should be controlled using objective measures and patients' reported symptoms within 2–4 weeks with validated tools such as Asthma Control Questionnaire [30] (Table 5.3). Measurement of baseline spirometry, coupled with PEFR measurements (twice/day in frequent symptom reporting patients), can help achieve this goal. For pregnant patients, an early ultrasound of the fetus (12–20 weeks) can provide a basis for subsequent development that can be compared. These patients should be followed up every 1–2 weeks till asthma control is achieved. Once asthma is well controlled, follow-up period can be lengthened to once a month.
2. Avoidance or control of triggering factors (Table 5.2).
3. Patient education: Patients should be educated to early recognize exacerbations with self-management tools and home-management plan [12]. Furthermore, despite evidence of adverse outcomes in uncontrolled asthma, pregnant patients are shown to reduce their asthma medications due to perceived threats of medications to fetus [16]. Physicians should emphasize importance of treatment and inform the patient on the risk of acute and chronic hypoxia both to mother and fetus. Another important goal of education is to instruct on correct use of inhalational technique [31].
4. Pharmacotherapy.

5.4.2 Pharmacotherapy

Guidelines [12, 23] and reviews of asthma management [1, 32] advise a stepwise approach in medications and titration of daily inhaler regimen (Table 5.4). According to this, the goal of the therapy is to encounter minimal or no chronic symptoms day/night and minimal or no exacerbations with no limitation of daily activity and to obtain normal lung functions. Although short-acting ß-2 agonist (SABA)—preferably albuterol 2–6 puffs repeatable in 20 min—may ensure a quick relief for symptoms, the main goal is to minimize its use. In this regard, the need for 1 canister of SABA/month should alert the physician to step up in treatment. Physicians are also urged to place a low priority on stepping down the treatment till delivery is concluded [12, 23].

Inhaled corticosteroids are the mainstay of therapy in maternal asthma with an established good safety track [33, 9, 34]. Majority of studies are with budesonide for which the US Food and Drug Administration (FDA) has categorized as B in drugs for pregnancy, yet other agents such as fluticasone or beclomethasone [35] have reassuring profile. Steps have defined ICS doses as low, medium, and high (Table 5.4). Daily drug doses of budesonide for comparison in low, medium, and high administration are 200–600, 600–1200, and >1200 mcg/day, respectively [32].

Short-acting ß-2 agonist (SABA) are rescue therapy for acute asthma exacerbations. In contrast, long-acting inhaled ß-2 agonists (LABA) are "add-on controller therapy" for patients whose symptoms cannot suppress with medium dose of ICS. They are not given as monotherapy, and their safety profile is expected to be like SABA due to shared similarities in pharmacology. LABA agents (namely, salmeterol and formoterol) are not different from each other regarding the risk of low birth weight [36]. However, there are concerns on bronchodilator use in pregnancy as they are linked with esophageal atresia [37], gastroschisis [38], orofacial defects [39], and cardiac abnormalities [40] in the newborn. Albuterol, formoterol, and

Table 5.4 Medical management of asthma: stepwise approach

Asthma severity	Preferred treatment	Alternative treatment
Step 1: mild intermittent	No daily medications required, possibility of severe exacerbation with long asymptomatic periods in between, a trial of systemic corticosteroids is recommended in such case	
Step 2: mild persistent	Low-dose inhaled corticosteroid	– Cromolyn, leukotriene receptor antagonist – Sustained release of theophylline to serum concentration of 5–12 mcg/mL
Step 3: moderate persistent	– Low-dose inhaled corticosteroid and long-acting inhaled ß-2 agonist (salmeterol) *or* – Medium-dose inhaled corticosteroid – If needed (particularly in patients with recurring severe exacerbations): medium-dose inhaled corticosteroid and long-acting inhaled ß-2 agonist	– Low-dose inhaled corticosteroid and either theophylline or leukotriene receptor antagonist – If needed: medium-dose inhaled corticosteroid and either theophylline or leukotriene receptor antagonist
Step 4: severe persistent	– High-dose inhaled corticosteroid and long-acting inhaled ß-2 agonist – If needed: systemic corticosteroids long term (2 mg/kg/ day, generally not to exceed 60 mg/day)	– High-dose inhaled corticosteroid and sustained-release theophylline to serum concentrations of 5–12 mcg/mL

Adapted from [32] and [12]

salmeterol are classified as in Category C by the FDA [41]. Still, evidence against ß-agonists should be treated with caution since their use is necessitated in severe exacerbations which by itself can cause fetal problems. Indeed, contrary to findings of previous studies, a large database review of could not find any evidence of increased risk of congenital malformations in patients exposed to asthma medication during gestation [42].

Leukotriene receptor antagonists montelukast and zafirlukast antagonize effects of leukotrienes C4, D4, and E4 on airway smooth muscle by suppressing inflammation and bronchoconstriction. There is a paucity of information regarding these agents. A small study with montelukast and zafirlukast could not find any relationship with their use and maternal (pregnancy loss, gestational diabetes, preeclampsia, or low maternal weight gain) or fetal (preterm delivery, low Apgar scores, reduced measures of birth length, or head circumference in the newborns) adverse events [43]. Unlike montelukast and zafirlukast which are shown in category B by the FDA, zileuton is shown to be unsafe in animal studies and not given to pregnant asthmatics [12].

Xanthine derivative theophylline and cromolyn are alternative treatments in persistent mild asthma as they have proven to be inferior to ICS [2]. Theophylline can also be an alternative add-on agent for moderate and severe persistent asthma (Step 3 and 4) for chronic administration as it is not effective in acute exacerbations [14]. Its use is limited due to adverse effects (insomnia, heartburn, palpitations, nausea) and narrow therapeutic range affected by concomitant medications (cimetidine, lorazepam, and erythromycin) and changes in pregnancy (decreased protein binding and decreased metabolism) resulting in the need for serum level controls [2].

Omalizumab is recombinant DNA-derived humanized immunoglobulin (Ig)G1k monoclonal antibody. It binds to human immunoglobulin E in the blood, reducing inflammation. Although this drug is Category B due to animal safety studies and no reported incidence of major congenital malformations, prematurity, or small-for-gestational-age births in its registry [44], it is not prescribed during pregnancy.

Lastly oral corticosteroids are reserved for severe asthma management in pregnancy as their use has been linked with preeclampsia, orofacial defects, congenital malformations, low birth weight, and preterm delivery [45, 46]. Once more, one cannot safely conclude whether these unwanted observations were due to corticosteroid exposure or were due to asthma severity. However, in severe persistent asthma, risk of uncontrolled disease to mother and fetus clearly outweighs aforementioned risks [29].

5.4.3   Management of Acute Exacerbation

Management of acute exacerbation during pregnancy at home and at health institutions is different from each other [32]. For brevity, the latter is displayed (Fig. 5.1).

Initial evaluation of the patient should aim in ensuring the well-being of the mother and fetus. In this regard, oxygen administration, left lateral positioning of the patient, initiating hydration, and avoiding hypotension are prioritized [1, 32].

In severely distressed patients who are not responsive to medical treatment and who exhibit acute respiratory failure with arterial pH <7.35, arterial carbon dioxide

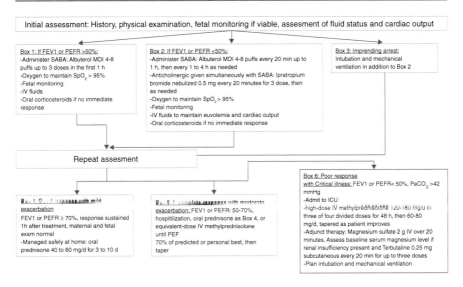

Initial assessment: History, physical examination, fetal monitoring if viable, assesment of fluid status and cardiac output

Box 1: If FEV1 or PEFR >50%:
-Administer SABA: Albuterol MDI 4-8 puffs up to 3 doses in the first 1 h
-Oxygen to maintain SpO₂ > 95%
-Fetal monitoring
-IV fluids
-Oral corticosteroids if no immediate response

Box 2: If FEV1 or PEFR <50%:
-Administer SABA: Albuterol MDI 4-8 puffs every 20 min up to 1 h, then every 1 to 4 h as needed
-Anticholinergic given simultaneously with SABA: Ipratropium bromide nebulized 0.5 mg every 20 minutes for 3 dose, then as needed
-Oxygen to maintain SpO₂ > 95%
-Fetal monitoring
-IV fluids to maintain euvolemia and cardiac output
-Oral corticosteroids if no immediate response

Box 3: Imprending arrest:
Intubation and mechanical ventilation in addition to Box 2

Repeat assesment

Box 4: Good response with mild exacerbation
FEV1 or PEFR ≥ 70%, response sustained 1h after treatment, maternal and fetal exam normal
-Managed safely at home: oral prednisone 40 to 60 mg/d for 3 to 10 d

Box 5: Incomplete response with moderate exacerbation: FEV1 or PEFR: 50-70%, hospitilization, oral prednisone as Box 4, or equivalent-dose IV methylprednisolone until PEF 70% of predicted or personal best, then taper

Box 6: Poor response with Critical illness: FEV1 or PEFR< 50%, PaCO₂ >42 mmHg
-Admit to ICU
-high-dose IV methylprednisolone 120-180 mg/d in three of four divided doses for 48 h, then 60-80 mg/d, tapered as patient improves
-Adjunct therapy: Magnesium sulfate 2 g IV over 20 minutes. Assess baseline serum magnesium level if renal insufficiency present and Terbutaline 0.25 mg subcutaneous every 20 min for up to three doses
-Plan intubation and mechanical ventilation

Fig. 5.1 It shows acute exacerbation treatment in pregnancy mirroring that in nonpregnant patients, adapted from [1] and [32]

partial pressure (PaCO₂) >42 mmHg, and arterial oxygen partial pressure (PaO₂) <70 mmHg, early intubation and mechanical ventilation must be considered. In such a case, ventilator settings should be carefully managed to avoid dynamic hyperinflation and auto-positive end-expiratory pressure (auto-PEEP) with air trapping. Dynamic hyperinflation not only leads to ineffective ventilation and increases risk of barotrauma but also causes hemodynamic instability. General goals for mechanical ventilation can be stated as low tidal volume (6–8 mL/kg), low respiratory rate (8–12 breaths/min), and high inspiratory flow rates (up to 100 L/min) to prolong expiratory time. In order to achieve these goals, hypercapnia is permitted in nonpregnant asthmatic patients, though permissive hypercapnia is controversial in pregnant patients due to fetal acidosis and reduced oxygenation of fetal hemoglobin. Yet, in a series of four patients, hypercapnia was well tolerated [47].

As a last resort, in patients in whom pharmacological treatment and mechanical ventilation have failed, extracorporeal membrane oxygenation (ECMO) may be considered. There are nonpregnant asthmatic patients reported in ECMO registry [48], but there is yet only one report of such a treatment in pregnant patient with successful results [49].

5.5   Obstetric Management

Several aspects of obstetric management need to be emphasized in asthmatic patients. Asthma medication continuation during labor and in the postpartum period is a must. There is also no contraindication to the use of prednisone, theophylline, cromolyn, inhaled corticosteroids, or ß-2 agonists during breastfeeding [23]. If the patient is on systemic corticosteroids, intravenous corticosteroid such as 100 mg hydrocortisone at 8-h intervals during labor should be given to prevent adrenal crisis. If the patient is on steroids, blood glucose levels should be monitored to avoid maternal hyperglycemia effects on fetus [25].

If there is preterm labor danger, magnesium and terbutaline may offer additional bronchodilator effects as tocolytic agents, but indomethacin should be avoided since it may cause bronchospasm specifically in aspirin-sensitive patients [25].

Agents that should be avoided also include bronchoconstricting drugs such as prostaglandin (PG) F2α (dinoprost), ergotamine, and other ergot derivatives. In contrast, PGE1 (misoprostol) and PGE2 (dinoprostone) are deemed safe to use [12, 50, 51]. Oxytocin should be preferred for labor induction and postpartum hemorrhage control [25].

Physicians should be cautious of low-dose aspirin prescription to prevent preeclampsia, as it may trigger bronchospasm in aspirin-sensitive patients. Labetalol, a combined α- and ß-receptor antagonist, commonly used to control blood pressure in preeclamptic patients, can also cause bronchospasm and should be avoided. Of note, vasodilator agents like calcium channel blockers, nitroprusside and nitroglycerin, or hydralazine are safe in terms of bronchoconstriction but have the potential to cause hypoxemia via disturbed hypoxic pulmonary vasoconstriction in asthmatic patients [52].

5.6   Anesthetic Management

Main aims of preoperative evaluation are stratifying risks, optimizing treatment, and minimizing complications of asthma. Patients should be carefully questioned for severity of the disease on symptom frequency, nighttime awakening, limitation of daily activity, and self-measured peak expiratory flow rate if they are measuring. In fact, a correlation between American Society of Anesthesiologists (ASA) physical status classification and asthma severity classification proposed by NAEPP (Table 5.3) [12] can be established with ASA Classes 2, 3, and 4 corresponding to mild, moderate, and severe disease, respectively, in nonpregnant patients [53]. Patients should also be interrogated about the course of the disease during pregnancy, compliance to their pharmacotherapy, date of last exacerbation, smoking habit if any, and any recent pulmonary infections. Patients with severe uncontrolled asthma will be at the highest risk for adverse outcomes [53].

Physical examination may reveal wheezing with or without prolonged expiratory time on chest auscultation. A simple way to understand if exhalation is prolonged is to auscultate the trachea while the patient is instructed to forcefully exhale [54]. If this forced expiratory time is longer than 6 s, it may correlate with decreased FEV_1/FVC ratio. Of note, if the patient is in severe stress with very limited airflow, wheezing may be inaudible. In such a condition, signs of respiratory distress such as increased respiratory rate, use of accessory respiratory muscles, and/or pulsus paradoxus (>20 mmHg) due to exaggerated intrathoracic pressure swings should be looked for [55].

If the patient is stable with no symptoms, there is no need for pulmonary function tests [56], as measurements return to normal values between the attacks. However, in case of a respiratory distress, chest X-ray, arterial blood gas analysis, and spirometry are essential in differential diagnosis and management. Chest X-ray may reveal pulmonary congestion, edema, or infiltrates for differential diagnosis, whereas hyperinflation of the lungs could support diagnosis of asthma. Arterial blood gas analyses in healthy pregnant women reveal a metabolically compensated respiratory alkalosis with $PaCO_2$ of ~30 (28–32) mmHg at term. A chronically elevated $PaCO_2$ in asthmatic pregnant patient may point out uncontrolled disease status [57]. Additionally, at early stages of acute respiratory distress, further decrease in $PaCO_2$ with signs of increased ineffective ventilation efforts can be observed. However, $PaCO_2$ accumulation >42 mmHg with progressive hypoxia, acidosis, and exhaustion should alert the clinician for aggressive precautions.

5.6.1 Anesthetic Management for Labor and Vaginal Delivery

For the asthmatic laboring parturient, analgesia gains a greater importance as pain could trigger disease symptoms. In patients whose symptoms are triggered by exercise or stress, it is also essential to prevent tachypnea and anxiety. Analgesia and relief of anxiety should be accomplished with minimal respiratory depression and sedation of the mother and fetus [58].

Systemic opioids, though inferior to neuraxial techniques in terms of analgesia, are long known to effectively suppress respiratory drive and cough reflex and prevent tachypnea. They may be of benefit in patients with contraindication to neuraxial anesthesia in whom hyperpnoea can be deleterious. In fact, recently opioid receptors in pulmonary neuroendocrine cells and sensory C-fibers are becoming attractive targets to relieve refractory dyspnea in cancer patients [59]. There is some concern for morphine as large boluses over a short period of time can cause histamine release and bronchoconstriction. This concern may not reflect truth as moderate dose of morphine was able to prevent bronchoconstriction in a bronchoprovocation volunteer study with mild asthma [59]. However, morphine is not a usually preferred systemic opioid for labor analgesia due to its difficulty in titration, long elimination half-life, and potent metabolite accumulation [59]. Synthetic opioids (fentanyl, remifentanil) may be preferred as systemic opioids in asthmatic patients [54], but the latter is associated with a significant risk for maternal respiratory depression and arterial desaturation when used in healthy laboring women [59]. Physicians should be aware of the fact that systemic opioid administration in an already respiratory-compromised patient may result in respiratory arrest.

Epidural or intrathecal opioid administration particularly in the first stage of labor can effectively maintain analgesia without any motor block. As stated in a comprehensive review about obstetric setting [60], maternal respiratory depression with neuraxial opioids is rare in doses used, and large doses of intrathecal lipophilic opioids (>10 mcg sufentanil or >50 mcg fentanyl) would only increase this risk without any increased analgesic effect. However, patients under risk (patients who have received systemic opioids or magnesium, patients with respiratory compromise) should be identified and closely monitored as respiratory depression is reported even in small doses [61].

Lumbar epidural local anesthetic administration in asthmatic laboring parturient can provide effective analgesia and suppress maternal hyperventilation caused by painful uterine contractions. Epidural analgesia using bupivacaine and fentanyl was reported to enhance effectiveness of bronchodilators in a case of laboring parturient in status asthmaticus [62]. Moreover, if emergency cesarean section is needed, presence of epidural catheter can facilitate epidural anesthesia avoiding the need for airway instrumentation. Epidural block extension higher than thoracic dermatomes could potentially lead problems in patients with respiratory compromise. But this is normally not a concern for labor analgesia, where dilute local anesthetics are used to aim an upper sensory block level of T10 dermatome.

5.6.2 Anesthetic Management for Cesarean Section

As mentioned above, regional anesthesia should be preferred for cesarean section to avoid airway instrumentation. Tracheal intubation has shown to evoke bronchoconstriction in volunteers with bronchial hyperreactivity [63]. This bronchoconstriction is an efferent response to reflex mechanism where stimulus is sensed via irritant receptors and carried by afferent parasympathetic fibers. In closed claims analysis of ASA in 1990, nearly all bronchospasm complaints were related with tracheal intubation [64]. Indeed, when similar procedures are compared, regional anesthesia is associated with fewer respiratory complications compared to general anesthesia [65].

Motor blockade of abdominal muscles during spinal anesthesia may decrease PEFR [66], but this is probably not important in asymptomatic asthma patients. It can become a point of concern when high and dense block in neuraxial anesthesia blocks accessory inspiratory muscles in patients who are dependent on these to sustain minute ventilation. However, some argue against such a possibility, as high epidural block did not result in significant vital capacity changes in respiratory-compromised mastectomy patients [67].

Second concern of high thoracic blockade is related to pulmonary sympathetic denervation with unopposed parasympathetic system causing bronchoconstriction. Yet, high thoracic epidural anesthesia did not result in such an outcome and even attenuated the response to provocation in a controlled study [68]. Still, albeit rare, there are reports of bronchospasm under regional anesthesia necessitating careful monitoring of block level [69]. Last concern is related to reduced output of adrenal medulla due to blockade of T6-L2 spinal segments. But this is not a valid theory. Although epinephrine is an effective bronchodilator, its release is not stimulated during bronchospasm [70].

General anesthesia, hence airway instrumentation, may be mandated in pregnant patients with contraindications to neuraxial anesthesia, or in patients with severe respiratory distress [71].

Need for awake intubation in obstetric anesthesia is very rare, but when indicated premedication with ß-2 agonist inhalation (even with patients' own inhaler) and local anesthetic (topical or airway blocks) can help in abolishing airway reflexes. In such a situation, risk of aspiration due to loss of reflexes should be taken into account. Intravenous lidocaine is also effective in blunting reflex response to intubation [63, 72].

Preoxygenation with adequate duration prior to induction is a must. Intubation is generally performed after rapid sequence induction with propofol and/or ketamine. Propofol has been shown to induce less bronchoconstriction than thiopentone [73, 74]. Similarly, ketamine, by directly acting on bronchial smooth muscle and potentiating catecholamine effects, has bronchodilator properties. Although there is one report of inhalation anesthesia induction [75], it is usually not preferred due to concerns of slow induction with possibility of aspiration.

For muscle relaxant choice, succinylcholine or rocuronium can be safely used for rapid sequence induction. Another alternative is vecuronium, but agents that cause histamine release such as atracurium and mivacurium should be avoided. An important point to remember is that reversal of neuromuscular agent with neostigmine at the end of the surgery could also increase secretions and trigger hyperreactivity. But this can be suppressed with atropine or glycopyrrolate. The use of sugammadex (a cyclodextrine derivative designed to encapsulate rocuronium and vecuronium) can present unique opportunities in reversing these agents at the end of operation in patients with respiratory diseases and are advocated for changes in rapid sequence induction in pregnancy [76–78]. Although an animal study on the effect of sugammadex on bronchial tonus could not demonstrate any negative effects [79], cases of laryngospasm and intraoperative anaphylaxis have recently been reported [80, 81].

Inhalational anesthesia with halogenated agents is typically used for general anesthesia maintenance, as they are effective bronchodilators also attenuating histamine-induced bronchospasm. Their effects are explained by increase intracellular c-AMP via ß-adrenergic stimulation [82]. Bronchodilator effects are dose-dependent and agent specific. There is animal data that sevoflurane inhibits allergic airway inflammation [83]. It may be preferred to desflurane as it has been shown to be superior in reducing respiratory resistance [84]. Desflurane has also been noted for bronchoconstricting effects in smokers [84]. One caveat with inhalational agents is their potential dose-dependent relaxation effect on uterine musculature [85].

Extubation and emergence is another discerning time period for asthmatic patients when bronchospasm could occur. Despite this, extubation in deep plane of anesthesia to avoid endotracheal tube stimulation carries aspiration risk.

Postoperative care should focus on adequate pain relief where trunk blocks could offer the benefit of decreasing opioid requirement. Administration of humidified oxygenation and short-acting bronchodilators may be necessary in postoperative care unit. If there is sustained exacerbation unresponsive to treatment, transfer to intensive care unit for noninvasive or invasive mechanical ventilation support may be required [32].

Key Learning Points

- Asthma is related with a series of maternal and fetal adverse outcomes. Therefore, severity and triggering factors in parturients should be assessed by a multidisciplinary team, and stepwise medical approach should be tailored according to individual needs.
- Patients should be informed that medication discontinuation, triggering agents, smoking, and/or respiratory viral infections could result in acute exacerbations with hazardous consequences.
- Anesthesiologists as well as obstetricians should avoid drugs or techniques that would provoke bronchoconstriction. In this regard, neuraxial analgesia/anesthesia—hence avoidance of airway instrumentation—should be preferred in stable patients.
- For unstable patients, rescue drugs as well as continued monitoring and possible need for mechanical ventilation should be anticipated.

References

1. Bonham CA, Patterson KC, Strek ME. Asthma outcomes and management during pregnancy. Chest. 2018;153(2):515–27.
2. Namazy JA, Schatz M. Pharmacotherapy options to treat asthma during pregnancy. Expert Opin Pharmacother. 2015;16(12):1783–91.
3. Zairina E, Stewart K, Abramson MJ, George J. The effectiveness of non-pharmacological healthcare interventions for asthma management during pregnancy: a systematic review. BMC Pulm Med. 2014;14(1):1–8.
4. Kwon HL, Belanger K, Bracken MB. Asthma prevalence among pregnant and childbearing-aged women in the United States: estimates from national health surveys. Ann Epidemiol. 2003;13(5):317–24.
5. Clifton VL, Engel P, Smith R, Gibson P, Brinsmead M, Giles WB. Maternal and neonatal outcomes of pregnancies complicated by asthma in an Australian population. Aust N Z J Obstet Gynaecol. 2009;49(6):619–26.
6. Baghlaf H, Spence AR, Czuzoj-Shulman N, Abenhaim HA. Pregnancy outcomes among women with asthma. J Matern Fetal Neonatal Med. 2017; https://doi.org/10.1080/14767058.2017.1404982.
7. Mendola P, Laughon SK, Männistö TI, Leishear K, Reddy UM, Chen Z, et al. Obstetric complications among US women with asthma. Am J Obstet Gynecol. 2013;208(2):127.e1–8. https://doi.org/10.1016/j.ajog.2012.11.007.
8. Blais L, Kettani FZ, Forget A. Associations of maternal asthma severity and control with pregnancy complications. J Asthma. 2014;51(4):391–8.
9. Murphy VE, Wang G, Namazy JA, Powell H, Gibson PG, Chambers C, et al. The risk of congenital malformations, perinatal mortality and neonatal hospitalisation among pregnant women with asthma: a systematic review and meta-analysis. BJOG. 2013;120(7):812–22.
10. Murphy VE, Mattes J, Powell H, Baines KJ, Gibson PG. Respiratory viral infections in pregnant women with asthma are associated with wheezing in the first 12 months of life. Pediatr Allergy Immunol. 2014;25(2):151–8.
11. Siston AM, Rasmussen SA, Honein MA, Fry AM, Seib K, Callaghan WM, et al. Pandemic 2009 influenza A (H1N1) virus illness among pregnant women in the United States. JAMA. 2010;303(15):1517–25.

12. National Heart Lung and Blood Institute. Expert panel report 3 (EPR-3): guidelines for the diagnosis and management of asthma-summary report 2007. J Allergy Clin Immunol. 2017;120(5 Suppl):S94–138.
13. Tamási L, Bohács A, Horváth I, Losonczy G. Asthma in pregnancy—from immunology to clinical management. Multidiscip Respir Med. 2010;5(4):259–63.
14. Hardy-Fairbanks AJ, Baker ER. Asthma in pregnancy: pathophysiology, diagnosis and management. Obstet Gynecol Clin N Am. 2010;37(2):159–72.
15. Juniper EF, Daniel EE, Roberts RS, Kline PA, Hargreave FE, Newhouse MT. Effect of pregnancy on airway responsiveness and asthma severity. Relationship to serum progesterone. Am Rev Respir Dis. 1991;143(3 Pt 2):S78.
16. Murphy VE, Gibson PG. Asthma in pregnancy. Clin Chest Med. 2011;32(1):93–110.
17. Bohács A, Pállinger E, Tamási L, Rigó J, Komlósi Z, Müller V, et al. Surface markers of lymphocyte activation in pregnant asthmatics. Inflamm Res. 2010;59(1):63–70.
18. Tamási L, Bohács A, Pállinger E, Falus A, Rigó J, Müller V, et al. Increased interferon-gamma- and interleukin-4-synthesizing subsets of circulating T lymphocytes in pregnant asthmatics. Clin Exp Allergy. 2005;35(9):1197–203.
19. Tamási L, Bohács A, Tamási V, Stenczer B, Prohászka Z, Rigó J, et al. Increased circulating heat shock protein 70 levels in pregnant asthmatics. Cell Stress Chaperones. 2010;15(3):295–300.
20. Bohács A, Cseh A, Stenczer B, Müller V, Gálffy G, Molvarec A, et al. Effector and regulatory lymphocytes in asthmatic pregnant women. Am J Reprod Immunol. 2010;64(6):393–401.
21. Tamási L, Horváth I, Bohács A, Müller V, Losonczy G, Schatz M. Asthma in pregnancy—immunological changes and clinical management. Respir Med. 2011;105(2):159–64.
22. Schatz M, Harden K, Forsythe A, Chilingar L, Hoffman C, Sperling W, et al. The course of asthma during pregnancy, post partum, and with successive pregnancies: a prospective analysis. J Allergy Clin Immunol. 1988;81(3):509–17.
23. Dombrowski MP, Schatz M, ACOG Committee on Practice Bulletins-Obstetrics. ACOG practice bulletin: clinical management guidelines for obstetrician-gynecologists number 90, February 2008: asthma in pregnancy. Obstet Gynecol. 2008;111(2 Pt 1):457–64.
24. Orzechowski KM, Miller RC. Common respiratory issues in ambulatory obstetrics. Clin Obstet Gynecol. 2012;55(3):798–809.
25. Vatti RR, Teuber SS. Asthma and pregnancy. Clin Rev Allergy Immunol. 2012;43(1–2):45–56.
26. Namazy JA, Schatz M. Asthma and pregnancy. J Allergy Clin Immunol. 2011;128(6):1384–1385.e2.
27. The National Institute for Health and Care Excellence (NICE). Asthma: diagnosis and monitoring of asthma in adults, children and young people. 2017. http://www.nice.org.uk/guidance/indevelopment/gid-cgwave0640/consultation. Accessed Feb 2018.
28. Murphy VE, Jensen ME, Mattes J, Hensley MJ, Giles WB, Peek MJ, et al. The breathing for life trial: a randomised controlled trial of fractional exhaled nitric oxide (FENO)-based management of asthma during pregnancy and its impact on perinatal outcomes and infant and childhood respiratory health. BMC Pregnancy Childbirth. 2016;16:111.
29. Reddel HK, Bateman ED, Becker A, Boulet L-P, Cruz AA, Drazen JM, et al. A summary of the new GINA strategy: a roadmap to asthma control. Eur Respir J. 2015;46(3):622–39.
30. Juniper EF, O'Byrne PM, Guyatt GH, Ferrie PJ, King DR. Development and validation of a questionnaire to measure asthma control. Eur Respir J. 1999;14(4):902–7.
31. Price DB, Román-Rodríguez M, McQueen RB, Bosnic-Anticevich S, Carter V, Gruffydd-Jones K, et al. Inhaler errors in the CRITIKAL study: type, frequency, and association with asthma outcomes. J Allergy Clin Immunol Pract. 2017; https://doi.org/10.1016/j.jaip.2017.01.004.
32. Alex Racusin D, Anneliese Fox K, Ramin SM. Severe acute asthma. Semin Perinatol. 2013;37(4):234–45.
33. Tegethoff M, Greene N, Olsen J, Schaffner E, Meinlschmidt G. Inhaled glucocorticoids during pregnancy and offspring pediatric diseases: a national cohort study. Am J Respir Crit Care Med. 2012;185(5):557–63.

34. Bjørn A-MB, Ehrenstein V, Nohr EA, Nørgaard M. Use of inhaled and oral corticosteroids in pregnancy and the risk of malformations or miscarriage. Basic Clin Pharmacol Toxicol. 2015;116(4):308–14.

35. de Aguiar MM, da Silva HJ, Rizzo JÂ, Leite DFB, Silva Lima MEPL, Sarinho ESC. Inhaled beclomethasone in pregnant asthmatic women – a systematic review. Allergol Immunopathol. 2014;42(5):493–9.

36. Cossette B, Beauchesne M-F, Forget A, Lemière C, Larivée P, Rey E, et al. Relative perinatal safety of salmeterol vs formoterol and fluticasone vs budesonide use during pregnancy. Ann Allergy Asthma Immunol. 2014;112(5):459–64.

37. Lin S, Munsie JPW, Herdt-Losavio ML, Druschel CM, Campbell K, Browne ML, et al. Maternal asthma medication use and the risk of selected birth defects. Pediatrics. 2012;129(2):e317–24.

38. Lin S, Munsie JPW, Herdt-Losavio ML, Bell E, Druschel C, Romitti PA, et al. Maternal asthma medication use and the risk of gastroschisis. Am J Epidemiol. 2008;68(1):73–9.

39. Munsie JW, Lin S, Browne ML, Campbell KA, Caton AR, Bell EM, et al. Maternal broncho-dilator use and the risk of orofacial clefts. Hum Reprod. 2011;26(11):3147–54.

40. Lin S, Herdt-Losavio M, Gensburg L, Marshall E, Druschel C. Maternal asthma, asthma medi-cation use, and the risk of congenital heart defects. Birth Defects Res A Clin Mol Teratol. 2009;85(2):161–8.

41. Kher S, Mota P. Maternal asthma: management strategies. Cleve Clin J Med. 2017;84(4):296–302.

42. Tata LJ, Lewis SA, McKeever TM, Smith CJP, Doyle P, Smeeth L, et al. Effect of maternal asthma, exacerbations and asthma medication use on congenital malformations in offspring: a UK population-based study. Thorax. 2008;63(11):981–7.

43. Bakhireva LN, Jones KL, Schatz M, Klonoff-Cohen HS, Johnson D, Slymen DJ, et al. Safety of leukotriene receptor antagonists in pregnancy. J Allergy Clin Immunol. 2007;119(3):618–25.

44. Namazy J, Cabana MD, Scheuerle AE, Thorp JM, Chen H, Carrigan G, et al. The Xolair Pregnancy Registry (EXPECT): the safety of omalizumab use during pregnancy. J Allergy Clin Immunol. 2015;135(2):407–12.

45. Namazy JA, Murphy VE, Powell H, Gibson PG, Chambers C, Schatz M. Effects of asthma severity, exacerbations and oral corticosteroids on perinatal outcomes. Eur Respir J. 2013;41(5):1082–90.

46. Chambers C. Safety of asthma and allergy medications in pregnancy. Immunol Allergy Clin N Am. 2006;26(1):13–28.

47. Elsayegh D, Shapiro JM. Management of the obstetric patient with status asthmaticus. J Intensive Care Med. 2008;23(6):396–402.

48. Yeo HJ, Kim D, Jeon D, Kim YS, Rycus P, Cho WH. Extracorporeal membrane oxygenation for life-threatening asthma refractory to mechanical ventilation: analysis of the extracorporeal life support organization registry. Crit Care. 2017;21(1):297.

49. Steinack C, Lenherr R, Hendra H, Franzen D. The use of life-saving extracorporeal membrane oxygenation (ECMO) for pregnant woman with status asthmaticus. J Asthma. 2017;54(1):84–8.

50. Rooney Thompson M, Towers CV, Howard BC, Hennessy MD, Wolfe L, Heitzman C. The use of prostaglandin E₁ in peripartum patients with asthma. Am J Obstet Gynecol. 2015;212(3):392.e1–3.

51. Towers CV, Briggs GG, Rojas JA. The use of prostaglandin E2 in pregnant patients with asthma. Am J Obstet Gynecol. 2004;190(6):1777–80.

52. Moudgil R. Hypoxic pulmonary vasoconstriction. J Appl Physiol. 2004;98(1):390–403.

53. Sisitki M, Bohringer CH, Fleming N. Anesthesia for patients with asthma. In: Bronchial asthma. New York: Springer; 2012. p. 345–59. Available from: http://link.springer.com/10.1007/978-1-4419-6836-4_15.

54. Woods BD, Sladen RN. Perioperative considerations for the patient with asthma and broncho-spasm. Br J Anaesth. 2009;103(Supp 1):57–65.

55. Hamzaoui O, Monnet X, Teboul JL. Pulsus paradoxus. Eur Respir J. 2013;42(6):1696–705.

56. Smetana GW. Preoperative pulmonary evaluation. N Engl J Med. 1999;340(12):937–44.

57. Kelly W, Massoumi A, Lazarus A. Asthma in pregnancy: physiology, diagnosis, and manage-ment. Postgrad Med. 2015;127(4):349–58.

58. Global Initiative for Asthma. Global strategy for asthma management and prevention. 2017. Available from: www.ginasthma.org. Accessed Sep 2017.
59. Eschenbacher WL, Bethel RA, Boushey HA, Sheppard D. Morphine sulfate inhibits broncho-constriction in subjects with mild asthma whose responses are inhibited by atropine. Am Rev Respir Dis. 1984;130(3):363–7.
60. Carvalho B. Respiratory depression after neuraxial opioids in the obstetric setting. Anesth Analg. 2008;107(3):956–61.
61. Kuczkowski KM. Respiratory arrest in a parturient following intrathecal administration of fen-tanyl and bupivacaine as part of a combined spinal-epidural analgesia for labour. Anaesthesia. 2002;57(9):939–40.
62. Younker D, Clark R, Tessem J, Joyce TH, Kubicek M. Bupivacaine-fentanyl epidural analgesia for a parturient in status asthmaticus. Can J Anaesth. 1987;34(6):609–12.
63. Groeben H, Schlicht M, Stieglitz S, Pavlakovic G, Peters J. Both local anesthetics and salbu-tamol pretreatment affect reflex bronchoconstriction in volunteers with asthma undergoing awake fiberoptic intubation. Anesthesiology. 2002;97(6):1445–50.
64. Cheney FW, Posner KL, Caplan RA. Adverse respiratory events infrequently leading to mal-practice suits. A closed claims analysis. Anesthesiology. 1991;75(6):932–9.
65. Groeben H. Strategies in the patient with compromised respiratory function. Best Pract Res Clin Anaesthesiol. 2004;18(4):579–94.
66. Arai Y-CP, Ogata J, Fukunaga K, Shimazu A, Fujioka A, Uchida T. The effect of intrathecal fentanyl added to hyperbaric bupivacaine on maternal respiratory function during cesarean section. Acta Anaesthesiol Scand. 2006;50(3):364–7.
67. Groeben H, Schafer B, Pavlakovic G, Silvanus M-T, Peters J. Lung function under high tho-racic segmental epidural anesthesia with ropivacaine or bupivacaine in patients with severe obstructive pulmonary disease undergoing breast surgery. Anesthesiology. 2002;96(3):536–41.
68. Groeben H, Schwalen A, Irsfeld S, Tarnow J, Lipfert P, Hopf HB. High thoracic epidural anes-thesia does not alter airway resistance and attenuates the response to an inhalational provoca-tion test in patients with bronchial hyperreactivity. Anesthesiology. 1994;81(4):868–74.
69. McGough EK, Cohen JA. Unexpected bronchospasm during spinal anesthesia. J Clin Anesth. 1990;2(1):35–6.
70. Emerman CL, Cydulka RK. Changes in serum catecholamine levels during acute broncho-spasm. Ann Emerg Med. 1993;22(12):1836–41.
71. Holland SM, Thomson KD. Acute severe asthma presenting in late pregnancy. Int J Obstet Anesth. 2006;15(1):75–8.
72. Adamzik M, Groeben H, Farahani R, Lehmann N, Peters J. Intravenous lidocaine after tra-cheal intubation mitigates bronchoconstriction in patients with asthma. Anesth Analg. 2007;104(1):168–72.
73. Wu RS, Wu KC, Sum DC, Bishop MJ. Comparative effects of thiopentone and propofol on respiratory resistance after tracheal intubation. Br J Anaesth. 1996;77(6):735–8.
74. Pizov R, Brown RH, Weiss YS, Baranov D, Hennes H, Baker S, et al. Wheezing during induc-tion of general anesthesia in patients with and without asthma. A randomized, blinded trial. Anesthesiology. 1995;82(5):1111–6.
75. Que JC, Lusaya VO. Sevoflurane induction for emergency cesarean section in a parturient in status asthmaticus. Anesthesiology. 1999;90(5):1475–6.
76. Amao R, Zornow MH, Cowan RM, Cheng DC, Morte JB, Allard MW. Use of sugammadex in patients with a history of pulmonary disease. J Clin Anesth. 2012;24(4):289–97.
77. McGuigan PJ, Shields MO, McCourt KC. Role of rocuronium and sugammadex in rapid sequence induction in pregnancy. Br J Anaesth. 2011;106(3):418–9.
78. Pühringer FK, Kristen P, Rex C. Sugammadex reversal of rocuronium-induced neuromuscular block in caesarean section patients: a series of seven cases. Br J Anaesth. 2010;105(5):657–60.
79. Yoshioka N, Hanazaki M, Fujita Y, Nakatsuka H, Katayama H, Chiba Y. Effect of sugammadex on bronchial smooth muscle function in rats. J Smooth Muscle Res. 2012;48(2–3):59–64.
80. Ue KL, Kasternow B, Wagner A, Rutkowski R, Rutkowski K. Sugammadex. An emerging trigger of intraoperative anaphylaxis. Ann Allergy Asthma Immunol. 2016;117(6):714–6.

81. McGuire B, Dalton AJ. Sugammadex, airway obstruction, and drifting across the ethical divide: a personal account. Anaesthesia. 2016;71(5):487–92.
82. Burburan SM, Xisto DG, M Rocco PR, de Ja Ro R. Anaesthetic management in asthma. Minerva Anestesiol. 2007;7373(357):357–65.
83. Shen Q-Y, Fang L, Wu H-M, He F, Ding P-S, Liu R-Y. Repeated inhalation of sevoflurane inhibits airway inflammation in an OVA-induced mouse model of allergic airway inflammation. Respirology. 2015;20(2):258–63.
84. Goff MJ, Arain SR, Ficke DJ, Uhrich TD, Ebert TJ. Absence of bronchodilation during desflurane anesthesia: a comparison to sevoflurane and thiopental. Anesthesiology. 2000;93(2):404–8.
85. Yoo KY, Lee JC, Yoon MH, Shin M-H, Kim SJ, Kim YH, et al. The effects of volatile anesthetics on spontaneous contractility of isolated human pregnant uterine muscle: a comparison among sevoflurane, desflurane, isoflurane, and halothane. Anesth Analg. 2006;103(2):443–7.

Anesthesia for the Pregnant Patient with Autoimmune Disorders

6

Rie Kato and Toshiyuki Okutomi

6.1 Systemic Lupus Erythematosus

Systemic lupus erythematosus (SLE) is a multisystem chronic inflammatory disease, with a heterogeneous presentation. It is most commonly recognized in women between 15 and 40 years of age. The main pathogenesis is thought to be autoimmunity against various cellular components, such as double-strand DNA [1].

6.1.1 Diagnosis

The diagnostic criteria by the American College of Rheumatology (ACR) are widely used for SLE (Table 6.1). Newly diagnostic criteria were developed in 2012 by Systemic Lupus International Collaboration group [4]. According to the comparative studies, two criteria have not indicated that one is superior to the other [4, 5].

6.1.2 Effects of Pregnancy on SLE

Lupus flares can occur at any time during pregnancy, as well as several months following delivery [6]. Such flares may be associated with immunological and hormonal changes caused by pregnancy [7]. A widely held perception is that the predominance of Th2 over Th1 cytokine, which enhances immunological tolerance to the fetus, is the main culprit of this exacerbation [7]. The serum concentrations of pro-inflammatory cytokines are increased by pregnancy in the general population. This is more prominent in SLE patients, especially during the active period [8].

R. Kato (✉) · T. Okutomi
Division of Obstetric Anesthesia, Center for Perinatal Care, Child Health and Development,
Kitasato University Hospital, Sagamihara, Japan
e-mail: rie.kato@nifty.com

© Springer International Publishing AG, part of Springer Nature 2018
B. Gunaydin, S. Ismail (eds.), *Obstetric Anesthesia for Co-morbid Conditions*,
https://doi.org/10.1007/978-3-319-93163-0_6

Table 6.1 Summary of diagnostic criteria for SLE by the American College of Rheumatology [2, 3]

1. Malar rash	
2. Discoid rash	
3. Photosensitivity	
4. Oral or nasopharyngeal ulceration	
5. Arthritis	Two or more peripheral joints
6. Serositis	Pleuritis or pericarditis
7. Renal disorder	Persistent proteinuria or cellular casts
8. Neurologic disorder	Seizures or psychosis
9. Hematologic disorder	Hemolytic anemia, leukopenia, lymphopenia, or thrombocytopenia
10. Immunologic disorder	Anti-DNA antibody, anti-Sm antibody, lupus anticoagulant, or false-positive syphilis test
11. Antinuclear antibody	

For identifying patients in clinical studies, presence of any 4 or more of the 11 criteria indicates systemic lupus erythematosus

Table 6.2 Symptoms and signs of pregnancy that mimic lupus activity [9, 10]

- Fatigue
- Dyspnea
- Backache
- Palmar erythema and a facial blush
- Mild anemia/thrombocytopenia
- Seizures in eclampsia

Estrogens and prolactin may interact with the immune system to amplify the inflammation. The risk of flares during pregnancy is seven times higher when the women had active disease 6 months prior to conception [6].

6.1.3 Flares

The recognition of an SLE flare during pregnancy can be difficult because its signs and symptoms often mimic those of normal pregnancy (Table 6.2). However, C3/C4 and anti-double-strand DNA can be useful tools to diagnose a flare. The serum levels of C3, C4, and C50 are increased during normal pregnancy due to increased production in the liver. But these complements are consumed and decreased by a flare. When the level of C3, C4, or C50 is below the normal range or falls by 25% during pregnancy, it should be attributed to SLE. Anti-double-strand DNA antibodies are a highly sensitive and specific test for SLE [9]. In nonpregnant patients, SLE activity scales, such as SLE Disease Activity Index (DAI) and Lupus Activity Index (LAI), are commonly used to evaluate the disease activity. Because of similarity of symptoms and signs between pregnancy and SLE, these scales have been modified to adapt to pregnancy. For example, LAI in pregnancy was validated in pregnant women and showed high sensitivity and specificity [9].

6.1.4   Flares and Preeclampsia

Differential diagnosis between lupus nephritis and preeclampsia is also challenging because hypertension, proteinuria, and edema are common features in both diseases. But the distinction is essential because not only the treatments but also anesthetic considerations are different. High level of serum uric acid and proteinuria without active urinary sediment are suggestive of preeclampsia rather than lupus nephritis. Whether SLE women are more likely to present with preeclampsia is controversial. When thrombocytopenia occurs in a pregnant woman with SLE, HELLP syndrome, pregnancy-induced thrombocytopenia, idiopathic thrombocytopenia, and thrombotic thrombocytopenia purpura should be ruled out. Elevated liver enzymes are suggestive of preeclampsia rather than deterioration of SLE. It should be noted that neurologic features of SLE include seizure, which can be confused with eclampsia.

6.1.5   Effects on Pregnancy Outcome

Pregnancies complicated with SLE are more likely to result in obstetric morbidities [11–13]. According to a large systematic review, fetal complications included spontaneous abortion (16%), intrauterine growth restriction (13%), still birth (4%), and neonatal deaths (2.5%). Among all live births, the premature birth rate was as high as 40% [14]. Disease activity at conception and the previous months is an important predictor of not only maternal outcome but also obstetrical complications. A study from Korea reported that 4 months' quiescence significantly reduced pregnancy loss, premature birth, and intrauterine growth restriction [15]. History of lupus nephritis and presence of antiphospholipid syndrome are also risk factors of obstetric outcomes [13, 16].

6.1.6   Effects on the Baby

When the mother is anti-SSA or -SSB antibody positive, a quarter of babies have developed neonatal lupus erythematosus (see Sjögren's syndrome). In the animal study, it has been suggested that exposure of maternal antibodies and cytokines to the fetus is an important risk factor for neurodevelopmental disorder. However, a very limited epidemiological data suggests that children born to women with SLE may have an increased risk of neurodevelopmental disorders compared to those born to non-SLE women [17].

6.1.7   Medical Treatment

Symptomatic treatments are the mainstay of management against SLE. The choice of medical agents depends on the severity and manifestations of the disease. The

European League Against Rheumatism has issued the recommendations for SLE management for the general population [18]. Glucocorticoids and antimalarial agents may be beneficial in patient without major organ manifestations. Nonsteroidal anti-inflammatory drugs (NSAIDs) may be used for short periods in patients at low risk for complications. Immunosuppressive agents (azathioprine, mycophenolate mofetil, methotrexate, and cyclophosphamide) should be considered in refractory cases or when steroid doses cannot be reduced to levels for long-term use. In pregnant patients, prednisolone, azathioprine, hydroxychloroquine (an antimalarial drug), and low-dose aspirin may be used. Dexamethasone and betamethasone have higher placental transfer rates than prednisolone and may lead to fetal growth restriction and abnormal neurodevelopment. Mycophenolate mofetil, methotrexate, and cyclophosphamide must be avoided due to their teratogenic effects [18]. Current data about the safety of belimumab, a human monoclonal antibody that inhibits B-cell-activating factor, for pregnant women are still very limited [19].

6.1.8   Anesthetic Considerations

Patients should be assessed early because SLE women are at high risk of preterm labor and further examination or treatment might be necessary before anesthesia. Preoperative assessment includes SLE flares, comorbidities, and medication history. Consultation with the rheumatologist will provide accurate information. SLE presents wide range of comorbidities. In the airway, cricoarytenoiditis, vocal cord paralysis, and epiglottitis have been reported. More commonly, ulceration in the mouth and nasopharynx may be observed. Pleuritis and interstitial pneumonia are relatively common pulmonary manifestations. Although rare, pulmonary hypertension is a well-documented complication. In the cardiovascular system, SLE patients are at higher risks of pericarditis, myocarditis, and coronary disease. Therefore, very careful anesthetic management is needed in some SLE cases. Neuropsychiatric SLE is consisted of wide range of pathologies: seizures, psychosis, myelopathy, and neuropathy. It may be prudent to avoid neuraxial anesthesia in such patients. As SLE may result in thrombocytopenia, platelet count should be checked before anesthesia, especially in the patient with a flare. Arthritis is not an uncommon manifestation. About 40% of SLE patient have antiphospholipid syndrome [20], which requires special anesthetic consideration (see antiphospholipid syndrome). SLE patients also have higher susceptibility to infection [1].

Choice of anesthetic method, monitoring, and drugs and fluid management must be tailored on individual cases, depending on types and severity of comorbidities. Corticosteroids should be replaced during anesthesia [1].

6.2   Antiphospholipid Syndrome

Antiphospholipid syndrome (APS) is an acquired autoimmune disorder that manifests as thrombosis or pregnancy morbidity. The mechanism of thrombosis is controversial but may include vascular endothelial and platelet activation by antiphospholipid antibody per se or resultant complement activation [21].

6.2.1 Clinical Features

Thrombotic events occur not only in the vein but also in the artery. Deep vein thrombosis of the lower extremities is common, but other veins may be affected, such as the pelvic, renal, and pulmonary veins. In the artery, cerebrovascular thrombosis is most frequently reported, followed by myocardial infarction [20]. The other characteristic feature of APL is pregnancy morbidity, which constitutes of a major part of diagnostic criteria of APS (Table 6.3). This includes miscarriage, intrauterine fetal demise, and preterm birth. Pregnant women with APL have higher incidence of hypertensive disorders of pregnancy, HELLP syndrome, and placental abruption [23]. The APS can be found in patients having neither clinical nor laboratory evidence of other definable condition (primary APS), or it may be associated with other disorders, such as other autoimmune diseases, infection, and cancer [24].

6.2.2 Diagnosis

Table 6.3 shows the international consensus criteria. APS is diagnosed by thrombosis or pregnancy morbidity, in the presence of antiphospholipid antibodies, namely, lupus anticoagulant, anticardiolipin antibody, or anti-beta-2 glycoprotein I antibody in plasma [22]. However, non-criteria obstetric APS, such as repetitive miscarriages less than 10 weeks in the presence of low anticardiolipin or anti-beta-2 glycoprotein antibody, is often treated as APS [25, 26].

Table 6.3 Summary of Sapporo (Sydney) classification criteria for the antiphospholipid syndrome [22]

Antiphospholipid antibody syndrome (APS) is diagnosed if at least one of the clinical criteria and one of the laboratory criteria are present
Clinical criteria
1. Vascular thrombosis
Thrombosis must be confirmed by objective validated criteria
2. Pregnancy morbidity
(a) One or more unexplained deaths of a morphologically normal fetus at or beyond the 10 weeks of gestation, with normal fetal morphology documented by ultrasound or by direct examination of the fetus
(b) One or more premature births of a morphologically normal neonate before the 34 weeks of gestation because of (1) eclampsia or severe preeclampsia defined according to standard definitions or (2) recognized features of placental insufficiency
(c) Three or more unexplained consecutive spontaneous abortions before the 10 weeks of gestation, with maternal anatomic or hormonal abnormalities and paternal and maternal chromosomal causes excluded
Laboratory criteria
1. Presence of lupus anticoagulant in plasma, on two or more occasions at least 12 weeks apart
2. Presence of anticardiolipin antibody in serum or plasma in medium or high titer on two or more occasions, at least 12 weeks apart
3. Presence of anti-b2 glycoprotein I antibody in serum or plasma, on two or more occasions, at least 12 weeks apart

6.2.3   Pathogenesis of Obstetric APS

As APS is a thrombotic disease, it is not surprising that the uteroplacental circulation is impaired. However, placental infarction is neither a universal nor a specific finding. Complement activation and chronic inflammation also play roles in the pregnancy loss [21].

6.2.4   Medical Treatments

Anticoagulant therapy is indicated in APS. Medications include antiplatelet agents (low-dose aspirin, dipyridamole, and ticlopidine) and anticoagulant (warfarin, unfractionated heparin, low-molecular-weight heparin) in the general population. During pregnancy, warfarin should be withheld because it is transferred to the fetus and might result in malformation. The rate of placental transfer of heparin is low. Heparin with or without low-dose aspirin should be considered for antenatal and postnatal thromboprophylaxis in pregnant women with APS [21, 27]. The dose of heparin depends on the severity of thrombotic events and other risk factors and should be individualized in each case [27, 28].

6.2.5   Anesthetic Considerations

Although APS is a thrombophilic disorder, APS patients often have prolonged aPTT. This is because lupus anticoagulant interferes with in vitro phospholipid that is required for the conversion of prothrombin to thrombin. Therefore, prolonged aPTT per se in lupus anticoagulant-positive patients is not a contraindication to neuraxial anesthesia. Monitoring anticoagulation can be very challenging. APTT is often used to monitor the anticoagulant effect of unfractionated heparin, but this is not feasible when aPTT is prolonged by lupus anticoagulant per se.

Prevention of thrombotic events is the main focus of anesthetic management. Compression stockings, avoiding dehydration, and early ambulation are highly recommended. Perioperative or peri-delivery anticoagulation plan should be discussed. Guidelines for neuraxial anesthesia in patients on anticoagulant agents have been published [13, 29]. However, they are based on data of nonpregnant patients. Pregnant women may have different pharmacokinetics and pharmacodynamics for anticoagulant agents. For example, pregnant women have attenuated response of aPTT to unfractionated heparin [30]. In addition, there is paucity of data regarding risks of neuraxial anesthesia in parturients on anticoagulant medication. Therefore, indication of neuraxial anesthesia and management of anticoagulation can vary markedly. Anesthetic plan also depends on other coexisting pathology. APS is often associated with SLE [22].

6.3   Sjögren's Syndrome

Sjögren's syndrome can present either alone (primary Sjögren's syndrome) or in association with another underlying autoimmune disease, most commonly rheumatoid arthritis or SLE (secondary Sjögren's syndrome) [31].

6.3.1   Clinical Features

The spectrum of clinical presentation extends from dryness of mucosal surfaces to systemic involvement (extraglandular manifestations). Dryness occurs because of immune-mediated inflammation causing secretory gland dysfunction. Chronic sialoadenitis and keratoconjunctivitis sicca are common glandular manifestations. Fatigue, chronic bronchitis, interstitial pneumonia, arthritis, and renal impairment are examples of extraglandular manifestation. Diagnostic criteria include presence of anti-SSA or anti-SSB antibody in the serum [32].

6.3.2   Effects on Pregnancy

Women with Sjögren's syndrome are likely to experience more complications during pregnancy compared with parturients without the disease. Several studies have reported an increased rate of spontaneous abortion and fetal loss associated with Sjögren's syndrome [31].

6.3.3   Neonatal Lupus Erythematosus

Neonatal lupus erythematosus is caused by the passive transfer of anti-SSA and anti-SSB antibodies from the mother. These antibodies begin to cross the placenta at the end of the first trimester and may exert the adverse effects on the fetal tissues. Clinical manifestation includes cutaneous lesions, cytopenias, hepatic abnormality, and atrioventricular block. The former three are more common and benign. They are transient and resolve spontaneously within 6 months of life, when maternal antibodies fade away from the baby. On the contrary, congenital atrioventricular block, which occur only 1–2% of anti-SSA antibody positive women, is mostly irreversible and can be life-threatening. The 10-year mortality rate of complete cardiac atrioventricular block reaches as high as 20–35% [33].

6.3.4   Treatments

Symptomatic treatments are given to the mother. For the fetus, there is no solid evidence about effectiveness of steroids against atrioventricular block. However, dexamethasone has been reported to reverse incomplete atrioventricular block and to improve fetal hemodynamics. Therefore, dexamethasone treatment is recommended if the block is recent or incomplete or if there is evidence of cardiac failure [33].

6.4 Rheumatoid Arthritis

Rheumatoid arthritis is an autoimmune disorder characterized classically as an erosive, symmetrical polyarthropathy. Typical presentation is painful joint swelling with morning stiffness. The small joints of the hand and wrist are usually affected. The spine, knee, and feet are also targets of the disease. It is a multisystem disease that may affect the function of other organs in the body. Rheumatoid arthritis commonly occurs in the fifth decade of life but can occur at the childbearing age [34].

6.4.1 Rheumatoid Arthritis and Pregnancy

It has long been recognized that the majority of rheumatoid arthritis patients experience remission during pregnancy and tend to have postpartum flares within a few months. However, it is currently indicated that for women with well-controlled rheumatoid arthritis, pregnancy outcomes are comparable with the non-rheumatoid arthritis parturients. But higher levels of rheumatoid arthritis disease activity are associated with an increased risk of preterm labor and small for gestational age [35].

6.4.2 Medical Treatment

Drugs for rheumatoid arthritis include NSAIDs, corticosteroids, synthetic disease-modifying antirheumatic drugs (DMARDs), and biologic DMARDs. NSAIDs are frequently used in rheumatoid arthritis. Nonselective NSAIDs can be used during the first and second trimester, but they should be avoided in the third trimester due to possible premature closure of the ductus arteriosus and fetal renal impairment. The safety of selective COX-2 inhibitors has not been established yet. Corticosteroids may be used during pregnancy at the lowest effective doses. Synthetic DMARDs, such as hydroxychloroquine, sulfasalazine, azathioprine, tacrolimus, and cyclosporine, should be continued during pregnancy. But methotrexate, mycophenolate, mofetil, and cyclophosphamide are teratogenic and should be discontinued before pregnancy. Among biologic DMARDs, TNF inhibitors should be considered. However, safety data is limited for other biologic DMARDs [36].

6.4.3 Anesthetic Considerations

As pathological change of rheumatoid arthritis increases over time, it is not common for parturients to have severe clinical presentation. Although neuraxial anesthesia is often preferred method in obstetrics, careful airway assessment and planning are crucial in parturients with rheumatoid arthritis. The range of motion can be restricted in the cervical spine. Atlanto-axial subluxation might exist. Therefore, gentle manipulation is needed when securing airway, during mask ventilation and laryngoscopy. If deformity of the cervical spine is severe, awake fiberoptic intubation may be indicated. Rheumatoid arthritis can also affect the temporomandibular joints. Patients with cricoarytenitis may be asymptomatic but also may have foreign body sensation in the oropharynx, dysphagia, and hoarseness. Respiratory presentation includes pleural effusions, pulmonary nodules, pulmonary fibrosis, and restrictive lung disease. Rheumatoid arthritis is associated with various cardiovascular diseases, including atherosclerosis, heart failure, valvular disease, arrhythmia, pericarditis, and vasculitis. Higher mortality rate of rheumatoid in the general population is attributed to coronary artery disease. The disease in rheumatoid arthritis patients is underdiagnosed partly because silent myocardial infarction is more common. Patients with arthritis should be carefully positioned under anesthesia and during delivery. Deformity of the spine can be a problem for neuraxial anesthesia. But the lumbar spine is less affected than the cervical spine, and neuraxial anesthesia is usually the choice of anesthetic method [37–39].

Key Learning Points
- The spectrum of autoimmune diseases is wide; they can affect various organs. Anesthetic management depends on types and severity of comorbidities.
- When the woman had active disease before pregnancy, the risk of SLE flares during pregnancy is increased.
- Symptoms of SLE flares and preeclampsia can be similar, but they should be differentiated.
- Women with SLE are at higher risk of premature delivery.
- SLE woman may develop thrombocytopenia.
- APS can result in repeated episodes of miscarriage.
- Since APS is a thrombotic disorder, anticoagulant therapy is indicated.
- Prolonged aPTT per se in lupus anticoagulant-positive patients is not a contraindication to neuraxial anesthesia.
- Anti-SSA/SSB causes neonatal lupus, of which atrioventricular can be fatal.
- Airway assessment and planning is crucial in rheumatoid arthritis.

References

1. Ben-Menachem E. Review article: systemic lupus erythematosus: a review for anesthesiologists. Anesth Analg. 2010;111:665–76.
2. Tan EM, Cohen AS, Fries JF, Masi AT, McShane DJ, Rothfield NF, et al. The 1982 revised criteria for the classification of systemic lupus erythematosus. Arthritis Rheum. 1982;25:1271–7.

3. Hochberg MC. Updating the American College of Rheumatology revised criteria for the classification of systemic lupus erythematosus. Arthritis Rheum. 1997;40:1725.
4. Petri M, Orbai AM, Alarcon GS, Gordon C, Merrill JT, Fortin PR, et al. Derivation and validation of the Systemic Lupus International Collaborating Clinics classification criteria for systemic lupus erythematosus. Arthritis Rheum. 2012;64:2677–86.
5. Pons-Estel GJ, Wojdyla D, McGwin G Jr, Magder LS, Petri MA, Pons-Estel BA, et al. The American College of Rheumatology and the Systemic Lupus International Collaborating Clinics classification criteria for systemic lupus erythematosus in two multiethnic cohorts: a commentary. Lupus. 2014;23:3–9.
6. Clowse ME, Magder LS, Witter F, Petri M. The impact of increased lupus activity on obstetric outcomes. Arthritis Rheum. 2005;52:514–21.
7. Jara LJ, Medina G, Cruz-Dominguez P, Navarro C, Vera-Lastra O, Saavedra MA. Risk factors of systemic lupus erythematosus flares during pregnancy. Immunol Res. 2014;60:184–92.
8. Bjorkander S, Bremme K, Persson JO, van Vollenhoven RF, Sverremark-Ekstrom E, Holmlund U. Pregnancy-associated inflammatory markers are elevated in pregnant women with systemic lupus erythematosus. Cytokine. 2012;59:392–9.
9. Stojan G, Baer AN. Flares of systemic lupus erythematosus during pregnancy and the puerperium: prevention, diagnosis and management. Expert Rev Clin Immunol. 2012;8:439–53.
10. Clowse ME. Lupus activity in pregnancy. Rheum Dis Clin N Am. 2007;33:237–52.
11. Moroni G, Ponticelli C. Pregnancy in women with systemic lupus erythematosus (SLE). Eur J Intern Med. 2016;32:7–12.
12. Lazzaroni MG, Dall'Ara F, Fredi M, Nalli C, Reggia R, Lojacono A, et al. A comprehensive review of the clinical approach to pregnancy and systemic lupus erythematosus. J Autoimmun. 2016;74:106–17.
13. Gogarten W, Vandermeulen E, Van Aken H, Kozek S, Llau JV, Samama CM. Regional anaesthesia and antithrombotic agents: recommendations of the European Society of Anaesthesiology. Eur J Anaesthesiol. 2010;27:999–1015.
14. Smyth A, Oliveira GH, Lahr BD, Bailey KR, Norby SM, Garovic VD. A systematic review and meta-analysis of pregnancy outcomes in patients with systemic lupus erythematosus and lupus nephritis. Clin J Am Soc Nephrol. 2010;5:2060–8.
15. Ko HS, Ahn HY, Jang DG, Choi SK, Park YG, Park IY, et al. Pregnancy outcomes and appropriate timing of pregnancy in 183 pregnancies in Korean patients with SLE. Int J Med Sci. 2011;8:577–83.
16. Andreoli L, Bertsias GK, Agmon-Levin N, Brown S, Cervera R, Costedoat-Chalumeau N, et al. EULAR recommendations for women's health and the management of family planning, assisted reproduction, pregnancy and menopause in patients with systemic lupus erythematosus and/or antiphospholipid syndrome. Ann Rheum Dis. 2017;76:476–85.
17. Vinet E, Pineau CA, Clarke AE, Fombonne E, Platt RW, Bernatsky S. Neurodevelopmental disorders in children born to mothers with systemic lupus erythematosus. Lupus. 2014;23:1099–104.
18. Bertsias G, Ioannidis JP, Boletis J, Bombardieri S, Cervera R, Dostal C, et al. EULAR recommendations for the management of systemic lupus erythematosus. Report of a Task Force of the EULAR Standing Committee for International Clinical Studies Including Therapeutics. Ann Rheum Dis. 2008;67:195–205.
19. Peart E, Clowse ME. Systemic lupus erythematosus and pregnancy outcomes: an update and review of the literature. Curr Opin Rheumatol. 2014;26:118–23.
20. Pons-Estel GJ, Andreoli L, Scanzi F, Cervera R, Tincani A. The antiphospholipid syndrome in patients with systemic lupus erythematosus. J Autoimmun. 2017;76:10–20.
21. Arachchillage DRJ, Laffan M. Pathogenesis and management of antiphospholipid syndrome. Br J Haematol. 2017;178:181–95.
22. Miyakis S, Lockshin MD, Atsumi T, Branch DW, Brey RL, Cervera R, et al. International consensus statement on an update of the classification criteria for definite antiphospholipid syndrome (APS). J Thromb Haemost. 2006;4:295–306.

23. Schreiber K, Radin M, Sciascia S. Current insights in obstetric antiphospholipid syndrome. Curr Opin Obstet Gynecol. 2017;29:397–403.
24. Gomez-Puerta JA, Cervera R. Diagnosis and classification of the antiphospholipid syndrome. J Autoimmun. 2014;48–49:20–5.
25. Arachchillage DR, Machin SJ, Mackie IJ, Cohen H. Diagnosis and management of non-criteria obstetric antiphospholipid syndrome. Thromb Haemost. 2015;113:13–9.
26. Keeling D, Mackie I, Moore GW, Greer IA, Greaves M, British Committee for Standards in H. Guidelines on the investigation and management of antiphospholipid syndrome. Br J Haematol. 2012;157:47–58.
27. Nelson-Piercy C, Maccallum P, Mackillop MA. Reducing the risk of venous thromboembolism during pregnancy and the puerperium. Green-top guideline. London: Royal College of Obstetricians & Gynaecologists; 2015.
28. Bates SM, Greer IA, Middeldorp S, Veenstra DL, Prabulos AM, Vandvik PO. VTE, thrombophilia, antithrombotic therapy, and pregnancy: antithrombotic therapy and prevention of thrombosis, 9th ed: American College of Chest Physicians evidence-based clinical practice guidelines. Chest. 2012;141:e691S–736S.
29. Horlocker TT, Wedel DJ, Rowlingson JC, Enneking FK, Kopp SL, Benzon HT, et al. Regional anesthesia in the patient receiving antithrombotic or thrombolytic therapy: American Society of Regional Anesthesia and Pain Medicine evidence-based guidelines (third edition). Reg Anesth Pain Med. 2010;35:64–101.
30. Butwick AJ, Carvalho B. Anticoagulant and antithrombotic drugs in pregnancy: what are the anesthetic implications for labor and cesarean delivery? J Perinatol. 2011;31:73–84.
31. Upala S, Yong WC, Sanguankeo A. Association between primary Sjogren's syndrome and pregnancy complications: a systematic review and meta-analysis. Clin Rheumatol. 2016;35:1949–55.
32. Shiboski CH, Shiboski SC, Seror R, Criswell LA, Labetoulle M, Lietman TM, et al. 2016 American College of Rheumatology/European League Against Rheumatism classification criteria for primary Sjogren's syndrome: a consensus and data-driven methodology involving three international patient cohorts. Ann Rheum Dis. 2017;76:9–16.
33. Klein-Gitelman MS. Neonatal lupus: what we have learned and current approaches to care. Curr Rheumatol Rep. 2016;18:60.
34. Isaacs JD, Moreland LW. Fast facts: rheumatoid arthritis. 2nd ed. Abington: Health Press; 2011.
35. Marder W, Littlejohn EA, Somers EC. Pregnancy and autoimmune connective tissue diseases. Best Pract Res Clin Rheumatol. 2016;30:63–80.
36. Gotestam Skorpen C, Hoeltzenbein M, Tincani A, Fischer-Betz R, Elefant E, Chambers C, et al. The EULAR points to consider for use of antirheumatic drugs before pregnancy, and during pregnancy and lactation. Ann Rheum Dis. 2016;75:795–810.
37. Aires RB, de Carvalho JF, da Mota LM. Pre-operative anesthetic assessment of patients with rheumatoid arthritis. Rev Bras Reumatol. 2014;54:213–9.
38. Samanta R, Shoukrey K, Griffiths R. Rheumatoid arthritis and anaesthesia. Anaesthesia. 2011;66:1146–59.
39. Hollan I, Dessein PH, Ronda N, Wasko MC, Svenungsson E, Agewall S, et al. Prevention of cardiovascular disease in rheumatoid arthritis. Autoimmun Rev. 2015;14:952–69.

Anesthesia for the Parturient with Intracranial and Spinal Surgery

7

Zerrin Ozkose Satirlar and Gozde Inan

7.1 Introduction

Neurosurgical disorders requiring neuroanesthesia during pregnancy are not common and still present a significant cause of morbidity and mortality in pregnant women [1, 2]. Decision regarding timing of neurosurgery and delivery is not straightforward and requires multidisciplinary discussion between the neurosurgeon, obstetrician, and anesthetist by assessing fetal maturity and the urgency to perform neurosurgical process. Conduct of anesthesia in a parturient presenting with a neurosurgical disorder is a major challenge. Physiological changes due to pregnancy can cause difficulty in any kind of surgery [3]. Moreover, airway, anesthetic, and hemodynamic management for neuroprotective interventions unique to neuroanesthesia should be used with caution in order to preserve fetal well-being. The literature on the evidence-based neuroanesthetic management of the pregnant patient is limited, and so decision-making should be based on general principles of both neurosurgical and obstetric anesthesia [4]. Maternal well-being without compromising fetal safety should remain a primary concern. The main goal is to provide a balance between some competing and even contradictory interventions unique for neuroanesthesia and obstetric anesthesia [5, 6].

7.2 Indications for Neurosurgery During Pregnancy

Essentially incidence of neurosurgical problems does not appear to be more in pregnant women than nonpregnant women. However, because of physiological and anatomical changes associated with pregnancy, pregnancy itself may promote or

Z. O. Satirlar (✉) · G. Inan
Department of Anesthesiology and Reanimation, Gazi University Faculty of Medicine,
Ankara, Turkey
e-mail: ozkose@gazi.edu.tr

© Springer International Publishing AG, part of Springer Nature 2018
B. Gunaydin, S. Ismail (eds.), *Obstetric Anesthesia for Co-morbid Conditions*,
https://doi.org/10.1007/978-3-319-93163-0_7

accelerate some certain neurosurgical diseases. The physiological changes related to pregnancy such as increased estrogen/progesterone levels and cardiac output in addition to edema formation and depressed immunotolerance are suspected to promote tumor growth [2].

Non-obstetric surgery during pregnancy is not uncommon; neurosurgical conditions encountered during pregnancy are cranial pathologies such as intracranial hemorrhage, hydrocephalus, intracranial tumors, spinal pathologies, trauma, and diagnostic and therapeutic interventions [1].

7.2.1 Cranial Pathologies

7.2.1.1 Brain Tumors

In general, a pregnant woman doesn't develop an intracranial tumor more than a nonpregnant woman [1, 3]. Exceptionally, choriocarcinoma is an aggressive gestational tumor, which is specifically associated with pregnancy [3].

The incidence of primary central nervous system tumor is approximately 6 per 100,000 pregnancies [4]. However, some tumors appear to manifest more rapidly because pregnancy seems to aggravate the natural history of tumor or become symptomatic during pregnancy. This exacerbation can be explained by increased blood volume, which increases the volume of vascular tumors; increased salt and water retention, which increases peritumoral edema and hence increases intracranial pressure (ICP); and hormonal influences of pregnancy that are associated with increased growth of meningiomas. Moreover, immunological tolerance, steroid-mediated growth, and hemodynamic changes are other factors contributed to tumors becoming symptomatic in the pregnant state [2].

Presentation, similar to nonpregnant, may include focal neurological defects, seizures, or signs of raised ICP such as headache, vomiting, seizures, and visual impairment. Differential diagnosis of raised ICP can be challenging during pregnancy because symptoms like headache and/or vomiting are common. Nevertheless, any pregnant patient with rapidly progressing headache, vomiting in the second or third trimester accompanied with new onset seizures and visual disturbances, should be evaluated accordingly [5]. Impending or actual cerebral herniation may be exacerbated with pregnancy at all gestations presenting with worsening headache, hypertension, deteriorating Glasgow coma scale, dilating ipsilateral pupil, bradycardia, and respiratory irregularity [3].

Meningiomas are the most common benign tumors, which may express estrogen or progesterone receptors and continue to grow in size during pregnancy [4, 5]. The incidence of meningioma is higher in women than in men. There is considerable relationship among menstrual cycle, pregnancy, and symptomatology of meningioma [1]. Treatment is mainly conservative unless they present with progressive neurological deficits. Pituitary adenomas and cerebellopontine angle tumors are other common types of intracranial tumors, and acute neurological deterioration of both tumors that warrant surgical resection during pregnancy has been reported [4].

Gliomas are the most common malignant tumors, which are rarely seen in pregnancy, but pose a risk for both mother and baby especially aggressive gliomas like glioblastoma multiforme grow rapidly and cause progressive neurological deficit [5]. So, definitive treatment should not be delayed. If the fetus is viable, neurosurgery can be performed after Cesarean section (C/S) or can be done at any time of gestation with adequate fetal monitoring. However, treatment should be individualized and tailored.

Imaging may be required to diagnose a new lesion or worsening of a previously known one. Magnetic resonance imaging (MRI) has been shown to be safe for detailed imaging in pregnancy. However, there are concerns on timing of imaging and contrast administration. In an acute setting, computed tomography (CT) is preferred, despite its risks.

Although evidence based strategy for the management of intracranial tumors during pregnancy is lacking, management can be summarized depending on the gestation as presented in Table 7.1.

If a brain tumor is diagnosed which is asymptomatic during pregnancy, then waiting and watching the patient is the advised approach [3]. Close observation of the mother and fetus is critical, since possible acute worsening may necessitate hospital admission. There is no evidence that C/S is advantageous over vaginal delivery in protecting from increased ICP in term parturients.

7.2.1.2 Hydrocephalus

In the treatment of hydrocephalus, which may be congenital or acquired, ventriculoperitoneal (VP) shunts are indicated. With advancing medical care in surgical

Table 7.1 Management of intracranial tumors during pregnancy

Preconceptual diagnosis
• Delay pregnancy: Treat as any other nonpregnant woman
• Continue pregnancy: Concerns on mother's prognosis and the potential risk of worsening during pregnancy
First and early second trimesters
• Fetus is not viable
• Hemodynamic changes of the pregnancy are not remarkable
• Stable patient: Permit gestational advancement to early second trimester for neurosurgery or adjuvant radiotherapy
• Unstable patient: Urgent neurosurgery
Late second and third trimesters
• At the end of the 2nd trimester due to the high maternal intravascular volume, increased risk of significant hemorrhage may occur during tumour resection
• Fetus is very premature
• Stable patient: Gestational advancement can be permitted. In a patient with worsening neurology, radiotherapy with appropriate radiation doses may be an option to delaying surgery
• Unstable patient: C/S under general anesthesia, followed immediately by surgical decompression
Term
• Stable patient: Vaginal delivery
• Unstable patient: C/S under general anesthesia, followed immediately by surgical decompression

technique and shunt technology, more women with shunts may survive to child-bearing age. During pregnancy, a woman with an in situ shunt or a woman who acquires the need for a shunt may present. Due to a combination of increased intra-abdominal pressure and anatomical changes, pregnancy is associated with an increased rate of complications such as VP shunt displacement or occlusion [3, 7]. The literature available to guide this group of patients' management is limited to case reports or case series. Management of VP shunt complications may be dependent upon symptoms and gestational age and guided by clinical status and imaging (Table 7.2).

7.2.1.3 Vascular Lesions and Intracranial Hemorrhage

Subarachnoid hemorrhage (SAH) occurs in 10–20:100,000 pregnancies with devastating consequences where maternal mortality rates range between 35 and 83% [8]. Presentation is the same as in the nonpregnant population with sudden onset severe headache. There is a spectrum of subsequent neurological sequel ranging from isolated cranial nerve lesions to a rapid reduction in Glasgow coma scale and unconsciousness. Most SAHs are thought to occur due to intracranial aneurysms. Rupture of intracranial aneurysms is believed to occur with a higher incidence during pregnancy. Additionally, the risk of aneurysmal rupture rises in each trimester, which

Table 7.2 Management of ventriculoperitoneal (VP) shunt complications during pregnancy

Preconceptual diagnosis
• In those considering pregnancy with a shunt already in situ, a CT or MRI of the brain, which acts as a baseline, should be performed
• The baby may also have a neural tube defect, if the indication for the shunt was for a neural tube defect. Genetic counseling may be required
During pregnancy
• Attention to developing symptoms and signs of increasing ICP (headache, nausea, vomiting, ataxia, and seizures)
• There is significant overlap with the presentation of preeclampsia
• Increase in ICP is suspected, a CT or MRI of brain should be undertaken and compared with the baseline
– If there is no change from preoperative imaging, the ICP should be measured and cerebrospinal fluid samples are collected for culture. If ICP is normal, and cultures are negative, physiological changes may be responsible. Treatment is bed rest. The shunt may be pumped to aid cerebrospinal fluid flow
– If there is an increase in ventricle size or if ICP is raised on shunt puncture, shunt revision is required. In the first and second trimesters, this may be performed as in the nonpregnant. In the third trimester, a VP shunt or third ventriculostomy may be considered as an alternative; however, risks of uterine trauma or induction of labor should be avoided
During labor and delivery
• Prophylactic extended antibiotic regimens
• No symptoms of increased ICP: Vaginal delivery is safe and may be the preferred option
• A shortened second stage is suggested, as increases in ICP may lead to functional shunt obstruction
• If patient becomes symptomatic during labor, C/S under general anesthesia is advised
• Epidural anesthesia is contraindicated in case of elevated ICP

reaches its highest in the third trimester. In a pregnancy, SAH is associated with 35% risk of poor feto-maternal outcomes [5].

There are no objective data to say vaginal delivery is associated with an increased incidence of aneurysmal rupture. However, valsalva maneuver might increase the chances of aneurysmal rupture. Hence, labor analgesia with epidural block should be provided to all patients planned for vaginal delivery [9]. Epidural analgesia is considered as safest because there is no dural breach or fall in ICP, unless an accidental dural puncture occurs. General anesthesia is reserved for fetal distress; care should be taken on hemodynamics throughout the surgery. Ruptured aneurysm in pregnant women is treated similar with nonpregnant women, where the patient is taken up for immediate craniotomy or coil embolization under general anesthesia. The safety and efficacy of coil embolization are established, and it is also an effective option in pregnant patients with a ruptured or unruptured aneurysm under sedation and local anesthesia or under general anesthesia [3].

Arteriovenous malformations (AVMs) are not more prevalent during pregnancy. Unlike intracerebral aneurysms, AVMs have the highest associated risk of bleeding in the second trimester because of the maximum changes in cardiovascular status [5]. There is an increased risk of rebleeding (25%) during the same pregnancy. In incidentally diagnosed unruptured or ruptured AVMs without new focal deficits and with stable neurological course, pregnancy can be continued, and definitive neurosurgical intervention is planned in the postpartum period. If a patient with ruptured AVM has progressive neurological dysfunction, an emergency craniotomy or endovascular procedure can be planned depending on the medical condition of the patient. At that point, maternal well-being becomes the primary concern compared to fetal outcomes. If a patient with unruptured AVM is scheduled to undergo C/S, neuraxial analgesia would be safer. However, if the same patient undergoes a sequential craniotomy and C/S, or it is an emergency situation, then general anesthesia is the preferred technique [10, 11].

7.2.2   Spinal Pathology

Low back pain is common during pregnancy, reported in over half of pregnant women [12]. However, symptomatic lumbar disc herniation is extremely rare, with an incidence of around 1:10,000 pregnancies [13]. Hormonal changes including increased concentrations of relaxin and altered body posture are argued to exacerbate previous spinal problems, but there is no increased risk of disc herniation in the pregnant group [14]. Back pain experienced during pregnancy is more severe than nonpregnant women. That disabling symptom attributed to sacroiliac is typically dull and radiates into the buttocks and thighs. Pain associated with lumbar disc herniation differs from backpain of pregnancy because nerve root compression may cause a sharp shooting pain in the dermatomal distribution of the nerve compressed. Therefore, neurological dysfunction of that nerve is evident on examination. Cauda equina syndrome, resulting from lumbar disc herniation and subsequent compression of the cauda equina, is extremely rare in pregnancy but presents a neurosurgical emergency [3]. Clinical features include lower back pain with or without sciatic nerve compression pain, sphincter disturbance, and numbness in the sacral region, motor weakness, and loss of ankle reflexes.

Diagnosis of lumbar disc herniation is made with a spinal MRI without contrast, and pregnancy does not preclude MRI. Neurosurgical management of these conditions in the pregnant woman is the same with the nonpregnant. Back pain of pregnancy resolves once pregnancy has completed. Therefore, surgery is not indicated. Conservative measures such as physiotherapy, bed rest, etc. along with simple analgesic medication are advised. It is also important to note that in those with symptomatic disc herniation due to nerve root compression, 85% of patients will get better with conservative management within 6 weeks [3]. In contrast, women presenting with worsening neurological deficit may require surgical intervention, and those with a cauda equine syndrome represent a surgical emergency.

In addition to disc herniation, parturients may present for surgery as a result of newly symptomatic spinal tumors or more rare complications such as vertebral canal hematoma (either spontaneous or following neuraxial procedures) and vertebral canal abscess or for vascular malformations. Spinal tumors may become symptomatic with hormonal effects. Bleeding from spinal tumors and spontaneous hematomas needing evacuation has been reported [15, 16].

Case reports have demonstrated that spinal surgery in the pregnant patient is safe [12]. The prone position is the preferred access for spinal surgery. During the first and early second trimester, surgery can be performed in the prone position as there is minimal aortocaval compression by the gravid uterus. Prone position for spinal surgery in pregnancy may cause difficulties with respect to fetal monitoring, emergent Cesarean delivery, and increased epidural venous bleeding. In this position, placental perfusion has been shown to increase in 23 pregnant women [17]. Three patients had successful lumbar spinal surgeries performed in the prone position under epidural anesthesia [12]. Some anesthesiologists do not prefer spinal surgery in the prone position if the spinal procedure follows C/S [18, 19].

7.2.3 Trauma

Maternal mortality due to obstetric causes is gradually decreasing due to better obstetric management however; non-obstetric causes of maternal mortality are increasing worldwide. Trauma is the leading non-obstetric cause of incidental maternal death during pregnancy [20]. Trauma itself complicates 6–7% of pregnancies and may involve cranial or spinal injuries that necessitate surgery [21, 22]. A multi-trauma will present significant clinical challenges in the care of mother and fetus, and early aggressive maternal resuscitation is the main priority. In life-threatening multi-trauma, C/S should be performed to improve maternal hemodynamics. Trauma carries worst outcome in the fetus. Fetal compromise is the result of the systemic effect of trauma on maternal physiology, mainly posttraumatic hypotension and hypoxia, hypovolemia, acidosis, or as a result of drugs used during the resuscitation process [23]. Head injury can increase the overall morbidity and mortality. If tracheal intubation and positive-pressure ventilation are indicated, a rapid sequence induction with thiopental or propofol and succinylcholine may be used. To avoid caval venous compression after 20 weeks' gestation, left lateral tilt of the whole body should be applied. Difficult intubation can be expected in 1 per 300 pregnant patients. Although there is no consensus on the best method of intubation in patients with cervical-spine injury, fiberoptic techniques may be preferable in a pregnant patient with cervical-spine injury because of the additional difficulty that may come from pregnancy and an unstable neck [24]. Treatment can be conservative or surgical. Progressive worsening of the symptoms is an indication for emergency surgery [5, 25].

7.2.4 Diagnostic and Therapeutic Neuroradiology

Diagnostic and therapeutic neuroradiology during pregnancy should be considered as a major procedure, and the management of anesthesia should be planned accordingly [4]. The interventional neuroradiology suite is a remote environment in where it is difficult to provide obstetric anesthesia. For both diagnostic and therapeutic interventions, concerns are fetal radiation exposure, anesthesia at remote location, anaphylaxis, and renal dysfunction due to contrast agents. Procedures can be done under sedation and local anesthesia at femoral cannulation site or can be done under general anesthesia. Both of the anesthesia techniques have their own advantages and disadvantages. Selected patients will need to be awake at important points of the procedure. Most interventions require invasive blood pressure monitoring. Levels of sedation should be carefully titrated [26]. Before femoral artery cannulation, precautionary steps should be taken, such as administration of aspiration prophylaxis and, for gestations over 20 weeks, uterine displacement [27]. Heparin is administered for interventional neuroradiology and may need reversal in the presence of emergency Cesarean delivery or obstetric hemorrhage. If fetal compromise is detected, neuroradiologic procedure may have to be stopped until the baby is delivered. In that circumstance, the intracranial catheters should be withdrawn and the femoral artery sheath left in situ, after which heparin can be reversed. Although fetal monitoring has not been shown to reduce fetal mortality or morbidity, Doppler monitoring has been advocated but poses its own practical difficulties in the radiology suite [28]. A small case series of patients treated with coiling after SAH suggests that sequential vaginal delivery is the safest choice [29].

7.3 Anesthesia for Neurosurgery in a Parturient

7.3.1 Timing

Pregnant women presenting for non-obstetric surgery represent a unique surgical and anesthetic challenge where the health of the mother is prioritized but equally careful consideration needs to be given to fetal well-being. If the conditions permit, it is recommended to wait until term. On the other hand, life-threatening, emergency neurosurgical conditions should be treated promptly [3].

Before 24 weeks' gestation, there is no option to deliver the baby, and neurosurgical intervention can proceed while maintaining the fetus in utero. Therefore, both optimizing maternal physiology and consideration for fetal well-being should be aimed and will result in the best outcomes. Subsequent fetal management following surgery can be then based on obstetric principles.

At gestational ages greater than 24 weeks, if the fetus is viable at the time of planned neurosurgery, consideration must be given to whether delivery is appropriate or not. There are three options:

- Neurosurgery during pregnancy: Continuous procedures; C/S proceeded by neurosurgery. Obstetric and neurosurgical anesthesia principles may need to be modified.
- Neurosurgery after delivery: C/S followed by later neurosurgery.
- Maintenance of pregnancy and proceeding with neurosurgery: Pregnancy in a parturient with a history of previous neurosurgical procedures or current neuropathology may have implications on the anesthetic management for later C/S, which is discussed below.

7.3.2   Concerns in Neuroanesthesia

Neuroanesthetic concerns include maintaining stable hemodynamics, hyperventilation, controlled hypotension, and ICP reduction [5]. Meanwhile, obstetric anesthetic concerns may be listed as potentially difficult intubation, rapid sequence induction, aspiration prophylaxis, maintenance of uteroplacental circulation, uteroplacental drug transfer, avoiding aortocaval compression, fetal monitoring, tocolysis, postpartum hemorrhage, dosage modifications, and teratogenicity. In recent years, major concerns on the neurotoxic effects of anesthetics, awareness during general anesthesia, and the airway management of pregnant women have arisen [6, 23].

One of the challenges is obtaining a balance between adequate cerebral perfusion pressure and uteroplacental perfusion pressure. Factors that precipitate fetal hypoxia and compromise uteroplacental perfusion can adversely affect fetal outcomes with poor Apgar scores. Hypotension and hypovolemia should be strictly avoided for better maternal and neonatal outcomes. In general, hemodynamic fluctuations should be avoided, anxiety and pain should be vigorously treated, and normoxemia, normoglycemia, and normothermia should be maintained to avoid fetal asphyxia at all times.

There is no evidence that premature labor is associated with types of the anesthetic drugs and anesthetic technique. Role of prophylactic use of tocolytics is controversial because of its own side effects. Nevertheless both intraoperative and postoperative tocolysis may be required in cases with high risk of preterm labor.

The use of fetal heart rate monitoring in the emergency setting is debatable. The decision to use fetal heart rate monitoring perioperatively should be individualized and based on consultation with obstetricians. It will only be of clinical utility if the woman is willing to accept intervention in the event of significant and uncorrected fetal compromise, if a person capable of interpreting the findings is present to avoid unnecessary intervention, and if immediate delivery is feasible [30, 31]. American Society of Anesthesiologists guideline on fetal monitoring during non-obstetric surgery suggests that surgery should be done at an institution including neonatal and pediatric services and an obstetric provider with C/S privileges and a qualified individual to interpret the fetal heart rate should be readily available during procedures [6]. Although fetal heart rate monitoring is possible after 16 weeks' gestation, changes in baseline are only predictive for neonatal mortality after 24 weeks' gestation, and baseline rate changes also occur in the healthy fetus, and drug-induced loss of variability is common during anesthesia, and so unnecessary premature delivery Is a significant risk [32]. In case of intraoperative severe fetal bradycardia, increase maternal arterial blood pressure by ensuring left lateral tilt and normoventilation to improve uteroplacental flow and fetal oxygenation.

Another challenge is the drug dosing due to pregnancy-related pharmacodynamic and pharmacokinetic changes in absorption, distribution, metabolism, and excretion of drugs and teratogenicity. Pregnancy is also associated with lower anesthetic requirements, with the minimum alveolar concentration of inhalational agent being reduced by up to 30%. Intravenous induction agents are also often required in lower doses. It is important to note that the incidence of awareness in the pregnant population is higher. This is in part due to the emergency nature of a large proportion of obstetric surgery, reduced induction to incision times to minimize fetal transfer, and a higher maternal cardiac output resulting in rapid redistribution of induction agents. Special care should be taken to avoid drugs, which cause fetal teratogenicity. Most of the anesthetic agents fall in the category of B and C in the Food and Drug Administration labeling system for drugs in pregnancy, that is, these can be used safely with caution. Controversy exists regarding the use of nitrous oxide and benzodiazepines. Cocaine is the only anesthetic agent known as teratogen, which is not even in use [5].

Furthermore, as there are a number of radiological investigations for imaging in neurosurgical conditions, concerns exist regarding fetal radiation exposure. Recommendations in relation to radiation exposure of the pregnant patient suggest a maximum acceptable dose of 1 rem (roentgen equivalent man = 10 mSivert) and a safe maximum fetal dose of 0.5 rem [4, 21]. Concerns of radiation-induced teratogenicity include microcephaly and childhood cancers. Fetal radiation effects are highly dependent on gestational age and dose that have the potential to cause early fetal loss or congenital abnormalities after exposure during the period of organogenesis. Exposure after organogenesis may cause growth restriction, microcephaly, and childhood cancer. A calculated fetal dose of 0.3 rem occurs during the endovascular closure of an intracranial aneurysm, and cerebral angiography delivers a dose of 0.1 rem to the fetus if the woman's abdomen is shielded with a lead apron [33].

7.3.3 Conduct of Anesthesia

The safe management of the parturient and the preservation of fetal well-being during anesthesia are closely linked to understanding the pregnancy-related physiological changes [34]. Individual management has to be tailored to the surgical and neuroanesthetic requirements and to the gestational age. The best approach is involvement of a coordinated multidisciplinary team with clear plans regarding timing of surgery, timing of delivery, and maternal and fetal management.

Relevant recommendations on obstetric practice in a non-obstetric surgery during pregnancy can be extracted from the American College of Obstetricians and Gynecologists Committee opinions [35].

Sedative premedication may be needed in an extremely anxious patient; however, the risk of hypoventilation, hypercarbia, and subsequent increases in ICP should be considered. Since pregnant patients are prone to gastric regurgitation and aspiration, medications to decrease gastric acidity and the volume of gastric contents are recommended. Inhibitors of gastric acid secretion, such as ranitidine 150–300 mg, may be given orally 1 h before anesthesia or as a 50 mg IV dose, once operation decision has been made [36]. Anticonvulsant therapy may need to be implemented or continued in the preoperative phase, and pregnancy-induced changes occur in the clearance, unbound fractions, and half-lives of some anticonvulsant drugs [37].

Pregnancy is associated with increased oxygen requirements and change in respiratory mechanics due to the effects of the gravid uterus and weight gain. Administration of oxygen is essential, as the reduction in functional residual capacity may lead to rapid maternal desaturation during hypoventilation or apnea. Pregnant women are considered more likely to be difficult to intubate, so careful airway planning for assessment and management is necessary. Intubation with smaller than usual tracheal tubes are better, additional equipment to manage a difficult airway should be readily available, and awake fiberoptic intubation should be considered when significant difficulty is anticipated. Although LMA has been successfully used for airway management during elective C/S in a large series of healthy parturients, its use in pregnant neurosurgical patients should not extend beyond emergency use as a rescue device for the unanticipated difficult intubation [38, 39].

The majority of neurosurgical procedures require general anesthesia, and rapid sequence induction is advisable early within the second trimester to reduce the risk of aspiration. For general anesthesia, either total IV anesthesia with propofol or balanced IV and volatile anesthesia are reasonable choices. The use of propofol for induction and maintenance of anesthesia for C/S is controversial because total IV anesthesia is associated with reduced neonatal neurobehavioral performance compared with thiopental and volatile maintenance. These effects, however, are of arguable clinical significance [40, 41].

Succinylcholine administration (1–1.5 mg/kg) may cause a transient increase in ICP. The choice of a non-depolarizing neuromuscular blocking drug for tracheal intubation is controversial because of increased risk in difficult intubation. Avoidance of responses to laryngoscopy is vital especially for SAH. Induction of anesthesia includes use of short-acting opioids. Magnesium sulfate can be used to blunt the response to laryngoscopy. Actually, it is the drug of choice in eclamptic and pre-eclamptic patients. The literature also describes the use of lignocaine (1 mg/kg) and short-acting beta-blockers such as esmolol (0.5–1 mg/kg). Lignocaine is found less effective than remifentanil, and beta-blockers have been associated with fetal bradycardia. Actually, in high doses ketamine increases uterine tone.

Volatile anesthetics suitable for anesthesia during pregnancy include isoflurane and sevoflurane, which are also favored in neuroanesthesia because they reduce cerebral metabolic rate, have the least effect on ICP, preserve cerebral autoregulation, and provide a level of cerebral protection in animal studies [42], and a degree of uterine relaxation because of their tocolytic effect. The MAC of volatile anesthetics is reduced by 25–30% during pregnancy. Nitrous oxide should be avoided in neuroanesthesia, since it increases ICP, increases cerebral blood flow and cerebral oxygen metabolic rate, impairs autoregulation, expands air bubbles, and may contribute to postoperative nausea and vomiting.

The effect of oxytocic drugs on ICP and cerebral blood flow has not been well studied, but safe use of synthetic oxytocin has been described in patients with intracranial tumors [43]. It should be noted that oxytocin causes transient hypotension and a significant increase in heart rate and cardiac output for several minutes [44]. Ergometrine is a potent venoconstrictor, producing a hypertensive response that may further elevate ICP in the presence of a disrupted blood-brain barrier and loss of autoregulation. The use of ergometrine in the presence of intracranial disease in pregnancy should be discussed with the neurosurgical team.

Maternal $PaCO_2$ implicates oxygen delivery to the fetus both in terms of uterine perfusion and the maternal oxygen-hemoglobin dissociation curve. Hyperventilation to manipulate maternal ICP remains an option although normocarbia is recommended [3].

Maintaining hemodynamic stability and avoiding fluctuation in blood pressure during the perioperative period are beneficial for maternal, fetal, and neurosurgical reasons. Therefore, it is advised to site invasive arterial pressure monitoring prior to induction. Hypertension related to laryngoscopy can be prevented by short-acting opioids. Magnesium sulfate given at induction is also effective, especially in preeclamptic states. Maternal positioning to avoid aortocaval compression is essential. Effective pelvic tilt of at least 15° to the left to minimize aortocaval compression is required after 20 weeks' gestation by means of either placing a hip wedge or a side-tilting table. Large-bore intravenous access is required, and central venous access should be sited if vasoactive substances or central venous pressure monitoring is required. Blood pressure should be maintained within normal limits. Ephedrine is no longer recommended for the vasopressor choice in the parturient [4]. Phenylephrine, a selective alpha agonist, is associated with better maternal cardiovascular stability and improved fetal acid-base status [45, 46]. Intravenous fluid therapy during cerebral and spinal neurosurgery should include isonatremic, isotonic, and glucose-free solutions to reduce the risk of cerebral edema and hyperglycemia [4].

A variety of measures to control ICP consists of slight head-up position, low tidal volumes during intermittent positive-pressure ventilation, and avoidance of vomiting. Mannitol and furosemide should be used cautiously. The administration of steroids to reduce peritumoral edema appears safe, as it accelerates fetal lung maturity at the same time [4].

It is worth remembering that fetal temperature is consistent with its mother's temperature and both maternal hyperthermia and hypothermia may be associated with increased morbidity in the presence of increased ICP [47]. Monitoring body temperature and preserving normal body temperature of the pregnant patient undergoing neurosurgery is beneficial [4].

Patient positioning is a particular problem for spinal surgery. Normally spinal surgery is carried out in the prone position. While prone position provides good uteroplacental perfusion, the mechanics are challenging in the pregnant population. There are a few case reports of spinal surgery carried out under regional anesthesia, where the women positioned themselves prone prior to surgery [12].

If the patient is going to be extubated following neurosurgery, similar with induction, care is required to prevent reflux and aspiration of gastric contents. Patients should be fully awake with intact airway reflexes. If abdominal pain occurs following surgery, onset of labor should be suspected, and tocodynamometric monitoring during the postoperative period is recommended [4]. Postoperative prophylactic pharmacologic tocolysis is only indicated to prevent premature labor if the risk of fetal loss is high.

After intracranial procedures, it is better to discharge the pregnant to an intensive care unit for close evaluation and further management. Good postoperative analgesia should be provided by a multimodal approach. Pregnancy is a hypercoagulable state and associated with increased risk of thromboembolism after surgery, so nonpharmacological prophylaxis (antithromboembolic stockings, calf stimulation, calf compressors, or pedal pumps) should be used perioperatively [4].

7.3.4 Anesthesia for Cesarean Delivery with Intracranial Pathology

Parturients with intracranial pathology are thought to have increased ICP, and so the risk of herniation due to an inadvertent dural puncture is cited as a contraindication for neuraxial anesthesia. Following key points may be helpful [1]:

- If the patient has new neurologic symptoms such as worsening headache, visual changes, seizure, and decreased level of consciousness, and there is imaging evidence of significant mass effect with midline shift, then the patient is likely at high risk of herniation.
- If the patient does not have neurologic symptoms but has imaging evidence of significant mass effect with midline shift, then the patient is likely at high risk of herniation.
- If the patient does not have neurologic symptoms but has imaging evidence of minimal mass effect, then do not proceed without neurological consultation; the patient is likely at mild-moderate risk.
- If the patient does not have neurologic symptoms and imaging evidence of mass effect, then search for an imaging evidence of hydrocephalus. If there is an

obstruction at or above the foramen magnum, then do not proceed without neurological consultation; the patient is likely at mild-moderate risk.
- If patient has none of the findings described above and also does not have any
clinical or imaging findings suggesting increased ICP, it may be reasonable to
proceed with neuraxial anesthesia. Patient is likely at minimal or no risk of
herniation.

7.3.5 Anesthesia for Cesarean Delivery After Recent Neurosurgery

Regional anesthesia may be appropriate to use when Cesarean delivery is performed
subsequent to recent successful and uncomplicated neurosurgery. The woman
should be alert, cooperative, and preferably have normal ICP. The potential for a
serious cerebral complication after dural puncture is of major concern if the ICP is
high, because a rapid decrease in spinal cerebrospinal fluid (CSF) pressure may
cause herniation or intracranial hemorrhage [48]. Intracranial subdural hematoma
formation after epidural anesthesia and SAH after spinal anesthesia have been
reported several times in the literature and are thought to result from acute CSF
pressure changes [49]. Wang and colleagues [4] suggest that intentional lumbar
dural puncture may be difficult to confirm under these circumstances. If epidural
techniques are used, care must be given to ensure the placement of an epidural catheter, and slow injection of incremental volumes of local anesthetic is also recommended [50]. Epidural infection is also a concern after previous spinal surgery,
especially with instrumentation, or in the presence of a ventriculoperitoneal shunt.

7.4 Maternal and Fetal Implications of Neuroanesthesia

Standard neuroanesthesia practices, including hyperventilation, intravenous fluid
management, and administration of mannitol and steroid, can challenge the general
obstetric principles of managing a parturient. Parturient may benefit from some
neuroprotective measures and interventions unique to neuroanesthesia, whereas
fetus may get harm. Avoiding maternal hypoxia, hypocarbia, and hypotension
remains as the primary goal to prioritize both maternal and fetal safety and avoid
preterm labor.

7.4.1 Induced Hypocapnia

As hyperventilation results in a fall in arterial carbon dioxide pressure ($PaCO_2$), thus
in cerebral vasoconstriction, induced hypocarbia is, therefore, one method used to
reduce ICP. In pregnancy, there is a progressive increase in minute ventilation lowering $PaCO_2$, and the set point for the cerebrovascular response to hyperventilation

is, thereby, reduced [1]. Attempts to lower ICP necessitate lowering the $PaCO_2$ to as low as 25 mmHg or less. However, this degree of hypokalemia may cause fetal hypoxia and acidosis by decreasing uterine blood flow and reducing release of oxygen secondary to left shift of the hemoglobin-oxygen dissociation curve [4]. For these reasons, maternal $PaCO_2$ should be maintained at around 30 mmHg.

7.4.2 Induced Hypotension

Induced hypotension is used to facilitate aneurysm clipping. Moreover, hypotension is a common side effect of certain neurosurgical practices, such as nimodipine and mannitol [3]. However, uterine blood flow is exquisitely sensitive to maternal systemic blood pressure. In the pregnant patient, maternal hypotension, and subsequent fetal hypoxia, should be avoided. Instead of inducing hypotension, temporary clipping of a vessel may be used to reduce intra-aneurysmal pressure [33].

7.4.3 Mannitol

Maternal administration of mannitol results in significant increases in maternal osmolality; as it crosses the placenta, it may accumulate in the fetus, leading to subsequent changes in fetal osmolality, fetal dehydration, and volume and the concentrations of various electrolytes [1, 3]. However, in dosages used in some case reports (0.25–0.5 mg/kg), mannitol is unlikely to cause severe fluid or electrolyte abnormalities in the fetus [28, 51]. If required to treat severe or life-threatening intracranial hypertension, moderate doses are recommended with judicious monitoring of blood pressure and treatment of any ensuing hypotension [4]. In human studies the effects on fetal outcome are unknown. Furosemide is an alternative but should also be used cautiously. Monitoring urine output is advised [4].

7.4.4 Steroids

Steroids decrease the vasogenic edema associated with tumor growth and improve the patient's symptoms [5]. It is safe to use steroids during pregnancy and have an additional advantage of promoting fetal lung maturity by increasing the fetal surfactant formation. However, maternal steroid administration may contribute to fetal adrenal hypoplasia [3]. Betamethasone has better neonatal outcomes than dexamethasone [52].

7.4.5 Antiepileptics

Antiepileptic drugs are used both for treatment and prophylaxis of seizures. Some of the antiepileptic drugs are teratogenic (e.g., phenytoin) [5, 53]. Therefore, their use in the first trimester requires careful consideration. Phenytoin is one of the most commonly used antiepileptic drugs in neurosurgical patients, which is poorly absorbed from the gastrointestinal tract and undergoes increased plasma clearance. So, appropriate dosing in pregnant women and monitoring plasma levels to achieve therapeutic plasma concentrations needs particular consideration [53].

7.4.6   Calcium Channel Blockers

There is limited evidence for the use of specific calcium channel blockers in pregnancy. Animal studies suggest that nimodipine may increase the risk of intrauterine growth retardation and congenital abnormalities but no comparative studies in humans are available. However, the known benefits of nimodipine in preventing spasm are likely to outweigh any potential risk to the fetus and should be administered as clinically indicated [4].

7.4.7   Chemotherapy, Radiotherapy, and Gamma Knife

Generalized chemotherapy is not an option in pregnancy; so localized chemotherapy with carmustine-impregnated wafers can be used [54]. Carmustine is an alkylating chemotherapeutic agent, which exerts its effects by alkylating the RNA and DNA. Systemic administration of carmustine is associated with systemic side effects and reduced efficacy; to overcome these problems, a localized delivery of the chemotherapeutic agent is desirable [55].

Radiotherapy is associated with teratogenicity and childhood cancers but still may be safely used if care is taken to decrease the dose of radiation and to provide adequate fetal shielding [56].

Gamma knife procedures during awake craniotomy provide local radiation and can be performed safely [57, 58].

> **Conclusion**
>
> Consequently compared to nonpregnant women, those who are pregnant are no more susceptible to neurosurgical interventions, nor routine neurosurgery is common during pregnancy. However, due to physiological changes of pregnancy, certain neuropathologies may be exacerbated, and standard neuroanesthesia practices may pose too many challenges. Care of the pregnant neurosurgical patient essentially follows the general principles of anesthesia for obstetrics and neurosurgery. On the other hand, anesthesiologists should be aware of various concerns from both neurosurgical and obstetric point of view discussed above. Most importantly, teamwork between the neurosurgeon, neuroanesthetist, obstetrician, and patient is crucial. The nature of neurosurgical conditions during pregnancy requires departments to be familiar with the management of pregnant patients. Protocols should be developed for such cases with close communication and referral between specialties, and thus, a decision will need to be made where the patient will be best cared for, in the neurosurgical or obstetric unit.

Key Learning Points

- Pregnant women presenting for non-obstetric surgery represent a unique surgical and anesthetic challenge where the health of the mother is prioritized but equally careful consideration needs to be given to fetal well-being.
- Even though neuroanesthesia is infrequently required during pregnancy, neurosurgical conditions encompasses anesthesia include cranial pathologies, intracranial hemorrhage, spinal pathologies, trauma, and diagnostic and therapeutic radiologic interventions.
- A multidisciplinary approach and careful consideration of the timing of both surgery and delivery are mandatory based on maternal outcome, assessment of fetal maturity and the urgency to perform neurosurgical process.
- The main goal is to provide a balance between some competing and even contradictory interventions unique for neuroanesthesia and obstetric anesthesia to accommodate the safety requirements of both the mother and the fetus.

References

1. Wlody DJ, Gambling DR, Griffiths TL. Anesthesia for neurosurgery in the pregnant patient. In: Cottrell JE, Patel P, editors. Cottrell and Patel's neuroanesthesia. New York: Elsevier; 2017. p. 433–44.
2. Nossek E, Ekstein M, Rimon E, Kupferminc MJ, Ram Z. Neurosurgery and pregnancy. Acta Neurochir. 2011;153:1727–35.
3. Ng J, Kitchen N. Neurosurgery and pregnancy. J Neurol Neurosurg Psychiatry. 2008;79:745–52.
4. Wang LP, Paech MJ. Neuroanesthesia for the pregnant woman. Anesth Analg. 2008;107:193–200.
5. Subramanian R, Sardar A, Mohanaselvi S, Khanna P, Baidya DK. Neurosurgery and pregnancy. Neuroanaesthesiol Crit Care. 2014;1:166–72.
6. Heesen M, Klimek M. Nonobstetric anesthesia during pregnancy. Curr Opin Anaesthesiol. 2016;29:297–303.
7. Chopra I, Gnanalingham K, Pal D, et al. A knot in the catheter—an unusual cause of ventriculoperitoneal shunt blockage. Acta Neurochir. 2004;146:1055–6.
8. Dias MS, Sekhar LN. Intracranial hemorrhage from aneurysms and arteriovenous malformations during pregnancy and the puerperium. Neurosurgery. 1990;27:855–65.
9. Wilson SR, Hirsch NP, Appleby I. Management of subarachnoid haemorrhage in a non–neurosurgical centre. Anaesthesia. 2005;60:470–85.
10. Nagamine N, Shintani N, Furuya A, et al. Anesthetic managements for emergency cesarean section and craniotomy in patients with intracranial haemorrhage due to ruptured cerebral aneurysm and arteriovenous malformation. Masui. 2007;56:1081–4.
11. Coskun D, Mahli A, Yılmaz Z, Cizmeci P. Anesthetic management of caesarean section of a pregnant woman with cerebral arteriovenous malformation: a case report. Cases J. 2008;1:327.
12. Brown MD, Levi AD. Surgery for lumbar disc herniation during pregnancy. Spine. 2001;26:440–3.
13. LaBan MM, Perrin JC, Latimer FR. Pregnancy and the herniated lumbar disc. Arch Phys Med Rehabil. 1983;64:319–21.

14. Fast A, Shapiro D, Ducommun EJ, Friedmann LW, Bouklas T, Floman Y. Low back pain in pregnancy. Spine. 1987;12:368–71.
15. Tanaka H, Kondo E, Kawato H, Kikukawa T, Ishihara A, Toyoda N. Spinal intradural hemorrhage due to a neurinoma in an early puerperal woman. Clin Neurol Neurosurg. 2002;104:303–5.
16. Szkup P, Stoneham G. Case report: spontaneous spinal epidural hematoma during pregnancy: case report and review of the literature. Br J Radiol. 2004;77:881–4.
17. Nakai Y, Mine M, Nishio J, Maeda T, Imanaka M, Ogita S. Effects of maternal prone position on the umbilical arterial blood flow. Acta Obstet Gynecol Scand. 1998;77:967–9.
18. Al-areibi A, Coveny L, Sing S, Katsiris S. Case report: anesthetic management for sequential caesarean delivery and laminectomy. Can J Anaesth. 2007;54:471–4.
19. Gunaydin B, Oncul S, Erdem M, Kaymaz M, Emmez H, Ozkose Z. General anesthesia for çesarean delivery followed by anterior and posterior spinal cord decompression of a parturient with symptomatic spine metastasis due to breast cancer. Turk J Med Sci. 2009;39:979–82.
20. Muench MV, Canterino JC. Trauma in pregnancy. Obstet Gynecol Clin N Am. 2007;34:555–83. xiii
21. Shah AJ, Kilcline BA. Trauma in pregnancy. Emerg Med Clin North Am. 2003;21:615–29.
22. Weinberg L, Steele RG, Pugh R, Higgins S, Herbert M, Story D. The pregnant trauma patient. Anaesth Intensive Care. 2005;33:167–80.
23. Chowdhury T, Chowdhury M, Schaller B, Cappellani RB, Daya J. Perioperative considerations for neurosurgical procedures in the gravid patient: continuing professional development. Can J Anaesth. 2013;60:1139–55.
24. Kuczkowsky KM, Fouha SM, Greenberg M, Benumof JL. Trauma in pregnancy: anaesthetic management of the pregnant trauma victim with unstable cervical spine. Anaesthesia. 2003;58:822.
25. Jain V, Chari R, Maslovitz S, Maternal Fetal Medicine Committee, et al. Guidelines for the management of a pregnant trauma patient. J Obstet Gynaecol Can. 2015;37:553–74.
26. Wang LP, Wolff J. Anesthetic management of severe chronic cardiopulmonary failure during endovascular embolization of a PICA aneurysm. J Neurosurg Anesthesiol. 2000;12:120–3.
27. Meyers PM, Halbach VV, Malek AM, et al. Endovascular treatment of cerebral artery aneurysms during pregnancy: report of three cases. Am J Neuroradiol. 2000;21:1306–11.
28. Tuncali B, Aksun M, Katircioglu K, Akkol I, Savaci S. Intraoperative fetal heart rate monitoring during emergency neurosurgery in a parturient. J Anesth. 2006;20:40–3.
29. Kizilkilic O, Albayram S, Adaletli I, et al. Endovascular treatment of ruptured intracranial aneurysms during pregnancy: report of three cases. Arch Gynecol Obstet. 2003;268:325–8.
30. Shaver SM, Shaver DC. Perioperative assessment of the obstetric patient undergoing abdominal surgery. J Perianesth Nurs. 2005;20:160–6.
31. Balki M, Manninen PH. Craniotomy for suprasellar meningioma in a 28-week pregnant woman without fetal heart rate monitoring. Can J Anaesth. 2004;51:573–6.
32. Burrus DR, O'Shea TM Jr, Veille JC, Mueller-Heubach E. The predictive value of intrapartum fetal heart rate abnormalities in the extremely premature infant. Am J Obstet Gynecol. 1994;171:1128–32.
33. Selo-Ojeme DO, Marshman LAG, Ikomi A, et al. Aneurysmal subarachnoid haemorrhage in pregnancy. Eur J Obstet Gynecol Reprod Biol. 2004;116:131–43.
34. Heidemann BH, McLure JH. Changes in maternal physiology during pregnancy. CEPD reviews. Br J Anaesth. 2003;3:65–8.
35. ACOG Committee on Obstetric Practice. ACOG Committee Opinion No. 474: nonobstetric surgery during pregnancy. Obstet Gynecol. 2011;117:420–1.
36. Rout CC, Rocke A, Gouws E. Intravenous ranitidine reduces the risk of acid aspiration of gastric contents at emergency caesarean section. Anesth Analg. 1993;76:156–61.
37. Anderson GD. Pregnancy-induced changes in pharmacokinetics. Clin Pharmacokinet. 2005;44:989–1008.
38. Han HT, Brimacombe J, Lee EJ, Yang HS. The laryngeal mask airway is effective (and probably safe) in selected healthy parturients for elective caesarean section: a prospective study of 1067 cases. Can J Anaesth. 2001;48:1117–21.

39. Preston R. The evolving role of the laryngeal mask in obstetrics (editorial). Can J Anaesth. 2001;48:1061–5.
40. Van de Velde M, Teunkens A, Kuypers M, Dewinter T, Vandermersch E. General anaesthesia with target controlled infusion of propofol for planned caesarean section: maternal and neonatal effects of a remifentanil-based technique. Int J Obstet Anesth. 2004;13:153–8.
41. Gregory MA, Gin T, Yau G, Leung RKW, Chan K, Oh TE. Propofol infusion anaesthesia for caesarian section. Can J Anaesth. 1990;37:514–20.
42. Koerner IP, Brambrink AM. Brain protection by anesthetic agents. Curr Opin Anaesthesiol. 2006;19:481–6.
43. Chang L, Looi-Lyons L, Bartosik L, Tindal S. Anesthesia for cesarean section in two patients with brain tumours. Can J Anaesth. 1999;46:61–5.
44. Thomas JS, Koh SH, Cooper GM. Haemodynamic effects of oxytocin given as i.v. bolus or infusion on women undergoing caesarean section. Br J Anaesth. 2007;98:116–9.
45. Ngan Kee WD, Lee A, Khaw KS, Ng FF, Karmakar MK, Gin T. A randomized double-blinded comparison of phenylephrine and ephedrine combinations given by infusion to maintain blood pressure during spinal anesthesia for cesarean delivery: effects on fetal acid-base status and hemodynamic control. Anesth Analg. 2008;107:1295–302.
46. Cooper DW, Carpenter M, Mowbray P, Desira WR, Ryall DM, Kokri MS. Fetal and maternal effects of phenylephrine and ephedrine during spinal anesthesia for caesarean delivery. Anesthesiology. 2002;97:1582–90.
47. Todd MM, Hindman BJ, Clarke WR, Tomer JC. Mild intraoperative hypothermia during surgery for intracranial aneurysm. N Engl J Med. 2005;352:135–46.
48. Kayacan N, Arici G, Karsli B, Erman M. Acute subdural haematoma after accidental dural puncture during epidural anaesthesia. Int J Obstet Anesth. 2004;13:47–9.
49. Eggert SM, Eggers KA. Subarachnoid haemorrhage following spinal anaesthesia in an obstetric patient. Br J Anaesth. 2001;86:442–4.
50. Chen SH, Sung YH, Chang PJ, Liu YC, Tsai YC. The management of labour using continuous lumbar epidural analgesia with 0.2% ropivacaine in a parturient with traumatic brain injury. Eur J Anaesthesiol. 2005;22:634–5.
51. Bharti N, Kashyap L, Mohan VK. Anesthetic management of a parturient with cerebellopontine-angle meningioma. Int J Obstet Anesth. 2002;11:219–21.
52. Lee BH, Stoll BJ, McDonald SA, Higgins RD, National Institute of Child Health and Human Development Neonatal Research Network. Adverse neonatal outcomes associated with antenatal dexamethasone versus antenatal betamethasone. Pediatrics. 2006;117:1503–10.
53. Klein AM. Epilepsy cases in pregnant and postpartum women: a practical approach. Semin Neurol. 2011;31:392–6.
54. Stevenson CB, Thompson RC. The clinical management of intracranial neoplasms in pregnancy. Clin Obstet Gynecol. 2005;48:24–37.
55. Lin SH, Kleinberg LR. Carmustine wafers: localized delivery of chemotherapeutic agents in CNS malignancies. Expert Rev Anticancer Ther. 2008;8:343–59.
56. Kal HB, Struikmans H. Radiotherapy during pregnancy: fact and fiction. Lancet Oncol. 2005;6:328–33.
57. Yu C, Jozsef G, Apuzzo ML, MacPherson DM, Petrovich Z. Fetal radiation doses for model C gamma knife radiosurgery. Neurosurgery. 2003;52:687–93.
58. Abd-Elsayed AA, Díaz-Gómez J, Barnett GH, et al. A case series discussing the anaesthetic management of pregnant patients with brain tumours. Version 2 F1000Res. 2013;2:92.

Anesthetic Management of Pregnant Patient with Neurological and Neuromuscular Disorders

8

Dominika Dabrowska

8.1 Neurological Disorders

8.1.1 General Considerations

Neurological diseases affecting pregnant patients can be classified into three main groups:

1. Pre-existing chronic neurological diseases such as epilepsy and multiple sclerosis
2. Disorders with onset predominantly during pregnancy such as cerebrovascular events
3. Neurological conditions which are specifically related to pregnancy such as eclampsia

This chapter focuses exclusively on the common pre-existing neurological comorbidities affecting obstetric patients and their anesthetic implications. Neurological disorders account for a significant cause of maternal morbidity and mortality.

According to the 2016 report by MBRRACE-UK (Mothers and Babies: Reducing Risks through Audits and Confidential Enquiries in the UK), neurological disorders represented the second most frequent cause of indirect maternal deaths in the UK [1]. As a result of the improvements in the therapeutic options for many neurological conditions over the past few decades, significant number of women with these disorders manages to become pregnant. In addition, more information is now available to help clinicians guide patients on which treatments need to be continued and how they should be administered.

D. Dabrowska
Chelsea and Westminster Hospital NHS Foundation Trust, London, UK

© Springer International Publishing AG, part of Springer Nature 2018
B. Gunaydin, S. Ismail (eds.), *Obstetric Anesthesia for Co-morbid Conditions*,
https://doi.org/10.1007/978-3-319-93163-0_8

Ideally, any woman with neurological disease who is pregnant or wishes to become pregnant should have a pre-pregnancy or early antenatal consultation with the obstetrician, neurologist, and obstetric anesthetist. The aim would be to assess the severity of the disease, review current medications, and advise the patient about any possible teratogenic effects. Neurological assessment should be performed during this consultation, and appropriate investigations, including neuroimaging and neurophysiological testing, should be arranged. Any pre-existing neurological deficit should be meticulously documented in view of the potential for exacerbation during pregnancy. As the physiological changes related to pregnancy also affect the central nervous system, the risk of neurological complications for patients with pre-existing disease can increase even further.

Anesthetic management of obstetric patients with neurological comorbidities can be challenging. Regional analgesia and anesthesia techniques offer many clinical benefits in the obstetric population but may be contraindicated in the presence of raised intracranial pressure, tethered spinal cord, or unstable disease. Moreover, abnormal anatomy such as kyphoscoliosis can make the insertion of epidural or spinal needle technically difficult or even impossible. The dose of the local anesthetic needs to be carefully titrated in all patients but especially in those at risk of respiratory depression related to their underlying neurological condition. If general anesthesia needs to be administered, this may carry significant risk due to associated rises in systolic blood pressure and its adverse effect on intracranial pressure. Therefore, rapid sequence induction should be modified by the addition of a short-acting opioid, such as remifentanil, in order to obtund the hypertensive response to laryngoscopy. In many neurological conditions, such as multiple sclerosis, increased sensitivity to depolarizing muscle relaxants is present. Succinylcholine may also cause hyperkalemia and cardiac arrest in those patients. In view of this, and the widespread availability of sugammadex as a reversal agent, succinylcholine should be replaced with sugammadex whenever appropriate. Volatile anesthetic agents such as isoflurane or sevoflurane are appropriate for the maintenance of anesthesia in view of their positive effect on preservation of the cerebral perfusion pressure and cerebral oxygen consumption.

Anesthetic complications which may occur during and after delivery, such as post-dural puncture headache or new-onset neurological deficit, can be difficult to distinguish from those related to the negative effects of pregnancy on the disease itself. A high index of suspicion should be present whenever new neurological symptoms are identified during the postnatal follow-up visit in order for appropriate investigations and clinical management to be commenced.

8.1.2 Specific Considerations

8.1.2.1 Multiple Sclerosis

Multiple sclerosis (MS) is a progressive neurological disease affecting the central nervous system, which causes a wide range of symptoms such as fatigue, visual disturbance, muscle weakness, sensory loss in the limbs, as well as bowel and bladder dysfunction. Its underlying mechanism is a demyelination of the nerve fibers with axonal damage and loss of myelin sheath causing disruption in conduction of the electrical impulse to and from the brain. The incidence of the disease is 3.6 cases per 100,000, and it is estimated that 2.5 million people in the world are affected by MS. The distribution of the disease is uneven, with the prevalence of the disorder increasing with the latitude. Women are twice as likely to be affected compared to men, and the diagnosis is frequently made during the second and third decades of their lives. Patients with MS are frequently treated with disease-modifying drugs (DMDs) such as interferon and/or glatiramer. Current advice is to stop treatment if they are planning to become pregnant due to limited data available to support safety of these agents in pregnancy. Symptoms of progressive disease such as spasticity bladder dysfunction, and depression are treated with baclofen, intermittent catheterization, and antidepressants.

Pregnancy itself has a protective effect on the course of the disease and is associated with a significant reduction in the frequency of the relapses, especially in the last trimester. A large prospective study of MS in pregnant women (PRIMS study) has demonstrated that the risk of relapses is significantly higher in the immediate postpartum period and all pregnant patients affected by MS should be adequately informed about this effect [2]. Multiple sclerosis does not have a negative impact on the course of the pregnancy, and therefore obstetric and neonatal outcomes do not differ between patients with MS and the general population.

The anesthetic management of the pregnant patient with multiple sclerosis has been a subject of controversy in the past. Some studies reported an increased rate in postpartum relapse in patients receiving spinal anesthetics due to unmasking of the silent demyelination effect [3]. However, in view of the increased frequency of the relapses in the immediate postdelivery period, this relationship can be purely casual. There is also some indirect evidence suggesting that epidural technique is of less risk compared to spinal block, probably in view of limited amount of local anesthetic getting in contact with cerebrospinal fluid.

However, these findings are based on experimental rather than clinical studies [4]. In the last decade, there have been several case reports in the literature reporting safe administration of spinal and epidural techniques for labor and delivery in patients with MS. A survey among the anesthetists in the UK showed that currently most anesthetist would not hesitate to proceed with neuraxial blocks in patients with MS [5]. Nevertheless, the demyelinated neurons are more susceptible to develop exaggerated block response and local anesthetic toxicity, and therefore lower concentrations of local anesthetics should be administered. Data describing use of regional and general anesthesia for cesarean section in parturients with multiple sclerosis is limited; however, current opinion considers both of them to be safe. Pastó et al. [6] investigated 423 pregnancies in 415 patients with multiple sclerosis. Cesarean section was performed in 155 patients, out of which 46 under regional anesthesia. No association has been found between the surgical mode of delivery, the type of anesthesia received, and the increased risk of the relapse in the postpartum period [6].

If general anesthesia is necessary due to patient's preferences or the surgical urgency, special attention needs to be emphasized on temperature control and the use of the muscle relaxants. Demyelinated nerves are very sensitive to increase in body temperature, which can translate into exacerbation of the symptoms, and therefore excessive warming should be avoided. Succinylcholine can produce severe hyperkalemia especially in patients with advanced disease and limb spasticity due to upregulation of the acetylcholine receptors, and this agent should be used with caution or avoided. Patients with MS may present unpredictable response to non-depolarizing muscle relaxants, and monitoring of the neuromuscular blockade should be routinely used if these drugs are given [7].

8.1.2.2 Epilepsy

Epilepsy is a common neurological disease with the prevalence rate of 4–8 per 1000. Seizures, which can be described as recurrent episodes of involuntary movements involving a part or the entire body, remain the main feature of this disorder. They may be accompanied by temporary loss of consciousness and control of the sphincters. Most of the epileptic female patients manage to become pregnant. The effect of the pregnancy on the course of the disease is variable: two-thirds of affected woman do not experience any deterioration of their condition, provided they are compliant with pharmacotherapy prior to the pregnancy [8]. In the remaining one-third of the patients, seizing activity can become more frequent and severe, mainly due to the pregnancy-related physical and emotional stress. On the other hand, epilepsy can affect pregnancy in a number of different ways. If seizures occur during pregnancy, they can cause decelerations in fetal heart rate and fetal hypoxia as well as direct injury to the fetus, placental abruption, and miscarriage. Some older antiepileptic drugs (AEDs) such as carbamazepine, valproate, and phenytoin may have a teratogenic effect and cause fetal abnormalities such as neural tube defects and congenital heart disease. Intrauterine growth restriction and preterm delivery have also frequently been described in pregnant patients receiving AEDs [9].

Anesthetic management of the parturient with epilepsy begins with the antenatal anesthetic assessment, which should focus on review of the anticonvulsive medication and prevention of the seizures. Patients with well-controlled epilepsy are not considered to be at higher risk. Optimal pain control is recommended for all epileptic women during labor and delivery in order to reduce the hyperventilation and stress, which can precipitate the seizure. Epidural analgesia has been used safely in majority of the patients, and the dose of the local anesthetic does not require to be modified [10].

If cesarean section is required, the choice of the anesthetic technique should be based on patient's preferences, any existing contraindications, and the grade of urgency. Regional techniques such as spinal and combined spinal-epidural are both suitable for epileptic patients. If general anesthesia is required, intravenous induction agents such as propofol and thiopental can be used. Monitoring of the neuromuscular blockade is necessary in view of the fact that some anticonvulsive drugs such as carbamazepine and phenytoin can antagonize non-depolarizing muscle relaxants.

The emergency management of the pregnant patient presenting with seizure should include supportive measures such as airway protection, supplemental oxygen, and monitoring of the vital signs. Intravenous access should be established as soon as it is safe for both patient and the clinician, in order to promptly terminate the seizure with pharmacological agents. Benzodiazepines are the drugs of choice. Second-line agents include phenytoin, valproate, and levetiracetam [11]. General anesthesia should be induced if the seizure cannot be terminated with other measures, and continuous fetal heart monitoring should be commenced and continued in the postictal period.

8.1.2.3 Chiari Malformation

A Chiari malformation, previously described as Arnold-Chiari malformation, is a congenital neurological defect resulting from the protrusion of the cerebellar tonsils and brain stem into the foramen magnum. Four main types of Chiari malformation have been identified, with Chiari 1 being the most common. Its incidence has been estimated to be 1 in 1000 births. Syringomyelia, a condition in which cyst filled with cerebrospinal fluid forms within the spinal cord, is present in up to 50% of patients with Chiari 1 [12]. Chiari 2 malformation is frequently associated with other defects of the neural tube such as myelomeningocele. Type 3 and 4 are very rare but more severe. Many patients with Chiari malformations are asymptomatic, and diagnosis is made incidentally. If symptoms occur, they include headache, neck pain, paresthesia in the upper extremities, blurred and double vision, muscle weakness, problems with balance and coordination, tinnitus, loss of hearing, insomnia, and depression. Treatment options depend on the severity of the symptoms and consist of painkillers and surgical procedures such as decompression surgery, electrocautery, and syringo-subarachnoid shunt.

The effect of pregnancy on the Chiari-related symptoms remains unknown due to the paucity of the data in the literature. Mueller et al. studied seven pregnant patients with Chiari malformation, and slight worsening of the symptoms was reported in most of them [13].

A review of the American national database performed between 2008 and 2011 showed a significant increase in the medical and obstetric complications such as stroke and cardiovascular accidents, preeclampsia, seizures, and sepsis in pregnant women with Chiari malformations [14].

Anesthetic management of parturients with Chiari malformation is challenging. There is a lack of evidence to suggest preference of general anesthesia over regional techniques. Although regional techniques are not contraindicated, they are considered unsuitable for patients with symptoms of increased intracranial pressure (ICP). Moreover, accidental dural puncture, a recognized complication of epidural technique, can lead to tentorial herniation and decreased cerebral perfusion pressure with its devastating consequences. On the other hand, rapid sequence induction and endotracheal intubation, essential elements of general anesthesia in obstetrics, can cause an increase in ICP with unfavorable effect on maternal and fetal outcomes. The uneventful use of spinal anesthesia in parturients with Chiari malformations has been described in several case reports [15, 16]. Epidural analgesia has been also successfully used in labor, provided that there were no signs of acute worsening of ICP [17]. Choi et al. reported safe use of combined spinal-epidural as effective pain relief method in a patient with Chiari 1 malformation [18].

The main goal in the management of general anesthesia is to avoid the increase in ICP, which can lead to the herniation and extension of the syrinx. In view of this, awake fiberoptic intubation with local airway anesthesia or modified rapid sequence induction with use of opioids should be considered [19, 20]. Patients with Chiari malformation and syringomyelia have increased sensitivity to muscle relaxants, and therefore careful monitoring of the neuromuscular blockade is recommended if these agents are administered. Regardless of the anesthetic technique selected, management of these patients requires caution, multidisciplinary approach, and individualized care plan in order to secure good outcomes for both mother and the baby.

8.1.2.4 Spina Bifida

Spina bifida is a congenital defect of the neural tube with an incomplete closing of the vertebrae and hernial protrusion of the meninges and of the spinal cord. The incidence of this malformation varies significantly by country from 0.1 to 5 per 1000 live births. Spina bifida can be classified into three main types: spina bifida occulta, meningocele, and myelomeningocele. Spina bifida occulta is the most common and the mildest type, presenting as a small gap in the spine with the hairy patch or dark spot on the skin of the back but no involvement of the spinal cord. This condition is usually asymptomatic but occasionally may be accompanied by scoliosis and cause back pain in some patients [21]. Meningocele occurs when a cystic herniation of the dura and arachnoid protrudes through the defect in the vertebral arch. It is described as myelomeningocele when it contains the spinal cord tissue. Myelomeningocele is the most severe form of spina bifida and is frequently associated with Chiari 2 malformation, hydrocephalus, and latex allergy. Other symptoms related to this defect include numbness and weakness in the legs and loss of bladder and bowel control. Spina bifida and other neural tube defects can be largely prevented by supplementation of the folic acid during pregnancy, and its incidence has decreased significantly since this preventing strategy has been implemented [22]. Pregnancy generally has a positive outcome in patients with spina bifida. Complications such as recurrent urinary infection and reduced mobility may occur in some patients [23].

There is a lack of specific guidelines in relation to the administration of the labor analgesia in patients with spina bifida. Neuraxial blocks are considered safe but vertebral abnormalities and scoliosis can make them technically difficult. An MRI of the lumbar spine should be obtained whenever possible to exclude the presence of the tethered spinal cord, a contraindication to regional techniques. Moreover, the incidence of the accidental dural tap is higher in patients with spina bifida [24]. In order to reduce the incidence of this complication, ultrasound can be used for locating of the intervertebral space and estimation of the depth of the epidural space. Excessive cranial spread of local anesthetic due to epidural insertion above the level of the defect as well as reduced volume of the epidural space may contribute to the high or patchy block, and therefore the dose of local anesthetic should be decreased

[25]. On the other hand, impaired caudal spread may lead to inadequate analgesia in the third stage of labor requiring additional methods such as pudendal block or insertion of a second epidural catheter below the level of the defect [26]. Valente et al. have described the use of patient-controlled analgesia using intravenous remifentanil, but a reduced analgesic effect has been reported in late stage of labor [27].

Regional techniques should be considered as a first choice if patient with spina bifida requires a cesarean section. If general anesthesia is necessary, there is an increased risk of difficult intubation, and this should be anticipated during preoperative assessment and planning [28].

8.1.2.5 Spinal Cord Injury

Spinal cord injuries (SCI) involve damage to the spinal cord, which may cause incomplete or complete loss of its sensory, motor, or autonomic function. Every year approximately 12,000 new spinal cord injuries are reported in the USA. Majority of the spinal cord injuries originate from direct trauma to the cord sustained during motor vehicle accidents, gunshots, falls, and sport-related accidents. Spinal cord can also be damaged as a result of tumors and due to infective and ischemic causes. The symptoms depend on the location and the severity of the damage with lesions below T1 resulting in paraplegia and lesions above T1 resulting in quadriplegia. Symptoms of autonomic dysreflexia such as headache, flushing, blurred vision, nausea, anxiety, and hypertension may frequently occur in lesions above T6 level [29].

There is no evidence to suggest that spinal cord injuries prevent female patients within their reproductive age from becoming pregnant. However, pregnancy may aggravate symptoms associated with those injuries such as pressure ulcers, constipation, bladder spasticity, urinary trait infections, deep venous thrombosis, and impaired lung function. Women with SCI have higher incidence of premature labor and instrumental or operative deliveries compared to healthy parturients [29].

Although patients with the spinal cord injury above the T10 level may perceive no pain during labor, epidural anesthesia should be considered in these patients in order to prevent complications related to autonomic dysreflexia. Distension and manipulation of the vagina, bladder, or bowels can all precipitate this complication, which may result in severe hypertension and fetal distress. If signs of autonomic dysreflexia occur before epidural is sited, other pharmacological agents such as labetalol, hydralazine, and magnesium sulfate should be administered [29].

If cesarean delivery is necessary, regional blocks should be offered as a first choice, but they may be technically difficult due to poor positioning and previous corrective surgery with metal work and bone deformities present. If general anesthesia is administered, difficult intubation should be anticipated in patients with fixed cervical injuries [29].

Profound hypotension can occur at induction since the sympathetic response is often absent, and it should be treated aggressively with vasopressors. Moreover, thermoregulation is frequently impaired in patients with SCI. Active warming should be established intraoperatively and continue into recovery period. Postoperatively a period of noninvasive ventilation may be necessary due to respiratory compromise frequently present in these patients [29].

8.2   Neuromuscular Disorders

8.2.1   General Considerations

Neuromuscular diseases consist of a heterogeneous group of disorders, which directly or indirectly affect the functioning of the muscles. They can be classified in different ways and subdivided in:

1. Hereditary or acquired
2. Pre-junctional or postjunctional
3. According to the anatomical structure affected, in:
   (a) Disorders of the motor neuron (such as amyotrophic lateral sclerosis and spinal muscular atrophy)
   (b) Disorders of the peripheral nerves (such as Guillain-Barré syndrome)
   (c) Disorders of the neuromuscular junction (such as myasthenia gravis)
   (d) Disorders of the muscles (such as muscular dystrophies, myotonic dystrophies, and myopathies)

Although the incidence of neuromuscular diseases in women of childbearing age is relatively low, they may present specific problems when occurring during pregnancy. In most cases, pregnancy has a negative effect on the course of the pre-existing neuromuscular disorder. Occasionally it can unmask an underlying condition of which the patient is unaware. In both cases the management of the obstetric patient with neuromuscular disease is challenging and should focus on adequate antenatal assessment and planning, multidisciplinary involvement, careful intrapartum monitoring, and postpartum follow-up. Weakness of the respiratory muscles, cardiac involvement, and severe scoliosis can be all frequently observed in mothers affected by neuromuscular diseases, and such patients should be considered high risk.

Involvement of the smooth uterine muscles and inability to push effectively may have adverse effects on labor and delivery, and the rate of instrumental or operative delivery is higher in these patients compared to general obstetric population. Several neuromuscular disorders, such as myasthenia gravis and myotonic dystrophy, may have a negative impact on both the fetus and the newborn. In view of this, all women with neuromuscular disease contemplating pregnancy should receive adequate pre-pregnancy counselling.

Management of pregnant patients with pre-existing neuromuscular disorders has many implications for obstetric anesthetists. A thorough antenatal examination aimed to assess the cardiorespiratory function and involvement of other organs is of particular importance. Respiratory complications can be frequently observed in these patients due to involvement of the diaphragm and respiratory muscles, spinal deformities, and difficult airways. Bearing this in mind, the 179th European Neuromuscular Centre (ENMC) workshop in 2010 recommended forced vital capacity (FVC), maximum inspiratory pressure (MIP), and peak cough flow (PCF) measurement at baseline and at least once in each trimester. In patients with FVC values less than 50% of predicted or less than 1 L, MIP less than 60 cm H_2O, or PCF less than 160 L/min, an additional arterial blood gas measurement and a sleep study should be performed. An echocardiogram is recommended in each trimester if ejection fraction is 45–60% and more frequently if ejection fraction is less than 45% [30].

Several general anesthetic medications are contraindicated or should only be used with caution in patients with neuromuscular disorders. Therefore, regional analgesic and anesthetic techniques offer significant advantages compared to general anesthesia.

Succinylcholine activates nicotinic acetylcholine receptors, which are upregulated in patients with denervated or dystrophic muscles. This may lead to excessive potassium influx and fatal hyperkalemia with rhabdomyolysis. In view of this succinylcholine should be avoided in majority of these disorders, with the exclusion of myasthenia gravis in which loss of receptors leads to a relative resistance to depolarizing muscle relaxants [31].

The vast majority of patients with neuromuscular disorders exhibit marked sensitivity to non-depolarizing neuromuscular blocking agents. Therefore, these drugs should be also avoided or given in reduced doses, and the level of the neuromuscular blockade should be closely monitored. Anticholinesterases are not recommended as a part of reversal of the neuromuscular block as they may cause hyperkalemia in muscular dystrophies as well as cholinergic crisis in myasthenia gravis. Sugammadex can be used instead of anticholinergics to reverse rocuronium-induced blockade. Volatile agents are considered safe in most of the patients with neuromuscular diseases. However, the postoperative shivering frequently associated with their use may lead to phenomenon of myotonia in patients with myotonic dystrophy. Intraoperative thermoregulation is extremely important in patients with neuromuscular diseases since they are vulnerable to both hypo- and hyperthermia. Hypothermia, exacerbated by reduced heat production from inactive muscles, may lead to myotonia, rhabdomyolysis, and prolonged neuromuscular block. Hyperthermia may occur during myotonic spasm or malignant hyperthermia and should be treated aggressively [31].

Historically, many neuromuscular diseases have been linked to increased risk of malignant hyperthermia and its life-threatening complications. However, recent improvements in the understanding of the pathophysiology of this condition have disproved this link with the exception of King-Denborough syndrome, central core disease, and hypokalemic periodic paralysis. The susceptibility to develop malignant hyperthermia in patients with those particular disorders derives from abnormalities in the ryanodine receptor (RYR1) gene which encodes calcium channel function in skeletal muscles [31].

Parturients with neuromuscular disease are at high risk of intra- and postpartum respiratory and cardiac complications. In addition, rhabdomyolysis may occur as a result of use of the depolarizing muscle relaxants or sustained muscle contraction in myotonic patients. Respiratory insufficiency is often due to progressive spine deformities and subsequent restrictive lung disease, in addition to respiratory muscles weakness. If general anesthesia is administered, severely affected patients may require a period of postoperative weaning or positive-pressure ventilation (CPAP) in an intensive care setting. Other postoperative complications such as chest infection may develop due to hypoventilation and aspiration in patients with impaired respiratory function and bulbar muscles involvement. Cardiac complications including cardiac failure and arrhythmias may occur as a consequence of cardio-depressive effect of anesthetic drugs or pre-existing cardiac conduction system abnormalities in patients with myotonic dystrophy. Frequency of death due to cardiac complications is second only to respiratory failure in affected patients [32].

Postoperative care of patients with neuromuscular disorders should focus on adequate pain control as well as respiratory monitoring and management, especially in patients with decreased respiratory muscle strength. Continuous infusion of local anesthetics via epidural catheters provides good analgesia while minimizing side effects such as hypoventilation. In the absence of epidural catheter in situ, especially in patients who underwent cesarean section under general anesthesia, peripheral nerve blocks such as transverse abdominis plane (TAP) block can be safely used to provide postoperative pain control and reduce use of opioids. Neuropathic pain, which is frequently present in patients with Guillain-Barré syndrome, can be treated with gabapentin [33].

Postoperative respiratory management is determined by the severity of the disease and preoperative respiratory function. Extubation should be postponed until the patient is able to achieve adequate tidal volumes and respiratory secretions are well controlled. Noninvasive ventilation strategies together with assisted cough techniques may provide adequate respiratory support and decrease the risk of re-intubation and tracheostomy.

8.2.2 Specific Considerations

8.2.2.1 Myasthenia Gravis

Myasthenia gravis is an autoimmune disease characterized by T cell-dependent and B cell-mediated production of antibodies directed against postsynaptic nicotinic acetylcholine receptors in skeletal muscles. It is considered the most common neuromuscular junction disorder with incidence of 15 in 100,000. Female patients in the second or third decade of their lives are more frequently affected than males. The main symptom of MG is weakness of the voluntary skeletal muscles, which typically gets worse with physical activity, stress, infection, heat, and emotions; all of these factors quite frequently present during pregnancy and labor. Other symptoms include ptosis, diplopia, dysphagia, dysarthria, and hypophonia as a result of the involvement of the ocular and bulbar muscles. Myasthenic crisis is a life-threatening complication, which may occur in about 20% of myasthenic patients. It is characterized by exacerbation of muscle weakness leading to respiratory failure which may require intubation and mechanical ventilation [34].

Treatment options for myasthenia include anticholinesterase agents such as pyridostigmine and immunosuppressive drugs such as corticosteroids, azathioprine, intravenous immunoglobulin, and plasmapheresis. Thymoma, a tumor originating from the epithelial cells of the thymus, occurs in 10–20% of patients, and its treatment may involve surgery [35].

The effect of pregnancy on the course of the disease is variable. Alpha-fetoprotein produced during pregnancy prevents acetylcholine receptors from binding to their postsynaptic ligands, and due to the relative immunosuppressive effect of the last two trimesters of the pregnancy, the disease remains unaffected in 70% of patients [36]. One-third of patients may deteriorate, especially in the postnatal period, and may require higher doses of oral steroids and period of CPAP at night. This occurs less likely in patients who had previous thymectomy [37].

Myasthenia may have several effects on pregnancy and birth. The risk of miscarriage is not increased, but a higher than normal incidence of premature rupture of membranes, preterm labor, and delivery as well as intrauterine growth restriction has been observed. Hoff et al. analyzed 127 births in mothers with myasthenia and demonstrated a high number of complications during delivery leading to increased risk of surgical interventions [38].

Maternal antibodies may cross the placenta and cause transitory neonatal MG or rarely neonatal arthrogryposis multiplex congenita with its typical nonprogressive contractures resulting from lack of fetal movements in utero [39].

The preoperative assessment of the pregnant patient affected by myasthenia should include the evaluation of the bulbar and respiratory muscle involvement and review of the anticholinesterase and corticosteroid therapy. Pulmonary function tests should be performed to evaluate respiratory reserve and to anticipate the need for postoperative mechanical ventilation. Factors such as FVC < 2.9 L, duration of the disease greater than 6 years, chronic respiratory disease, and doses of pyridostigmine greater than 750 mg/day are all associated with the prolonged period of postoperative ventilation [40].

The anesthetic management should focus on the avoidance of the factors enhancing the blockade at the neuromuscular junction level such as hypothermia, hypokalemia, and hypophosphatemia in order to facilitate the transmission of the compromised signal.

Regional analgesia and anesthesia are techniques of choice since several general anesthetic drugs may have direct negative effect on the neural transmission and muscular power. The duration of action of the ester local anesthetics, metabolized by cholinesterase, is prolonged in patients receiving anticholinesterases, and therefore ester local anesthetics should be avoided, and amide-type local anesthetics should be used instead.

Patients with MG show relative resistance to depolarizing muscle relaxants such as succinylcholine, probably due to loss of receptors. The ED95 of succinylcholine in MG patients is 2.6 times that in non-myasthenic ones, and therefore the dose of this drug should be adjusted accordingly [41]. On the other hand, myasthenic patients present marked sensitivity to non-depolarizing muscle relaxants. Long-acting muscle relaxants are best avoided, and intermediate- and short-acting should be used, together with careful monitoring of neuromuscular transmission. Anticholinesterase drugs such as neostigmine administered as a part of the reversal may produce cholinergic crisis and therefore should be administered slowly and cautiously. Sugammadex in combination with neuromuscular monitoring can be used to reverse rocuronium-induced neuromuscular blockade [42]. Numerous drugs frequently used in peripartum period may cause exacerbation of myasthenia. Myasthenic crisis can be precipitated by several antibiotics, antimalarial drugs, beta-blockers, calcium channel blockers, magnesium, gabapentin, and phenytoin. Management of the severe preeclampsia in the myasthenic patient is particularly challenging since magnesium, nifedipine, and labetalol are all contraindicated. Methyldopa and hydralazine are considered safe and should be used to control the hypertension. A UK multispecialty working group recommended that magnesium sulfate should be used only in the setting of eclamptic seizure with extreme caution and in consultation with obstetric anesthetist as intubation and ventilation may be required [43].

8.2.2.2 Muscular Dystrophies

Muscular dystrophies are a group of inherited genetic disorders affecting skeletal muscles which can result in progressive weakness and atrophy. In some types of muscular dystrophies, cardiac muscle may also be affected. Nine main categories of muscular dystrophies have been identified, and they contain more than 30 specific types. The most common types are Duchenne muscular dystrophy (DMD) and Becker muscular dystrophy; however, they typically affect male patients and therefore are rarely observed during pregnancy. The other categories include facioscapulohumeral muscular dystrophy (FSHD), limb-girdle muscular dystrophy, oculopharyngeal muscular dystrophy (OPMD), distal muscular dystrophy, Emery-Dreifuss muscular dystrophy, and myotonic dystrophy.

There is currently no definitive cure for these disorders, and the treatment options such as corticosteroids, physiotherapy, and corrective surgery aim to reduce symptoms and prevent complications.

The majority of the patients with muscular dystrophies experience worsening of the symptoms during pregnancy. However, vaginal delivery may be attempted in the absence of the obstetric contraindications. Anesthetic management of patients with muscular dystrophies involves adequate antenatal assessment with assessment of the cardiac and respiratory function. Regional techniques should be deployed whenever possible: epidural, spinal, and combined spinal-epidural blocks are considered safe provided that the dose of the local anesthetic is carefully titrated in order to avoid high block and cardiovascular and respiratory compromise. Succinylcholine can cause rhabdomyolysis and hyperkalemia due to the expression of the extrajunctional postsynaptic acetylcholine receptors and therefore should be avoided. Moreover, the sensitivity to the non-depolarizing muscle relaxants is increased in these patients. If restrictive lung disease is present, the period of postoperative ventilation may be required.

8.2.2.3 Myotonic Dystrophy

Myotonic dystrophy, also known as dystrophia myotonica (DM) or Steinert's disease, is a multi-organ genetic disorder inherited with autosomal dominant pattern. It represents the most common type of muscular dystrophy with an onset in adulthood, and its estimated prevalence is 0.5–18.1 per 100,000 [44]. Smooth and skeletal muscles are both affected, and symptoms include progressive muscle weakness, wasting, and "myotonia," inability of the muscles to relax after contraction. Resulting muscular atrophy may lead to significant deterioration in cardiorespiratory function and cardiomyopathy. Other symptoms are present and include heart conduction abnormalities, insulin resistance, cataracts, and intellectual disability. Due to the smooth muscles involvement, dysphagia, constipation, and gallstones can occur. Uterine smooth muscles may behave abnormally leading to complications in pregnancy and during labor. Two distinct genetic forms of myotonic dystrophy have been identified: myotonic dystrophy type 1 (DM1 or Steinert's disease) and myotonic dystrophy type 2 (DM2 or proximal myotonic myopathy). Type 1 is caused by a mutation in DMPK gene located on the chromosome 19, which consist of an abnormal expansion of the cytosine-thymine-guanine (CTG) trinucleotide repeat. Type 2 is caused by a mutation in the CNBP gene located on chromosome 3. The symptoms of both forms tend to overlap, but type 1 appears to be more severe [44].

Pregnancy may cause exacerbation of the muscle weakness, myotonia, and muscle wasting especially in the last trimester. In view of the smooth uterine muscle involvement, patients with myotonic dystrophy have an increased risk of miscarriage, prolonged first stage of labor, malpresentation, placenta previa, preeclampsia, and uterine atony [45]. Fetus may develop congenital myotonia and hypotonia. This can lead to decreased fetal movements and decreased swallowing of the amniotic fluid with the resulting polyhydramnios and consequently increased risk of premature rapture of membranes, preterm labor, and postpartum hemorrhage [46].

The anesthetic management of parturients with myotonic dystrophy can be complex. Serious complications such as loss of airway, aspiration, and life-threatening arrhythmias may occur in only mildly affected patients. In view of this, regional techniques should be performed whenever possible. If general anesthesia is required, succinylcholine should be avoided due to its potential to precipitate myotonic spasm. Also, non-depolarizing muscle relaxants should be avoided or used with caution, and neuromuscular block should be monitored with peripheral nerve stimulator. Patients with myotonic dystrophy present an increased sensitivity to thiopental and propofol with marked cardiovascular instability during induction of anesthesia. All type 1 DM patients require cardiac monitoring during labor and delivery in view of the potential arrhythmias and sudden death. There is also higher than usual risk of aspiration due to hyperglycemia, bulbar palsy, and reflux. Myotonia, the inability of the muscles to relax, occurs as a result of an intrinsic change in the muscle, not in the nerve or neuromuscular junction, and therefore cannot be abolished by peripheral nerve blockade or use of the muscle relaxants. If laryngeal and respiratory muscles are involved, intubation may be difficult or impossible. Factors such as hypothermia, electrical scalpel, nerve stimulator and some pharmacological agents such as anticholinesterases and succinylcholine can all cause myotonic contraction and should be avoided. Sugammadex can be used for reversal of the rocuronium-induced muscle relaxation. Use of volatile agents is controversial since postoperative shivering which is often associate with their use can

precipitate myotonia. Admission to the intensive care for postoperative management should always be considered given the increased risk of serious complications
that may occur.

8.2.2.4 Guillain-Barré Syndrome

Guillain-Barré syndrome (GBS) is a rare acute autoimmune polyneuropathy. It
occurs with the estimated incidence of 1.2–1.9 cases per 100,000 annually. The
main symptoms of this disorder include progressive muscle weakness, tingling sensation in the extremities, and respiratory difficulty. It may evolve rapidly and cause
symmetrical flaccid paralysis. The underlying mechanism is an autoimmune inflammatory process which causes demyelination of the peripheral nerves. It can be triggered by an infection, vaccination and surgery. Treatment includes plasmapheresis,
intravenous immunoglobulin, and supportive care. A period of mechanical ventilation may be necessary if signs of respiratory failure are present. This condition is
usually self-limiting and majority of the patients make good functional recovery but
residual weakness may be present in about 30% of patients after 3 years.

Guillain-Barré syndrome is rare during pregnancy but may be associated with
high maternal morbidity. The management of the pregnant patient with GBS does
not differ from the nonpregnant population and includes maintenance of fluid and
electrolyte balance, nutritional support, thromboprophylaxis, and supportive care.
Plasmapheresis and intravenous immunoglobulin may be necessary in severe cases
of GBS requiring mechanical ventilation.

The mode of delivery and the choice of the anesthetic technique depend on the
patient's clinical condition [47]. Regional analgesic and anesthetic techniques are
not contraindicated in patients with GBS, but marked sensitivity to local anesthetics
can be present with the possibility of profound hypotension and bradycardia [48].

Autonomic dysfunction and hyperreflexia can be precipitated by physical stimulation, and epidural analgesia may be useful to minimize this complication. Directly
acting adrenergic agent should be used instead of indirect ones, due to the unpredictable effect associated with their use. In patients requiring general anesthesia,
succinylcholine can cause hyperkalemia leading to cardiac arrest and should be
avoided. As in other demyelinating disorders, there is an increased sensitivity to
non-depolarizing muscle relaxants, and therefore those agents should be avoided or
used with caution. Patients with respiratory muscle weakness may require a period
of postoperative ventilation in the intensive care setting.

8.2.2.5 Spinal Muscular Atrophy

Spinal muscular atrophy (SMA) is a neurodegenerative disorder of spinal anterior
horn cells which most important symptom is a skeletal muscle weakness. It is genet-
ically inherited with the autosomal recessive pattern and represents second most
common autosomal recessive disorder after cystic fibrosis. It is caused by a mutation in the survival motor neuron 1 (SMN1) gene located on chromosome 5 which
results in the lack of functional SMN protein.

The incidence of SMA is estimated to be 1 in 10,000 with a carrier frequency of 1 in 50–80. The main feature of this life-limiting illness is a progressive muscle weakness, which affects the ability to walk, swallow, and breathe. Four types of SMA have been identified based on the age at which symptoms occur and the severity of the disease, with type 1 being the most severe and with life expectancy limited to few weeks. So far, nusinersen is the only existing therapeutic option, and it became approved for treatment of SMA recently [49].

Spinal muscular atrophy accounts for a leading cause of infant mortality, and women affected by this disorder who become pregnant should receive genetic counselling. In view of high carrier frequency and the severity of the disease, the American College of Medical Genetics has recommended routine carrier screening for SMA in all pregnant patients.

Pregnancy causes exacerbation of the muscle weakness especially in the second trimester. Elsheikh et al. in a recent study investigated 32 patients with SMA and reported that 74% of them experienced increased weakness during pregnancy, which persisted after delivery in 42% of them [50]. In addition to this pulmonary function can worsen due to reduction in lung capacities. Overall there is a high rate of complicated pregnancies and deliveries in patients affected by SMA. Rudnik-Schöneborn et al. studied 17 deliveries in 12 patients and found that 76% of them presented obstetric problems such as premature and prolonged labor [51]. Weak abdominal muscles and ineffective contractions increase the need of instrumental delivery and cesarean section. In the absence of severely compromised respiratory function, vaginal delivery is possible, but postpartum recovery is prolonged in most of the patients.

Anesthetic management can be problematic whether regional or general anesthesia is chosen. Regional techniques should be considered whenever possible, but scoliosis and corrective surgery may affect the anatomy and make them technically difficult. Altered epidural space can cause unpredictable distribution of local anesthetic and therefore patchy or unilateral block. The dose of local anesthetic needs to be carefully titrated in order to avoid high block and respiratory compromise. In view of that, both CSE and spinal catheter appear to be a better choice than single-shot spinal. If general anesthesia needs to be administered, intubation can result difficult due to bulbar weakness and limited cervical spine mobility. Ventilation can also result difficult if restrictive lung disease is present. Succinylcholine may cause severe hyperkalemia and should be avoided. Patients with SMA are very sensitive to non-depolarizing muscle relaxants. In view of this, intubation without muscle relaxants is a good alternative whenever possible. Short-acting opioids are better suited for analgesia purposes in order to avoid respiratory depression. Finally, due to respiratory muscles weakness, there are increased requirements for postoperative ventilatory support in patients with SMA.

Key Learning Points

- Neurological and neuromuscular diseases affect obstetric patients occasionally but account for significant maternal morbidity and mortality.
- In a vast majority of cases, pregnancy has a negative effect on the course of the disease.
- Thorough antenatal assessment, multidisciplinary involvement, and awareness of conditions that may precipitate complications are vital to achieve good outcomes.
- Regional analgesia and anesthesia are techniques of choice but may be technically difficult due to scoliosis or contraindicated in the presence of raised intracranial pressure or tethered spinal cord.
- Succinylcholine may cause life-threatening hyperkalemia in many neuromuscular disorders and should be avoided. Patients with myasthenia gravis are relatively resistant to succinylcholine.
- Patients with neurological and neuromuscular disorders have increased sensitivity to non-depolarizing muscle relaxants, and these agents should be avoided or used with caution.
- Regional techniques are not contraindicated in patients with multiple sclerosis, but the rate of postpartum relapse is high.
- Hypothermia, electrical scalpel, nerve stimulator, anticholinesterases, and succinylcholine can cause myotonic spasm in patients with myotonic dystrophy and should be avoided.
- Patients with central core disease and King-Denborough syndrome are susceptible to malignant hyperthermia.
- Respiratory and cardiac complications occur frequently in postpartum period. Postoperative ventilatory support may be required in patients with respiratory muscle weakness and restrictive lung disease.

References

1. Knight M, Nair M, Tuffnell D, Kenyon S, Shakespeare J, Brocklehurst P, et al., editors. On behalf of MBRRACE-UK. Saving lives, improving mothers' care—surveillance of maternal deaths in the UK 2012–14 and lessons learned to inform maternity care from the UK and Ireland confidential enquiries into maternal deaths and morbidity 2009–14. Oxford: National Perinatal Epidemiology Unit, University of Oxford; 2016.
2. Confavreux C, Hutchinson M, Hours MM, Cortinovis-Tourniaire P, Moreau T. Rate of pregnancy-related relapse in multiple sclerosis. Pregnancy in Multiple Sclerosis Group. N Engl J Med. 1998;339:285–91.
3. Bamford C, Sibley W, Laguna J. Anesthesia in multiple sclerosis. Can J Neurol Sci. 1978;5:41–4.
4. Bader AM, Hunt CO, Datta S, Naulty JS, Ostheimer GW. Anesthesia for the obstetric patient with multiple sclerosis. J Clin Anesth. 1988;1:21–4.
5. Drake E, Drake M, Bird J, Russell R. Obstetric regional blocks for women with multiple sclerosis: a survey of UK experience. Int J Obstet Anesth. 2006;15:115–23.

6. Pastó P, Portaccio E, Ghezzi A, Hakiki B, Giannini M, Razzolini M, et al. Epidural analgesia and cesarean delivery in multiple sclerosis post-partum relapses: the Italian cohort study. BMC Neurol. 2012;12:165. https://doi.org/10.1186/1471-2377-12-165.

7. Brett RS, Schmidt JH, Gage JS, Schartel SA, Poppers PJ. Measurement of acetylcholine receptor concentration in skeletal muscle from a patient with multiple sclerosis and resistance to atracurium. Anesthesiology. 1987;66:837–9.

8. RCOG. Epilepsy in pregnancy. Green-top Guideline No. 68, June 2016. https://www.rcog.org.uk/en/guidelines-research-services/guidelines/gtg68/.

9. Hvas CL, Henriksen TB, Ostergaard JR, Dam M. Epilepsy and pregnancy: effect of antiepileptic drugs and lifestyle on birthweight. BJOG. 2000;107:896–902.

10. Griffiths S, Durbridge JA. Anaesthetic implications of neurological disease in pregnancy. Continuing education in anaesthesia. Crit Care Pain. 2011;11(5):157–61. https://doi.org/10.1093/bjaceaccp/mkr023.

11. Perlas A, Cheema S, Mohanraj R, Anaesthesia and epilepsy. Br J Anaesth. 2012;108:562–71. https://doi.org/10.1093/bja/aes027.

12. Milhorat TH, Chow MW, Trinidad EM, Kula RW, Mandell M, Wolpert C, et al. Chiari I malformation redefined: clinical and radiographic findings for 364 symptomatic patients. Neurosurgery. 1999;44:1005–17.

13. Mueller DM, Oro' J. Chiari I malformation with or without syringomyelia and pregnancy: case studies and review of the literature. Am J Perinatol. 2005;22:67–70.

14. Orth T, Babbar S, Porter B, Lu G, Gerkovich M. Maternal and pregnancy complications among women with Arnold-Chiari malformation: a national database review. Am J Obstet Gynecol. 2015;212 https://doi.org/10.1016/j.ajog.2014.10.922.

15. Landau R, Giraud R, Delrue V, Kern C. Spinal anesthesia for cesarean delivery in a woman with a surgically corrected type I Arnold Chiari malformation. Anesth Analg. 2003;97:253–5.

16. Kuczkowski KM. Spinal anesthesia for Cesarean delivery in a parturient with Arnold-Chiari type I malformation. Can J Anesth. 2004;51:639.

17. Chantigan RC, Koehn MA, Ramin KD, Warner MA. Chiari I malformation in parturients. J Clin Anesth. 2002;14:201–5.

18. Choi CK, Tyagaraj K. Combined spinal-epidural analgesia for labouring parturient with Arnold-Chiari type I malformation: a case report and a review of the literature. Case Rep Anesthesiol. 2013;2013:512915. https://doi.org/10.1155/2013/512915.

19. Ghaly RF, Candido KD, Sauer R, Knezevic NN. Anesthetic management during cesarean section in woman with residual Arnold-Chiari malformation type I, cervical kyphosis and syringomyelia. Surg Neurol Int. 2012;3:26.

20. Penney DJ, Smallman JM. Arnold Chiari malformation and pregnancy. Int J Obstet Anesth. 2001;10:139–41.

21. Gambling D, Douglas M, McKay R. Obstetric anaesthesia and uncommon disorders. 2nd ed. Cambridge: Cambridge University Press; 2008. Section 3: Nervous system disorders. p. 167–89.

22. Center for Disease Control and Prevention. Use of folic acid for prevention of spina bifida and other neural tube defects 1983-1991. MMWR Morb Mortal Wkly Rep. 1991;40:513–6.

23. Arata M, Grover S, Dunne K, Bryan D. Pregnancy outcome and complications in women with spina bifida. J Reprod Med. 2000;45:743–8.

24. McGrady EM, Davis AG. Spina bifida occulta and epidural anaesthesia. Anaesthesia. 1998;43:867–9.

25. Vaagenes P, Fjaerestad I. Epidural block during labour in a patient with spina bifida cystica. Anaesthesia. 1981;36:299–301.

26. Tidmarsh MD, May AE. Epidural anaesthesia and neural tube defects. Int J Obstet Anesth. 1998;7:111–4.

27. Valente A, Frassanito L, Natale L, Draisci G. Occult spinal dysraphism in obstetrics: a case report of caesarean section with subarachnoid anaesthesia after remifentanil intravenous analgesia for labour. Case Rep Obstet Gynecol. 2012;2012:472482. https://doi.org/10.1155/2012/472482.

28. Degler SM, Dowling RD, Sucherman DR, Leighton BL. Awake intubation using an intubating laryngeal mask airway in a parturient with spina bifida. Int J Obstet Anesth. 2005;14:77–8.
29. Petsas A, Drake J. Perioperative management for patients with a chronic spinal cord injury. BJA Educ. 2015;15:123–30.
30. Norwood F, Rudnik-Schöneborn S. 179th ENMC international workshop: pregnancy in women with neuromuscular disorders 5-7 November 2010, Naarden, The Netherlands. Neuromuscul Disord. 2012;22:183–90.
31. Litman RS, Griggs SM, Dowling JJ, Riazi S. Malignant hyperthermia susceptibility and related diseases. Anesthesiology. 2018;128:159–67. https://doi.org/10.1097/ALN0000000000001877.
32. Ishikawa Y, Bach JR, Sarma RJ, Tamura T, Song J, Marra SW, et al. Cardiovascular considerations in the management of neuromuscular disease. Semin Neurol. 1995;15:93–108.
33. Pandey CK, Bose N, Garg G, Singh N, Baronia A, Agarwal A, et al. Gabapentin for the treatment of pain in Guillain-Barre syndrome: a double-blinded, placebo-controlled, crossover study. Anesth Analg. 2002;95:1719–23.
34. Spillane J, Higham E, Kullman DM. Myasthenia gravis. BMJ. 2012;345:e8497. https://doi.org/10.1136/bmj.e8497.
35. Lucchi M, Ricciardi R, Melfi F, Duranti L, Basolo F, Palmiero G, et al. Association of thymoma and myasthenia gravis: oncological and neurological results of the surgical treatment. Eur J Cardiothorac Surg. 2009;35:812–6.
36. Brenner T, Beyth Y, Abramsky O. Inhibitory effect of alpha-fetoprotein on the binding of myasthenia gravis antibody to acetylcholine receptor. Proc Natl Acad Sci U S A. 1980;77:3635–9.
37. Roth TC, Raths J, Carboni G, Rosler K, Schmid RA. Effect of pregnancy and birth on the course of myasthenia gravis before or after transsternal radical thymectomy. Eur J Cardiothorac Surg. 2006;29:231–5.
38. Hoff JM, Daltveit AK, Gilhus NE. Myasthenia gravis: consequences for pregnancy, delivery and the newborn. Neurology. 2003;61:1362–6.
39. Hoff JM, Midelfart A. Maternal myasthenia gravis: a cause for arthrogryposis multiplex congenita. J Child Orthop. 2015;9:433–5. https://doi.org/10.1007/s11832-015-0690-8.
40. Leventhal SR, Orkin FK, Hirsh RA. Prediction of the need for postoperative mechanical ventilation in myasthenia gravis. Anesthesiology. 1980;53:26–30.
41. Eisenkraft JB, Book WJ, Mann SM, Papatestas AE, Hubbard M. Resistance to succinylcholine in myasthenia gravis: a dose-response study. Anesthesiology. 1988;69:760–3.
42. de Boer HD, van Egmond J, Driessen JJ, Booij LH. A new approach to anesthesia management in myasthenia gravis: reversal of neuromuscular blockade by sugammadex. Rev Esp Anestesiol Reanim. 2010;57:181–4.
43. Norwood F, Dhanjal M, Hill M, James N, Jungbluth H, Kyle P, et al. Myasthenia in pregnancy: best practice guidelines from a U.K. multispecialty working group. J Neurol Neurosurg Psychiatry. 2014;85:538–43. https://doi.org/10.1136/jnnp-2013-305572.
44. Theadom A, Rodrigues M, Roxburgh R, Balalla S, Higgins C, Bhattacharjee R, et al. Prevalence of muscular dystrophies: a systematic literature review. Neuroepidemiology. 2014;43:259–68.
45. Johnson NE, Hung M, Nasser E, Hagerman KA, Chen W, Ciafaloni E, et al. The impact of pregnancy on myotonic dystrophy: a registry-based study. J Neuromuscul Dis. 2015;2:447–52.
46. Zaki M, Boyd PA, Impey L, Roberts A, Chamberlain P. Congenital myotonic dystrophy: prenatal ultrasound findings and pregnancy outcome. Ultrasound Obstet Gynecol. 2007;29:284–8.
47. Kocabas S, Karaman S, Firat V, Bademkiran F. Anesthetic management of Guillain-Barré syndrome in pregnancy. J Clin Anesth. 2007;19:299–302.
48. McGrady EM. Management of labour and delivery in a patient with Guillain-Barré syndrome. Anaesthesia. 1987;42:899–900.
49. Chiriboga CA. Nusinersen for the treatment of spinal muscular atrophy. Expert Rev Neurother. 2017;17:955–62.
50. Elsheik h BH, Zhang X, Swoboda KJ, Chelnick S, Reyna SP, Kolb SJ, et al. Pregnancy and delivery in women with spinal muscular atrophy. Int J Neurosci. 2017;127:953–7.
51. Rudnik-Schöneborn S, Zerres K, Ignatius J, Rietschel M. Pregnancy and spinal muscular atrophy. J Neurol. 1992;239:26–30.

Anesthetic Management of Pregnant Patient with Renal Disease

9

Gulay Ok

9.1 Introduction

Changes in hormonal activity, increased metabolic requirements of the growing fetus and placenta, and mechanical obstruction of the growing uterus lead to reversible anatomic and physiological changes during pregnancy in the renal system [1]. A detailed awareness of renal physiology is of crucial importance in the perioperative evaluation of a kidney disease. There are basically two points to be considered:

1. Effect of pregnancy on maternal kidney disease
2. Maternal and fetal effects of kidney disease

Careful monitoring of both of these two key points in the preoperative and perioperative period will ensure proper planning and implementation of the anesthetic approach.

9.1.1 Changes Encountered in the Renal System During Pregnancy

During normal pregnancy, the size of the kidney grows up to 1 cm. Ureters and renal pelvis are initially dilated by progesterone-related atony followed by mechanical pressure exerted due to the growing uterus starting from the 12th week of pregnancy until the term. Prevention of urinary output from the kidneys and the bladder caused by that mechanical pressure effect increases the risk of urinary system infections which might further precipitate preterm birth.

G. Ok
Manisa Celal Bayar University School of Medicine, Department of Anesthesiology and Reanimation, Manisa, Turkey

© Springer International Publishing AG, part of Springer Nature 2018
B. Gunaydin, S. Ismail (eds.), *Obstetric Anesthesia for Co-morbid Conditions*,
https://doi.org/10.1007/978-3-319-93163-0_9

In addition to these changes, there is a 20% decrease in systemic vascular resistance, while blood volume and cardiac output increase 40% and 50%, respectively [2]. Considering the important role of the kidney in maintaining homeostasis of fluid and blood pressure, the resulting cardiovascular changes have significant effects on renal function. During pregnancy, renal blood flow increases by 80%, while glomerular filtration rate (GFR) increases approximately by 50% [3]. Reabsorption of water and electrolytes from the tubes also increases, thus allowing liquid and electrolyte balance to be maintained. Blood urea nitrogen (BUN) and serum creatinine levels in healthy pregnancies are about 50% of a nonpregnant woman where normal reference range for BUN is 8–9 mg/dl and for serum creatinine is 0.4–0.6 mg/dl [3]. Therefore, the creatinine clearance is increased. Glomerular permeability is partially increased in pregnancy, and proteinuria (normal up to 300 mg/day) is encountered [3].

Maternal hyperventilation-related arterial carbon dioxide pressure decrease results in respiratory alkalosis. Subsequently compensatory changes characterized by a decrease in serum bicarbonate and basal negativity can be also encountered. Reduction in glucose reabsorption capacity and glycosuria may be observed secondary to the already-affected tubular functions during pregnancy. It is a physiological condition for the pregnant woman to gain weight up to 12 kg on average due to sodium and water retention. Plasma osmolality is also reduced by 10 mOsm/kg. These changes are related to the altered response of the antidiuretic hormone in the renal tubule. In addition, many vitamins that are not normally excreted in the urine are lost during pregnancy.

Evaluation of these changes during pregnancy is very important in the perioperative evaluation for proper planning of the perioperative anesthetic approach of the pregnant woman.

The values considered normal in a non-pregnant woman when occur in a pregnant woman indicates that her renal function is impaired. In pregnancy, serum creatinine levels of 0.8 mg/dl or BUN level ≥ 16 mg/dl or proteinuria more than 300 mg/day are considered as abnormal [2].

9.2   Anesthetic Approach to Pregnant Women with Kidney Disease

An anesthesiologist may come across with pregnant women with kidney diseases which have different diagnoses. Kidney diseases during pregnancy are listed below:

1. Acute renal failure (ARF)
2. Chronic renal failure (CRF)
3. Cases on dialysis treatment
4. Pregnancy after renal transplantation

The severity of kidney disease, biochemical test results, and accompanying comorbid diseases serve as a guideline in determining the anesthesia technique.

Fluid resuscitation to be performed perioperatively for the pregnant women with acute renal failure differs from the pregnant women with chronic renal failure [4]. For that reason, after overview of physiopathological conditions of the pregnant women, anesthesia choices for the pregnant women with acute or chronic renal failures and/or receiving hemodialysis treatment and pregnant women with kidney transplant will be addressed.

9.2.1   Acute Renal Failure and Pregnancy

Acute renal failure (ARF) is rare during pregnancy. The prognosis is usually better than in non-obstetric cases [4]. Frequently hyperemesis gravidarum-induced hypovolemia and uterine hemorrhage cause prerenal failure. Sudden hypovolemia resulting in acute tubular necrosis results in azotemia [5].

One of the causes of acute renal failure in pregnancy is *renal cortical necrosis*. Septic abortion, amniotic fluid embolism, acute tubular necrosis, drug-induced acute interstitial nephritis, acute glomerulonephritis, acute pyelonephritis, HELLP (hemolysis, elevated liver enzymes, and low platelets) syndrome, acute fatty liver of pregnancy, and idiopathic postpartum renal failure may cause renal cortical necrosis which can occur in both early and late stages of pregnancy [4, 6]. Acute renal failure due to renal cortical necrosis is irreversible because there is bilateral, symmetric, and ischemic necrosis in the cortex of the kidneys. Patients may present a patchy necrosis despite the fact that the cortex involvement is often diffuse in the majority of the cases. Once diffuse cortical necrosis is developed, patients can survive by dialysis or have cure after transplantation. Renal functions still go on by decreasing in function in the patchy cortical necrosis, but these patients also require dialysis after a while. If prepregnancy azotemia is present, both maternal and fetal renal functions are negatively affected [7].

Rapid deterioration of renal function is observed in 35% of those with creatinine levels of ≥ 1.6 mg/dl [8]. Likewise, in those with reflux nephropathy, pregnancy accelerates the progression to end-stage renal failure [8, 9].

Acute renal failure may develop because of postrenal causes such as urolithiasis, pressure exerted by growing uterus to ureter, or tubo-ovarian masses [6].

9.2.1.1 Preeclampsia and Renal Failure

In preeclamptic pregnant women, renal blood flow and GFR are reduced by about 30–40%, as opposed to healthy pregnant women [9–11]. The serum creatinine and BUN levels are similar to those of healthy pregnancies. However, as the severity of preeclampsia increases, renal perfusion deteriorates, creatinine clearance decreases, and proteinuria increases. If the preeclampsia with acute renal failure is treated properly, renal function returns to normal after delivery.

The nephrotic syndrome rarely occurs in pregnancy and is usually caused by preeclampsia [12]. In the first trimester, intrinsic renal disease is present, and perinatal mortality is reported to be greater than 40% [12].

In addition to impaired renal function, risk of disseminated intravascular coagulation is of note in eclamptic pregnancies.

HELLP syndrome develops in 10–20% of parturients with severe preeclampsia and/or eclampsia. These cases are manifested with a clinical proteinuria (86–100%), hypertension (82–88%), right upper quadrant/epigastric pain (40–90%), nausea and/or vomiting (29–84%), headache (33–61%), or visual changes (10–20%) [12, 13].

9.2.1.2 The Approach to Pregnant Patients with Acute Renal Failure

In pregnancies with prerenal failure, to prevent renal damage and ensure renal perfusion, volume resuscitation at early stage should be considered to maintain adequate intravascular volume. Invasive arterial pressure monitoring may be needed to provide optimal intravascular volume for controlling the blood pressure. Diuretics should be used if heart failure is seen as a result of an increase in intravascular volume. If hypovolemia due to blood loss and subsequent acute renal failure develops, appropriate blood and blood product replacement should be performed.

Dialysis is started if serum creatinine level is >3.5 mg/dl or GFR <20 mL/min in pregnancies with renal disease [4]. Better fetal outcomes are observed after long-term and more frequent hemodialysis. The most important point is to avoid hypotension during hemodialysis because of its fetal negative effects resulting from uteroplacental failure. Although the prevalence of spontaneous abortus and preterm delivery during pregnancy is high, fetal survival in ongoing pregnancies is nearly 71% [7]. Intrauterine fetal growth retardation is a problem especially in developing countries [4].

Daily intake of protein, potassium, and phosphate should be limited in pregnancies with ARF. In eclamptic pregnant women for seizure prophylaxis, intravenous loading dose of 4 g of $MgSO_4$ in 10–15 min followed by an infusion of 1 g/h.

Besides the general treatment for pregnant women with acute renal failure, it is also important to terminate the pregnancy at the best available fetal maturity by evaluating severity of preeclampsia and maternal and fetal well-being.

9.2.1.3 Anesthesia Management

Changes in intravascular volume status, electrolyte imbalance, coagulopathy, thrombocytopenia, platelet dysfunction, and altered drug clearance should be considered in determining the anesthesia type. Platelet dysfunction may occur in patients with preeclampsia particularly receiving low-dose aspirin therapy. Although corticosteroid use is controversial, there are some reports that corticosteroids increase platelet count and fetal lung maturation in pregnancies with HELLP syndrome [14, 15]. If there is no coagulopathy, thrombocytopenia, or platelet dysfunction, regional anesthesia could be preferred after obtaining the patient's consent.

In cases where hemodynamics is not stable, invasive pressure monitoring may be necessary. The GFR should be monitored when administering intravenous anesthetics, inhalation agents, opioids, muscle relaxants, and perioperative antibiotics. Drugs with short duration of action and nontoxic to the kidney or having less metabolism (such as desflurane, propofol, atracurium/cisatracurium, remifentanil) should be preferred [12]. Neuromuscular monitoring is recommended. Follow-up in post-operative intensive care unit in pregnancies with acute renal failure reduces morbidity and mortality.

9.2.2 Chronic Renal Failure and Pregnancy

Chronic renal failure (CRF) is seen in 0.03–0.12% of all pregnancies [4]. In pregnancies with CRF, the live birth rate varies depending on the severity of renal failure and the presence of hypertension [16]. Nephrologists do not recommend pregnancy to women with severe renal failure (if serum creatinine ≥2.5 mg/dL); these cases are usually infertile.

It has been found that approximately 20% of the pregnant women who developed early preeclampsia had most probably previously unknown chronic renal disease [4, 17]. The risk of developing preeclampsia in chronic renal failure cases increases according to the degree of impairment in renal function. It is 20% in patients with mild renal impairment, 60–80% in severe renal failure, and approximately 5% in the general population and is often associated with hypertension and proteinuria present before the pregnancy [18]. Gestational course and results are usually good in women who have mild renal failure with a serum creatinine level of <1.4 mg/dl.

Women with diabetic nephropathy and normal serum creatinine levels do not experience deterioration in kidney functions during pregnancy, but the risk of preeclampsia and preterm labor is increased. For that reason, the metabolic status before and during pregnancy should be well monitored, and antihypertensive treatment with low-dose aspirin is required starting from the 12th week of pregnancy [19].

Systemic lupus erythematosus (SLE) is often seen in women of childbearing age and leads to lupus nephritis. Women with SLE are advised to conceive before their renal functions worsen (at least after 6 months of remission phase). Presence of an active disease, impaired renal function, hypertension, and antiphospholipid antibodies has increased maternal and fetal morbidity and mortality [20].

Pregnant women with chronic renal failure cannot maintain the required GFR increase in normal pregnancy in addition to vitamin D3, erythropoietin, and renin production increases. This leads to normochromic normocytic anemia, a decreased plasma volume, and vitamin D deficiency. In preeclampsia due to reduced plasma volume, resulting prerenal failure and this cause more renal damage. Venous thromboembolism risk is increased in the pregnancies with severe proteinuria (3 g/day), and it requires prophylaxis with low molecular weight heparin [12]. Mild kidney dysfunction is observed in the majority of chronic renal failure pregnancies. In these cases, kidney function is not affected negatively from pregnancy. However, a rapid deterioration of renal function may be seen in the presence of proteinuria and hypertension prior to pregnancy. Maternal and fetal morbidity and mortality are increased in pregnancies with severe renal failure. Therefore, these cases should be evaluated before pregnancy, and they should be informed about the possible risks and warned about their medications. Thus, it has been reported that both maternal and fetal risks such as spontaneous abortion, prematurity, and intrauterine growth retardation (IUGR) can be minimized [4, 21]. Anemia, hypertension, and proteinuria presenting with CRF should be treated.

Low-dose aspirin (50–150 mg/day) in the early period of gestation (12th week) reduces the risk of preeclampsia and the subsequent renal damage observed [4]. Angiotensin-converting enzyme inhibitors and angiotensin II receptor blockers should not be used as an antihypertensive due to their teratogenic effects. If the diastolic blood pressure is above 90 mmHg, it causes renovascular injury and low blood pressure values also limiting fetal growth and causes IUGR [11].

Another important finding of chronic renal failure is anemia. Therefore ferritin levels should be assessed; iron and erythropoietin therapy should be initiated to maintain hemoglobin level between 10 and 11 g/dl [4]. Until 30th week of gestation every 2–3 weeks and after weekly, hemoglobin levels should be checked. Antenatal tests showing fetal growth should be initiated at week 28 and should be closely monitored against the risk of IUGR.

9.2.2.1 Anesthesia Management

Pregnant patients with CRF should be carefully evaluated before anesthesia. These patients should be evaluated in terms of the accompanying medical conditions or diseases (such as anemia, hypertension) and the drugs they use. The physiological anemia of the pregnancy becomes even more prominent due to such reasons as erythropoietin deficiency in CRF and shortened erythrocyte life.

A multidisciplinary team approach including nephrologists, anesthesiologists, and obstetricians is a must. Monitoring of changes in plasma volume and electrolyte balance in pregnant patients with CRF is of critical importance in determining the appropriate need for any replacement and to choose the most proper anesthesia modality.

Presence of left ventricular hypertrophy and decreased left ventricular ejection fraction as a consequence of uremic cardiomyopathy will negatively affect hemodynamics in the perioperative period [22]. *Fluctuations* in hemodynamic may threaten both maternal and fetal life because of the sympathetic block caused by regional anesthesia in these pregnancies. Central blocks should be avoided in cases with cardiomyopathy.

Gastric emptying is further reduced in pregnant patients with CRF compared to nonpregnants. Therefore, aspiration prophylaxis using H_2 receptor blocker must routinely be performed [4]. Metoclopramide is best avoided because of the reduced clearance and the prolonged elimination half-life.

Invasive arterial blood pressure monitoring is required for anticipated hemodynamic fluctuations. Central venous pressure should also be monitored in pregnancies with cardiomyopathy.

Due to the hypoalbuminemia, free fractions of drugs are increased leading to reduced dose requirements of drugs that are bound to albumin, e.g., benzodiazepine and thiopental sodium. The pharmacokinetics of propofol does not change [4, 23]. Alfentanil can be a safe option because it has short duration of action and its metabolism does not change. Remifentanil is a better choice because of its rapid metabolism by plasma esterases. Meperidine hydrochloride is avoided because it has an active metabolite (normeperidine) which is neurotoxic that may cause convulsions [4]. Atracurium and cisatracurium are the preferred safe non-depolarizing muscle relaxants because they are metabolized by Hoffman elimination independently from the liver or kidney [1]. Succynilcholine should be avoided in pregnancies with hyperpotassemia. Hypermagnesemia and metabolic acidosis may prolong the duration of action of all non-depolarizing neuromuscular blockers. Neuromuscular monitoring is necessary in these cases [12, 22]. The duration of action of rocuronium is prolonged in these cases. Sugammadex (4 mg kg^{-1}) rapidly and safely reverses profound rocuronium induced neuromuscular blockade [24].

Although inhalation agents lead to reversible renal dysfunction by reducing renal blood flow, GFR, and urinary output, the uptake and distribution of these drugs remain almost unchanged in cases with CRF [4]. Sevoflurane is not preferred in case of using low-flow anesthesia. Desflurane is a good choice in the pregnancies with CRF. Normovolemia should be preserved by replacing with appropriate fluids (0.9% NaCl). Potassium-containing fluids should be avoided [11].

Of note, thrombocytopenia, platelet function, and coagulation abnormalities are taken into account when selecting anesthesia method.

Hydration before neuraxial blockade should be done in order not to decrease the renal perfusion pressure. During neurological blockade, sensory block starts more quickly and reaches higher levels. Excessive hemodynamic fluctuations associated with autonomic neuropathy or neuraxial blockade are not rare [4]. Epidural anesthesia should be preferred to spinal anesthesia. Invasive hemodynamic monitoring is recommended to avoid hypotension and to maintain renal perfusion with available vasopressors (phenylephrine or ephedrine).

9.2.3 Dialysis and Pregnancy

Successful pregnancies can be observed in patients undergoing peritoneal dialysis. After peritoneal dialysis, uremia is reduced, and rapid fluid balance changes are prevented. As pregnancy progresses, the growing uterus may reduce peritoneal blood flow and prevent adequate fluid to make effective peritoneal dialysis.

Pregnancy is not uncommon in women under hemodialysis. The live infant rate in hemodialysis-dependent pregnancies is around 60% [25]. Investigations have reported a positive correlation between more frequent and intense hemodialysis and better neonatal outcome [4, 26].

It is necessary to immediately initiate continuous renal replacement therapy (CRRT) in the presence of refractory hyperkalemia/metabolic acidosis and encephalopathy or severe uremia that could result in pericarditis [18]. Since it does not lead to hemodynamic fluctuations, it is applied safely both in terms of maternal and fetal well-being.

Hypokalemia/hypophosphatemia should be avoided in pregnant women dependent to hemodialysis. As in other pregnancies, hypotension may cause fetal distress by reducing uteroplacental perfusion. Therefore, hypotension should be avoided at all times, and fetal monitoring should be performed during hemodialysis [4]. The time elapsed since last dialysis is crucial because severe hypotension may occur during anesthesia induction or in the perioperative period in the cases of patients who underwent hemodialysis. In addition, heparin use during hemodialysis may trigger clotting disorders. Hemoglobin, biochemistry, and coagulation tests should be repeated after hemodialysis in these cases.

If coagulation parameters are observed to be normal and platelet dysfunction is absent, peripheral nerve blocks can be safely used.

9.2.4 Pregnancy After Renal Transplantation

In reproductive age renal transplant patients, pregnancy rate is 2% [4, 27]. Pregnancies following renal transplantation, the risk of preterm delivery, premature rupture of membranes, spontaneous abortion, low birth weight, and IUGR are high.

Preoperative anesthetic evaluation is important in these cases. Due to the immunosuppressive drugs (prednisolone, azathioprine, cyclosporine) affecting the kidney and liver function, biochemical parameters should be evaluated carefully [18]. Asepsis is extreme in these immunosuppressed patients.

Additional corticosteroids should be administered to these pregnant women who are currently receiving corticosteroid therapy in the perioperative period.

As with other pregnancies, perioperative hypovolemia/hypotension should be avoided.

Nonsteroidal anti-inflammatory drugs should not be used for postoperative analgesia; instead, non-nephrotoxic simple analgesics such as paracetamol can be administered [12].

> **Key Learning Points**
> - Pregnancy leads to anatomical and physiological changes in the renal system most of which are reversible.
> - During pregnancy, renal blood flow and GFR increase by approximately 50%. Serum creatinine and BUN levels are nearly 50% of a nonpregnant woman.
> - If the serum creatinine level in the pregnancy is 0.8 mg/dl or BUN level is ≥16 mg/dl, or proteinuria is more than 300 mg/day, it is considered as abnormal.
> - The management of anesthesia for the pregnancies with ARF is different from the pregnancies with CRF.
> - Anesthetics drugs with short duration of action and metabolized independently from the kidney (atracurium/cisatracurium, remifentanil, etc.) should be preferred.
> - Aspiration prophylaxis using H2 receptor blocker should be performed in patients with CRF.
> - Neuraxial anesthesia is preferred if there is no coagulopathy, thrombocytopenia, and platelet dysfunction.
> - Central blocks should be avoided in patients with uremic cardiomyopathy.

References

1. Bajwa SJ, Kwatra IS, Bajwa SK, Kaur M. Renal diseases during pregnancy: critical and current perspectives. J Obstet Anesth Crit Care. 2013;3(1):7–15.
2. Baylis C. Impact of pregnancy on underlying renal disease. Adv Ren Replace Ther. 2003;10:31–9.
3. Cheung KL, Lafayette RA. Renal physiology of pregnancy. Adv Chronic Kidney Dis. 2013;20(3):209–14.
4. Baidya DK, Maitra S, Chhabra A, Mishra R. Pregnancy with renal disease-pathophysiology and anaesthetic management. Trends Anaesth Crit Care. 2012;2(6):281–6.
5. Basile DP, Anderson MD, Sutton TA. Pathophysiology of acute kidney injury. Compr Physiol. 2012;2(2):1303–53.
6. Reid RW. Renal disease. In: Chestnut David M, editor. Obstetric anaesthesia principles and practice. 2nd ed. Amsterdam: Elsevier; 2004. p. 904–13.
7. Sahay M. Acute kidney injury in pregnancy. In: Basic nephrology and acute kidney injury; 2012. p. 151–72.
8. Fischer MJ, Lehnerz SD, Hebert JR, et al. Kidney disease is an independent risk factor for adverse fetal and maternal outcomes in pregnancy. Am J Kidney Dis. 2004;43:415–23.
9. Karumanchi SA, Maynard SE, Stillman IE, et al. Preeclampsia: a renal perspective. Kidney Int. 2005;67:2101–13.
10. Moran P, Baylis PH, Lindheimer MD, et al. Glomerular ultrafiltration in normal and pre-eclamptic pregnancy. J Am Soc Nephrol. 2003;14:648–52.
11. Mirza FG, Cleary KL. Pre-eclampsia and the kidney. Semin Perinatol. 2009;33(3):173–8.
12. Hofmeyr R, Matjila M, Dyer R. Preeclampsia in 2017: obstetric and anaesthesia management. Best Pract Res Clin Anaesthesiol. 2017;31(1):125–38.
13. Haddad B, Barton JR, Livingston JC, Chahine R, Sibai BM. Risk factors for adverse maternal outcomes among women with HELLP (hemolysis, elevated liver enzymes, and low platelet count) syndrome. Am J Obstet Gynecol. 2000;183(2):444–8.
14. O'Brien JM, Shumate SA, Satchwell SL, et al. Maternal benefit of corticosteroid therapy in patients with HELLP (hemolysis, elevated liver enzymes, and low platelet count) syndrome: impact on the rate of regional anesthesia. Am J Obstet Gynecol. 2002;186(3):475–9.
15. Woudstra DM, Chandra S, Hofmeyr GJ, et al. Corticosteroids for HELLP (hemolysis, elevated liver enzymes, low platelets) syndrome in pregnancy. Cochrane Database Syst Rev. 2010;9:CD008148.
16. Ramin SM, Vidaeff AC, Yeomans ER, Gilstrap LC. Chronic renal disease in pregnancy. Obstet Gynecol. 2006;108:1531–9.
17. Davison J, Baylis C. Renal disease. In: De Swiet M, editor. Medical disorders in obstetric practice. 3rd ed. Oxford: Blackwell; 1995. p. 226–305.
18. Hall M, Brunskill NJ. Renal disease in pregnancy. Obstet Gynaecol Reprod Med. 2010;20(5):131–7.
19. Mathiesen ER, Ringholm L, Feldt-Rasmussen B, Clausen P, Damm P. Obstetric nephrology: pregnancy in women with diabetic nephropathy e role of antihypertensive treatment. Clin J Am Soc Nephrol. 2012;7:2081–8.
20. Smyth A, Garovic VD. Systemic lupus erythematosus and pregnancy. Minerva Urol Nefrol. 2009;61:457–74.
21. Bramham K, Lightstone L. Pre-pregnancy counselling for women with chronic kidney disease. J Nephrol. 2012;25:450–9.
22. Palevsky PM. Perioperative management of patients with chronic kidney disease or ESRD. Best Pract Res Clin Anaesthesiol. 2004;18:129–44.
23. Baxi V, Jain A, Dasgupta D. Anaesthesia for renal transplantation: an update. Indian J Anaesth. 2009;53:139–47.
24. de Souza CM, Tardelli MA, Tedesco H, Garcia NN, Caparros MP, Alvarez-Gomez JA, et al. Efficacy and safety of sugammadex in the reversal of deep neuromuscular blockade induced by rocuronium in patients with end-stage renal disease: a comparative prospective clinical trial. Eur J Anaesthesiol. 2015;32(10):681–6.

25. Chao AS, Huang JY, Lien R, Kung FT, Chen PJ, Hsieh PC. Pregnancy in women who undergo long term haemodialysis. Am J Obstet Gynecol. 2002;187:152–6.
26. Luciani G, Bossola M, Tazza L, Panocchia N, Liberatori M, De Carolis S, et al. Pregnancy during chronic hemodialysis: a single unit experience with five cases. Ren Fail. 2002;24:853–62.
27. Lindheimer MD, Grunfeld JP, Davison JM. Renal disorders. In: Barron WM, Lindheimer MD, editors. Medical disorders during pregnancy. 3rd ed. St. Louis: Mosby; 2000. p. 39–70.

Anesthesia for Pregnant Patient with Psychiatric Disorders

10

Oya Yalcin Cok

10.1 Introduction

Psychiatric diseases during pregnancy are considered to be one of the main causes of maternal morbidity and mortality in parturients with non-obstetric systemic diseases [1, 2]. The increasing number of women with perinatal mental illness has been requiring obstetric anesthesia care. However, regarding anesthetic management in this particular population, the evidence-based knowledge filtered from randomized and controlled trials are very scarce. The main point of view is to gather the knowledge and the experience in the management of pregnant patients with mental illnesses and use this information at the operating theater where both groups intersect. The purpose of this chapter is to summarize perinatal psychiatric illnesses and their implications on obstetric anesthesia.

10.2 Common Perinatal Mental Disorders

Perinatal mental illness is a complication of pregnancy and postpartum period. These disorders refer to conditions that are prevalent during pregnancy and/or 1 year after delivery, as well as the disorders which were present before pregnancy [3]. These conditions include mood, anxiety, psychotic, substance use, eating, and personality disorders. The most prevalent ones are mood and anxiety conditions [4].

O. Yalcin Cok
Baskent University, School of Medicine, Department of Anesthesiology
and Reanimation, Adana, Turkey

© Springer International Publishing AG, part of Springer Nature 2018
B. Gunaydin, S. Ismail (eds.), *Obstetric Anesthesia for Co-morbid Conditions*,
https://doi.org/10.1007/978-3-319-93163-0_10

10.2.1 Perinatal Depression

Perinatal depression is described as a consistent low mood along with biological and cognitive symptoms for two consecutive weeks either during pregnancy or within the first year of delivery [4]. Its prevalence rate varies between 5 and 33% at a considerably high rate, especially in low-income settings.

This condition should be differentiated from *postpartum (or baby) blues* which is a normal variation in emotions in a negative aspect such as irritability, anxiety, and mood lability on the fourth or fifth day postpartum. Postpartum blues is expected to peak between day 3 and day 5 and to resolve in ten days without medical intervention.

10.2.2 Anxiety Disorders

Perinatal anxiety disorders include, but not limited to, generalized anxiety disorder, posttraumatic stress disorder, panic disorder, obsessive-compulsive disorder, and phobias such as tokophobia (phobia of childbirth) and needle phobia. The prevalence rates vary between 4 and 15% [4]. These conditions can be diagnosed by self-report measures [5].

10.2.3 Bipolar Affective Disorder and Psychotic Disorders

The bipolar affective disorder is characterized by repeated and/or consecutive periods of depression, mania, or mixed states. Childbirth is often related to the initial onset of bipolar affective disorder [6]. The risk of perinatal relapse is as high as 50% in patients with this condition. Psychotic disorders present with mood fluctuations, emotional blunting, insomnia, confusion, cognitive impairment, bizarre behavior, and hallucinations. These patients may even believe that they can save their children by killing them as a consequence of psychotic episode.

Obsessive-compulsive disorder is also very challenging for differentiating it from postpartum psychosis. Obsessions include intrusive thoughts and images which are bizarre but not hallucinating. Pregnant patients with major depression may also have obsessional thoughts of harm to their babies [7].

The main concern about psychotic disorders during pregnancy is the discontinuation of medical treatment [4]. It has been suggested that pregnancy may have a retarding effect on bipolar disorder symptoms during the drug-free period [8]. However, a gap in the treatment may trigger a relapse and may cause anesthetists to meet mentally challenging parturients during clinical practice.

10.2.4 Substance Abuse

Nicotine (tobacco), alcohol, caffeine, opioids, marijuana, cocaine, amphetamines, hallucinogens, and toluene-based solvents are the most commonly abused substances during perinatal period [9]. Polysubstance abuse is also very common.

Mainly, the obstetricians have an ethical obligation to screen and assess the patients with substance abuse disorders and to consult them with specialized physicians. However, obstetric anesthetists who may be the first ones to suspect illicit substance use should also be aware of the related responsibility and actions at the setting or the country they work. Lack of prenatal care and history of premature labor should be warning signs for suspected substance abuse in parturients. Other than their effects on fetal and neonatal health, the abused substances also pose unexpected alterations in maternal physiology and metabolism that intervene in anesthesia management. Especially an opioid-using pregnant patient requires more attentive care during the perioperative period [10]. The patients with substance abuse benefit more from regional anesthesia techniques to avoid systemic drug interactions [11].

10.3   Anesthetic Implications

10.3.1 Preoperative Evaluation

Preoperative evaluation of the patients with known or suspected psychiatric disease should include an understanding of type and severity of the mental disorder. The treatments including behavioral and drug therapies should be questioned in detail but in a nonjudgmental manner, to ease the management of the patient in the perioperative period. The knowledge of the drug regimen is essential to understand the effects of the psychotropic medications and avoid anesthetic interactions. However, confidentiality is the mainstay of management in every stage of care.

Simple screening measures such as questionnaires or scales may be used to foresee possible related consequences during the perioperative period if any condition such as perinatal depression is suspected during preoperative period. However, patients with undiagnosed conditions with serious implications should be consulted with dedicated psychology service since psychiatric emergencies such as self-harming or suicidal intentions justify hospitalization [3]. Parturients using illicit drugs or substances should be further questioned about acute use or state of intoxication to optimize pain management for labor and delivery and anesthetic care.

The patients with known psychiatric diseases who are willing to conceive often quit using mood stabilizers, since these drugs, especially antidepressants, are linked to maternal and fetal negative outcomes such as spontaneous abortion, stillbirth, hypoglycemia, jaundice, gestational diabetes, convulsions, low birth weight, and cardiac septal defect. These patients who quitted medical therapies frequently present to anesthesia clinic or operating theater with relapsed psychiatric conditions such as depression, hypomania, mania, and psychotic episodes [12].

Another issue that should be addressed during pre-anesthetic assessment is the patient's ability to consent to anesthetic interventions [1]. On an individual basis, a patient with the psychiatric disease may not lack the capacity to decide or to refuse an anesthetic intervention or to consent [13]. If the current condition of the parturient is not suitable for giving consent, a legal guardian should be present to complete obligatory documents. Cooperation issues which are especially important during regional techniques should also be assessed during preoperative visit.

10.3.2 Intraoperative Management

Intravenous access may pose difficulty in patients with cooperation issues or history of substance abuse. The possibility of drug abuse should be seriously considered when any unexpected reactions occur during any otherwise uneventful anesthesia course since the prevalence of substance abuse is higher than clinically assumed [11].

10.3.2.1 General Versus Regional Anesthesia

General anesthesia is the appropriate option if the patient's psychiatric disorder involves neuromuscular system. Involuntary movements and tics may hinder the performance of regional techniques and, even, surgery [14]. Also, the patients who are at the extremes of the psychiatric conditions, such as delirium, catatonia, unconsciousness, and severe agitation, are natural candidates for general anesthesia [15]. Patients with severe needle phobia mostly demand general anesthesia, and the appropriate practice is to place an intravenous line following inhalational induction via mask ventilation; however, this brings its own risks in this special situation [16, 17].

The patients with stable mental status should be encouraged to have regional anesthesia due to well-known benefits of techniques during obstetric anesthesia. Many pregnant patients with psychological diseases such as borderline personality disorder may undergo procedures with spinal, epidural, or combined spinal-epidural anesthesia uneventfully under the supervision of an experienced obstetric anesthetist [18]. The patients with a history of chronic substance abuse benefit more from regional anesthesia techniques to avoid systemic drug interactions [11]. Benzodiazepine or other sedatives such as zolpidem use should be administered attentively due to the unexpectedly deep level of sedation and respiratory depression in patients on opioid-agonist treatment.

If general anesthesia is to be employed in parturients with drug dependency, associated hepatic and cardiac disorders, hypovolemia, and hypoalbuminemia should be assessed. If chronic alcohol abuse is considered, the increased requirement for barbiturates and volatile anesthetics is arguable, and increased use may lead to significant cardiovascular depression. However, anesthetic requirements are decreased in patients who are acutely intoxicated with alcohol, but the risk of aspiration is increased [9].

Any anesthetic drug hasn't been promoted for any particular psychiatric disorder in the medical literature. Ketamine with its promising features for depression has unfortunately been found to be ineffective for postpartum depression [19].

10.3.2.2 Drug Interactions

The drugs used for the treatment of psychological diseases are mainly very active ingredients on the central and autonomic nervous systems which are also target systems for general anesthetics. Although many of these drugs are abruptly abandoned by the patients when they are aware of their pregnancy or adjusted under the supervision of a physician, patients may continue to use them unintentionally or in emergency conditions [20]. Coexistence of psychiatric and anesthetic drugs in the body may end up with significant interactions and exaggerated effects. For example, monoamine oxidase inhibitors used for depression may interact with opioids and sympathomimetic drugs leading to excitatory or depressive effects and exaggerated hypertension, respectively.

Tricyclic antidepressant drugs cause exaggerated hypertension when administered together with sympathomimetic drugs. Volatile anesthetic use along with tricyclic antidepressant drugs trigger arrhythmias. Serotonin and norepinephrine reuptake inhibitors (SNRIs) and selective serotonin reuptake inhibitors (SSRIs) are the drugs used for depression and many other indications such as anxiety disorders, obsessive compulsive disorders, and neuralgias. SSRIs provoke hepatic enzyme induction and rarely increase bleeding time. The main consideration with SSRI and SNRIs is the serotonin syndrome triggered with concurrent use of opioids, especially pethidine.

Serotonin syndrome is a potentially life threatening syndrome that is precipitated by the use of serotonergic drugs and over-activation of both the peripheral and central postsynaptic 5HT-1A and 5HT-2A receptors [21]. Actually, it is due to accumulation of high levels of serotonin. The symptoms can range from mild to severe ones such as sweating, shivering, headache, diarrhea, agitation or restlessness, muscle twitching or rigidity, rapid heart rate, high blood pressure, arrhythmias, dilated pupils, confusion, seizures, and unconsciousness. When these symptoms are observed in a patient, anticholinergic syndrome, malignant hyperthermia, neuroleptic malignant syndrome, and severe alcohol withdrawal should also be considered for differential diagnosis for the well-being of the parturient and the fetus.

Antipsychotic drugs, mainly used for perinatal psychosis and schizophrenia, also interact with opioids. The anticipated consequences during concurrent use of antipsychotic drugs and opioids are exaggerated respiratory depression, deep level of sedation, and prolonged analgesic effects. Many of antipsychotic medications have alpha-adrenergic antagonist properties that may cause cardiovascular implications. Risperidone has been associated with exaggerated hypotension during a spinal anesthetic for cesarean delivery [22]. Lithium used for bipolar disorder causes neuromuscular blocking drugs and anesthetic agents to have prolonged and more potent effects [23].

10.3.3 Postoperative Care

Any consequence of surgery or anesthesia such as anxiety, pain, confusion, or drugs may deteriorate the patient's mental status or stability [1].

Postoperative pain management should be planned carefully in opioid-dependent patients, especially when they are recovering from addiction [24]. A multidisciplinary approach involving obstetricians, anesthetists, and staff of the Drug and Alcohol Service has been advised [11]. The patients who use opioids may be hypersensitive to pain and have tolerance to opioids, and they may experience opioid withdrawal symptoms if non-opioids or mixed opioid antagonist-agonist drugs are used for acute postoperative pain management [24]. A multimodal pain management plan including acetaminophen, nonsteroid analgesics, neuraxial opioids such as morphine, and abdominal wall blocks such as transversus abdominis plane block should be employed. Patient-controlled analgesia should be arranged in an on-demand manner without continuous infusion, especially for patients who had neuraxial opioids. Some patients may be maintained on opioid-agonist pharmaco-therapy with methadone or buprenorphine throughout perinatal period. These drugs present in low levels in breast milk, but this level is reported to be compatible with breastfeeding [25]. A withdrawal syndrome to any abused substance may be observed in 6–48 h postoperatively since the substance significantly decreased or abruptly discontinued. Acute withdrawal symptoms such as tremor, hypertension, tachycardia, arrhythmias, nausea, vomiting, confusion, and agitation should imme-diately be recognized and differentiated from possible anesthetic complications [9]. Delirium tremens is a more complicated condition and a medical emergency which should be managed immediately especially in alcohol addicted patients.

Parturients with perinatal mental illness continue to have a risk of maternal self-harm and suicide in the postoperative period, and close monitoring should be employed until the mental status of the patient is stabilized.

10.3.4 Anesthetic Complications and Adverse Drug Effects that Mimic Psychiatric Disorders During Pregnancy

An acute psychotic episode is a rare, but possible, complication of combined spinal-epidural anesthesia for labor analgesia. A fluctuating behavioral dysfunction, emo-tional lability, disinhibition, and impulsivity may be observed due to intracranial hypotension secondary to dural puncture and CSF leakage [26]. Chronic subdural hematoma following epidural anesthesia may mimic puerperal psychosis [27].

A possible adverse drug effect to indomethacin has been reported to mimic psy-chiatric disorders with the symptoms of anxiety, fear, agitation, affective lability, depersonalization, paranoia, and hallucinations occurring in postpartum patients who had no past psychiatric history [28].

10.4   Interventions

10.4.1 Labor Analgesia

Labor analgesia with epidural intervention has been associated with low risk of postpartum depression when compared with non-epidural labor analgesic methods. Furthermore, absence of labor epidural analgesia is associated with the develop-ment of postpartum depression [29].

It is difficult to predict the interaction of the drugs abused and routine medications used to provide labor analgesia in patients with substance abuse disorder. Patients who are *opioid-dependent* as well as tobacco-abusing parturients may benefit well from epidural or combined spinal/epidural analgesia [9, 30]. What is recommended for these neuraxial techniques in this particular group of patients is to initiate them early in labor to grab control over pain as early as possible. Adequate hydration and vasopressors such as phenylephrine should be used for hemodynamic stability, and small doses of benzodiazepines should be spared for ceasing agitation [24].

10.4.2 Cesarean Section

Patients with severe mental illness require induction of labor, assisted vaginal birth, or emergency cesarean delivery more than their mentally healthy peers [31]. Furthermore, pregnant women with active eating disorders appear to be at greater risk for delivery by cesarean section; these patients may also have electrolyte imbalance which may affect anesthetic management [32].

Psychiatric disorders require general anesthesia for cesarean delivery when the patient is in a state of uncontrolled agitation or in need of a subsequent, emergent electroconvulsive therapy [15]. However, the patients with acute psychosis have also been reported to receive spinal anesthesia for cesarean delivery while they were on haloperidol therapy [33, 34]. Neuraxial anesthesia is preferred for cesarean delivery in patients who are *opioid-dependent*. However, the patient should be cooperative and alert during utilizing these techniques. The patients who are in the toxic state, not breathing adequately, or not able to protect airway stability aren't good candidates for regional techniques. General anesthesia should be reserved for these latter patients or in emergency situations [24].

10.4.3 Electroconvulsive Therapy

Electroconvulsive therapy (ECT) is a management modality used for the patients with bipolar disorder, atypical psychosis, and depression when drug therapies are insufficient or unsuitable. ECT is reported to be an effective method for pregnant patients, and it has low fetal and maternal risks and side effects [12]. The suggested anesthesia method during ECT is either sedation or general anesthesia. Propofol (1 mg kg^{-1}, intravenously) and succinylcholine (1 mg kg^{-1}, intravenously) have been reported to be used uneventfully [35]. Propofol provides faster postictal recovery, and succinylcholine isn't significantly transferred across the placenta to have an effect on the fetus [34]. When the patient has a difficult airway, the use of airway equipment such as ProSeal laryngeal mask airway has been suggested for securing airway initially and for controlled ventilation [35]. The recommended staff includes an anesthesiologist capable of anesthesia care at a remote setting and advanced life support, an obstetrician who can monitor the well-being of the fetus, and the parturient and the psychiatrist who can cope with deleterious and catastrophic events such as status epilepticus [36]. The general cautions such as adequate monitoring both for the mother and the fetus, non-particulate antacid administration prior to anesthesia, elevating the right hip of the patient, and avoiding excessive hyperventilation should be considered [37–39].

10.5 Summary

Pregnant patients with psychiatric disorders present as challenging cases for obstetric anesthetists. An obstetric anesthetist should be aware of legal, ethical, and medical aspects of the conditions and solve each problem on an individualized basis.

Preoperative assessment and the preparation should be adjusted according to the type of patient's disorder. Choice of anesthetic technique should actively be dependent on the mental status of the patient, and postoperative care should be attentively managed regarding pain relief and continuation of medical therapy for the psychiatric disease.

Key Learning Points
- Perinatal mental illness is a complication of pregnancy and postpartum period.
- The confidentiality is the mainstay of management in every stage of care. If the current condition of the parturient is not suitable for giving consent, a legal guardian should be present to complete obligatory documents.
- The drugs used for the treatment of psychological diseases are mainly very active ingredients on the central and autonomic nervous systems which are also target systems for general anesthetics.
- General anesthesia is the appropriate option if the patient's psychiatric disorder involves neuromuscular system and the patient is at delirium, catatonia, unconsciousness, or severe agitation.
- The patients with stable mental status should be encouraged to have regional anesthesia due to well-known benefits of techniques during obstetric anesthesia.
- The possibility of drug abuse should be seriously considered when any unexpected reactions occur during any otherwise uneventful anesthesia course.

References

1. Reide PJW, Yentis SM. Anaesthesia for the obstetric patient with (non-obstetric) systemic disease. Best Pract Res Clin Obstet Gynaecol. 2010;24:313–26. http://linkinghub.elsevier.com/retrieve/pii/S1521693409001515.
2. Oates M. Suicide: the leading cause of maternal death. Br J Psychiatry. 2003;183:279–81.
3. O'Hara MW, Wisner KL. Perinatal mental illness: definition, description and aetiology. Best Pract Res Clin Obstet Gynaecol. 2014;28:3–12.
4. Paschetta E, Berrisford G, Coccia F, Whitmore J, Wood AG, Pretlove S, et al. Perinatal psychiatric disorders: an overview. Am J Obstet Gynecol. 2014;210:501–U258.
5. Stuart S, Couser G, Schilder K, O'Hara MW, Gorman L. Postpartum anxiety and depression: onset and comorbidity in a community sample. J Nerv Ment Dis. 1998;186:420–4.
6. Munk-Olsen T, Laursen TM, Meltzer-Brody S, Mortensen PB, Jones I. Psychiatric disorders with postpartum onset: possible early manifestations of bipolar affective disorders. Arch Gen Psychiatry. 2012;69:428–34. http://archpsyc.jamanetwork.com/article.aspx?doi=10.1001/archgenpsychiatry.2011.157.
7. Hudak R, Wisner KL. Diagnosis and treatment of postpartum obsessions and compulsions that involve infant harm. Am J Psychiatry. 2012;169:360–3. http://psychiatryonline.org/doi/abs/10.1176/appi.ajp.2011.11050667.

8. Grof P, Robbins W, Alda M, Berghoefer A, Vojtechovsky M, Nilsson A, et al. Protective effect of pregnancy in women with lithium-responsive bipolar disorder. J Affect Disord. 2000;61:31–9. http://www.ncbi.nlm.nih.gov/pubmed/11099738.
9. Kuczkowski KM. Labor analgesia for the tobacco and ethanol abusing pregnant patient: a routine management? Arch Gynecol Obstet. 2005;271:6–10.
10. Ashley OS, Marsden ME, Brady TM. Effectiveness of substance abuse treatment programming for women: a review. Am J Drug Alcohol Abuse. 2003;29:19–53. http://www.ncbi.nlm.nih.gov/pubmed/12731680.
11. Ludlow J, Christmas T, Paech MJ, Orr B. Drug abuse and dependency during pregnancy: anaesthetic issues. Anaesth Intensive Care. 2007;35:881–93.
12. Bulbul F, Copoglu US, Alpak G, Unal A, Demir B, Tastan MF, et al. Electroconvulsive therapy in pregnant patients. Gen Hosp Psychiatry. 2013;35:636–9.
13. McCullough LB, Chervenak FA, Coverdale JH. Managing care of an intrapartum patient with agitation and psychosis: ethical and legal implications. AMA J Ethics. 2016;18:209–14.
14. Sener EB, Kocamanoglu S, Ustun E, Tur A. Anesthetic management for cesarean delivery in a woman with Gilles de la Tourette's syndrome. Int J Obstet Anesth. 2006;15:163–5.
15. Vermersch C, Smadja S, Amselem O, Gay O, Marcellin L, Gaillard R, et al. Cesarean section and sismotherapy in a severe psychotic parturient: a case report. Ann Fr Anesth Reanim. 2013;32:711–4.
16. McAllister N, Elshtewi M, Badr L, Russell IF, Lindow SW. Pregnancy outcomes in women with severe needle phobia. Eur J Obstet Gynecol Reprod Biol. 2012;162:149–52.
17. Hillermann T, Breitenstein C, Soll C. Kasuistik: Patientin mit Nadelphobie zur Sectio caesarea – Nicht ganz wie im Lehrbuch. Anasthesiol Intensivmed Notfallmed Schmerzther. 2015;50:388–91.
18. Nakanishi R, Nishimura S, Kimura M, Miyazaki Y, Hamada T, Mori T. Cesarean section in a morbidly obese parturient with borderline personality disorder under combined spinal and epidural anesthesia. Masui. 2008;57:628–30.
19. Xu Y, Li Y, Huang X, Chen D, She B, Ma D. Single bolus low-dose of ketamine does not prevent postpartum depression: a randomized, double-blind, placebo-controlled, prospective clinical trial. Arch Gynecol Obstet. 2017;295:1167–74.
20. Wakil L, Perea E, Penaskovic K, Stuebe A, Meltzer-Brody S. Exacerbation of psychotic disorder during pregnancy in the context of medication discontinuation. Psychosomatics. 2013;54:290–3.
21. Volpi-Abadie J, Kaye AM, Kaye AD. Serotonin syndrome. Ochsner J. 2013;13:533–40. http://www.pubmedcentral.nih.gov/articlerender.fcgi?artid=3865832&tool=pmcentrez&rendertype=abstract.
22. Williams JH, Hepner DL. Risperidone and exaggerated hypotension during a spinal anesthetic. Anesth Analg. 2004;98:240–1.
23. Blake LD, Lucas DN, Aziz K, Castello-Cortes A, Robinson PN. Lithium toxicity and the parturient: case report and literature review. Int J Obstet Anesth. 2008;17:164–9.
24. Jones HE, Deppen K, Hudak ML, Leffert L, McClelland C, Sahin L, et al. Clinical care for opioid-using pregnant and postpartum women: the role of obstetric providers. Am J Obstet Gynecol. 2014;210:302–10. http://linkinghub.elsevier.com/retrieve/pii/S0002937813010582.
25. Jones HE, Heil SH, Baewert A, Arria AM, Kaltenbach K, Martin PR, et al. Buprenorphine treatment of opioid-dependent pregnant women: a comprehensive review. Addiction. 2012;107:5–27.
26. Loures V, Savoldelli GL, Alberque C, Haller G. Post-dural puncture cerebrospinal fluid leak presenting as an acute psychiatric illness. Br J Anaesth. 2012;108:529–30.
27. Campbell DA, Varma TRK. Chronic subdural haematoma following epidural anaesthesia, presenting as puerperal psychosis. BJOG. 1993;100:782–4.
28. Clunie M, Crone L-A, Klassen L, Yip R. Psychiatric side effects of indomethacin in parturients. Can J Anaesth. 2003;50:586–8.

29. Suhitharan T, Pham TPT, Chen H, Assam PN, Sultana R, Han NLR, et al. Investigating analgesic and psychological factors associated with risk of postpartum depression development: a case-control study. Neuropsychiatr Dis Treat. 2016;12:1333–9.
30. Cassidy B, Cyna AM. Challenges that opioid-dependent women present to the obstetric anaesthetist. Anaesth Intensive Care. 2004;32:494–501.
31. Frayne J, Lewis L, Allen S, Hauck Y, Nguyen T. Severe mental illness and induction of labour: outcomes for women at a specialist antenatal clinic in Western Australia. Aust N Z J Obstet Gynaecol. 2014;54:132–7.
32. Franko DL, Blais MA, Becker AE, Delinsky SS, Greenwood DN, Flores AT, et al. Pregnancy complications and neonatal outcomes in women with eating disorders. Am J Psychiatry. 2001;158:1461–6.
33. Birnbach DJ, Bourlier RA, Choi R, Thys DM. Anaesthetic management of caesarean section in a patient with active recurrent genital herpes and AIDS-related dementia. Br J Anaesth. 1995;75:639–41.
34. Soltanifar S, Russell R. Neuraxial anaesthesia for caesarean section in a patient with narcolepsy and cataplexy. Int J Obstet Anesth. 2010;19:440–3.
35. Ozgul U, Erdogan MA, Sanli M, Erdil F, Begec Z, Durmus M. Anaesthetic management in electroconvulsive therapy during early pregnancy. Turk J Anaesthesiol Reanim. 2014;42:145–7.
36. Bakı ED, Akıcı ÖÇ, Güzel Hİ, Kokulu S, Ela Y, Sıvacı RG. Nossa experiência em anestesia durante terapia eletroconvulsiva em pacientes grávidas. Braz J Anesthesiol. 2016;66:555.
37. Balki M, Castro C, Ananthanarayan C. Status epilepticus after electroconvulsive therapy in a pregnant patient. Int J Obstet Anesth. 2006;15:325–8.
38. Ivascu Brown N, Fogarty Mack P, Mitera DM, Dhar P. Use of the ProSeal™ laryngeal mask airway in a pregnant patient with a difficult airway during electroconvulsive therapy. Br J Anaesth. 2003;91:752–4.
39. Rabheru K. The use of electroconvulsive therapy in special patient populations. Can J Psychiatr. 2001;46:710–9.

Anesthesia for Pregnant Patient with Coagulation Disorders

11

Semra Karaman and Zeynep Cagiran

11.1 Introduction

The mechanism of the coagulation cascade is a complex biochemical chain reaction involving several pathways. Obstetric patients undergo several physiological changes that impact hemostasis to improve reserve for the anticipated blood loss at the time of delivery [1, 2]. Changes in coagulation affect the course of pregnancy and change the mode of delivery and approach to anesthesia type. The goal of this chapter is to discuss the physiological changes on coagulation in pregnancy and the common inherited and non-inherited hemostatic disorders that occur in pregnancy and their implications for neuraxial anesthesia.

11.2 Coagulation Systems in the Parturient

While plasma volume itself increases up to 40%, red blood cell volume level increases by only 25% leading to a decrease in hemoglobin concentration known as the physiological anemia of pregnancy [3]. There is also a decrease in platelet count due to hemodilution and its consumption by the uteroplacental unit. In addition to these hematologic changes, normal pregnancy is associated with several alterations in coagulation factors as listed in Table 11.1 [4–7].

Although it seems like the net results of these changes in pregnancy create a hypercoagulable and hypofibrinolytic state, occasionally, comorbidities and complications of pregnancy itself can cause tendency to bleeding.

S. Karaman (✉) · Z. Cagiran
Ege University, School of Medicine, Izmir, Turkey

© Springer International Publishing AG, part of Springer Nature 2018
B. Gunaydin, S. Ismail (eds.), *Obstetric Anesthesia for Co-morbid Conditions*,
https://doi.org/10.1007/978-3-319-93163-0_11

Table 11.1 Hemostatic changes during normal pregnancy

	Increase (↑)	Decrease (↓)	No significant change (↔)
Fibrinogen	↑ (more than 100%)		
FVII	↑ (up to 1000%)		
FVIII	↑		
FX	↑		
FXII	↑		
VWF	↑		
FII			↔
FV			↔
FIX			Variable
FXI			↔
FXIII		↓	

F factor, *VWF* von Willebrand factor

11.3 Acquired Coagulopathies

11.3.1 Platelet Disorders

Thrombocytopenia is the most common platelet disorder in pregnancy with an incidence of 10% of all pregnancies. Thrombocytopenia is defined as a count of less than 150×10^9/L. The platelet count may decline by approximately 10% during pregnancy [8]. It is generally (99%) related to hypertensive disorders, gestational thrombocytopenia (GT), or idiopathic thrombocytopenic purpura (ITP) [9].

11.3.1.1 Gestational Thrombocytopenia
The GT is the most common cause of thrombocytopenia during pregnancy, which occurs in 5–8% of all pregnant women and comprises 75% of pregnancy-associated thrombocytopenia cases [10]. The platelet counts are in the lower range of normal and can be as low as 100×10^9/L. It usually rises in the third trimester of the pregnancy which can be detected incidentally. Platelet count returns to normal range within 7 days of delivery. It is thought to be due to hemodilution and/or accelerated platelet clearance. Monitoring the platelet count is necessary during pregnancy. If the platelet count falls under 100×10^9/L, the diagnosis must be rechecked. Epidural anesthesia is thought to be safe when platelet count is higher than 80×10^9/L. Delivery should be planned according to the obstetric indications.

11.3.1.2 Idiopathic Thrombocytopenic Purpura
The incidence of pregnant women with ITP is 1–2/1000; ITP comprises 5% of pregnancy-related thrombocytopenia cases, and 15% of pregnant women with ITP have platelet count lower than 50×10^9/L at the time of delivery [8]. It is the most common cause of significant thrombocytopenia in the first trimester. It is an autoimmune disorder, which is associated with the production of antibodies mainly to

platelet glycoproteins and other determinants, resulting in coating platelets with IgG antibodies [11]. Women with previously diagnosed ITP often experience an exacerbation in pregnancy. The clinical signs of altered coagulation are minor bruises, petechiae, epistaxis, gingival bleeding, or rarely fatal intracranial bleeding. The diagnosis of ITP is a process of exclusion; other causes of thrombocytopenia must be considered before making this diagnosis. A complete blood count is generally normal except thrombocytopenia. There are larger, immature platelets in the periphereal smear. The treatment depends on assessment of the risk of significant maternal hemorrhage. Platelet count generally falls in the developing months, and it achieves the lowest values in the third trimester.

Treatment of ITP during pregnancy is not indicated if the patient is asymptomatic and platelet count is higher than 20×10^9/L. But they should be closely followed up. Near term, platelet counts $\geq 50 \times 10^9$/L are required for normal vaginal delivery, and those with $>80 \times 10^9$/L are safe for cesarean delivery under spinal or epidural anesthesia.

Treatment includes supplementation with steroids, high-dose intravenous immunoglobulin (IVIg), and splenectomy. Corticosteroids are the first line of treatment [12]. Corticosteroids increase pregnancy-induced hypertension and gestational diabetes and may cause premature rupture of the fetal membranes. The IVIg is generally used as an alternative due to concerns about the potential adverse maternal effects of corticosteroids and for individuals refractory to steroids [13]. Approximately 15% of individuals with ITP have platelet count less than 50×10^9 at the time of delivery. In case of low platelet count, either before cesarean delivery or acute postpartum hemorrhage, platelet transfusion may be required.

11.3.1.3 Secondary Autoimmune Thrombocytopenia

Antiphospholipid Syndrome
Antiphospholipid syndrome (APS) is associated with autoimmune thrombocytopenia in 20–40% of cases [14]. Thrombocytopenia is generally not severe though; some patients with APS have no evidence of any definable associated disease, while in others, APS occurs in association with SLE or another rheumatic or autoimmune disorder. Asymptomatic individuals who have positive laboratory tests do not require specific treatment [15]. If the pregnant patient has the history of both thrombosis and APS, antenatal and postpartum thrombosis prophylaxis is indicated [16].

Systemic Lupus Erythematosus
Systemic lupus erythematosus (SLE) is an autoimmune disease affecting diverse organs of the body and cause chronic inflammation. Thrombocytopenia is common in SLE, and it is known as one of the hematological criteria of SLE. Severe thrombocytopenia is uncommon; less than 5% of cases have a platelet count$<30 \times 10^9$/L during the course of the disease. Isolated thrombocytopenia associated with SLE in pregnancy is treated like ITP. The type of delivery in SLE is related to obstetrical indications. Postpartum period is the most critical time for thrombosis. Heparin

should be continued until the sixth week postpartum. To avoid neural tube defects, folic acid may be given to patients who use metotrexat before the gestation [17, 18].

HIV-Associated Thrombocytopenia

Chronic thrombocytopenia is common in patients infected with the human immunodeficiency virus (HIV). The incidence is 5–9% in patients who have HIV infection and 21–40% in those with AIDS. Although often asymptomatic, the thrombocytopenia may be associated with a variety of bleeding abnormalities [19]. The clinical presentation and response to therapy are similar to that of ITP.

11.3.1.4 Drug-Induced Thrombocytopenia

Drug-induced thrombocytopenia (DIT) is an increasingly common cause of isolated thrombocytopenia, a fact that should not be surprising considering today's everexpanding pharmacopeia. The reasons of the disease are immune- or nonimmunemediated platelet destruction or suppression of platelet production. Both are uncommon in pregnancy but should be considered and excluded because DIT typically appears suddenly, is often severe, and can cause major bleeding and death [20]. Drugs commonly associated with DIT are rifampin, trimethoprimsulfamethoxazole, cephalosporins, para-aminosalicylic acid, acyclovir, interferon, carbamazepine, phenytoin, valproate, prednisone, procainamide, hydrochlorotiazide, sulfasalazine, quinidine, cimetidine, gold salts, and abciximab.

11.3.1.5 Heparin-Induced Thrombocytopenia

There are two types of heparin-induced thrombocytopenia (HIT). Type 1 HIT is a nonimmune disorder which appears within the first 2 days after exposure to heparin, and the platelet count normalizes with continued heparin therapy [21]. Type 2 HIT is an immune-mediated disorder that typically occurs 4–10 days after exposure to heparin and has life-threatening thrombotic complications. In general, the term HIT refers to type 2 HIT. HIT results from an autoantibody directed against platelet factor 4 (PF4) in complex with heparin. HIT antibodies activate platelets and can cause catastrophic arterial and venous thrombosis with a mortality rate as high as 20%. It occurs in 1–5% of patients receiving unfractionated heparin but is considerably less common in patients treated with LMWH. HIT must be suspected when a patient who is receiving heparin has a decrease in the platelet count, particularly if the fall is over than 50% of the baseline count. Clinical symptoms of HIT are skin lesions at heparin injection sites or acute systemic reactions (e.g., chills, fever, dyspnea, chest pain) after administration of an intravenous bolus of heparin. Unlike other forms of thrombocytopenia, venous thromboembolism is the most common complication. Less often, arterial thrombosis (e.g., myocardial infarction) may occur. So it is sometimes termed as HIT and thrombosis (HITT). If HIT is suspected, heparin products should be immediately discontinued. In case of thrombotic events, alternative anticoagulants such as direct thrombin inhibitor (DTI) must be added. Argatroban is an approved DTI for prophylaxis and treatment of thrombosis in patients with HIT. Fondaparinux which is an indirect factor Xa inhibitor is not approved for use in HIT, but there are some reports of its successful use in pregnant women [22]. Another indirect factor Xa inhibitor, danaparoid, has been used in pregnant women successfully [23].

11.3.1.6 Thrombocytopenia with Microangiopathy

It is generally associated with either preeclampsia and HELLP syndrome or thrombotic thrombocytopenic purpura (TTP) or hemolytic-uremic syndrome (HUS).

Preeclampsia and HELLP Syndrome

Preeclampsia affects 2–8% of all pregnancies and remains a leading cause of maternal and perinatal morbidity and mortality worldwide. Visual disturbances, headache, epigastric pain, thrombocytopenia, and abnormal liver function are the other clinical signs of the disease. These clinical manifestations result from mild to severe microangiopathy of target organs. It is caused by placental and maternal vascular dysfunction and always resolves after delivery. Preeclampsia causes about 20% of cases of thrombocytopenia in pregnancy. Thrombocytopenia is sometimes the only initial sign of this condition, predating all the other laboratory changes [24]. Coagulation tests are usually in normal ranges, but D-dimer and thrombin-antithrombin complexes are elevated. In severe cases prolongation in clotting test times and a fall in plasma fibrinogen can be seen.

HELLP syndrome complicates 10–20% of cases of severe preeclampsia. It is the most common cause of severe liver disease in pregnant individuals. Microangiopathic hemolytic anemia, aspartate aminotransferase more than 70 U/I, and a platelet count of $<10 \times 10^9$/L are the diagnostic criteria of HELLP syndrome. Thrombocytopenia associated with the HELLP syndrome is approximately 12%. Decreased platelet count in the HELLP syndrome is due to their increased consumption. Platelets are activated and adhere to damaged vascular endothelial cells, resulting in increased platelet turnover with shorter life span. Supportive treatment is recommended in these situations; however, platelet transfusion should be considered if there is severe thrombocytopenia, acute hemorrhage, or plan for a cesarean delivery. Transfused platelets have diminished survival in preeclampsia [8]. But maternal platelet counts tend to recover spontaneously within 24–48 h of delivery.

Thrombotic Thrombocytopenic Purpura and Hemolytic Uremic Syndrome

These are characterized by microangiopathic hemolytic anemia, thrombocytopenia, fever, and neurologic and renal abnormalities. Neurological disorder is more common in TTP, whereas renal insufficiency is more frequent in HUS. HUS is seen especially in childhood and adolescence. In the pathogenesis of both diseases, there is a marked decrease in the metalloproteinase enzyme called ADAMTS13 which is responsible for cleaning von Willebrand factor (VWF) multimers, because of either congenital deficiency or acquired autoantibodies. As a consequence platelet aggregation contributing to systemic is promoted by these multimers [25]. Levels of ADAMTS 13 decrease during normal pregnancy period, and it contributes to a predisposition of thrombotic microangiopathy during pregnancy. It may be difficult to distinguish these diseases from the other pregnancy-associated microangiopathies. HUS and TTP are not associated with hypertension like preeclampsia and HELLP syndrome. But the degree of hemolysis is greater in HUS and TTP according to preeclampsia and HELLP syndrome. The time of onset and their response to delivery are also important. TTP is seen usually in the second trimester, HUS in the postpartum period, and preeclampsia and the HELLP syndrome in the third trimester. After delivery preeclampsia and HELLP syndrome generally improve, but clinical symptoms do not change in TTP and HUS. So pregnancy termination is not recommended [26].

Plasmapheresis should be considered urgently for the treatment of TTP and should be continued daily until at least 48 h after complete remission is obtained. The repetition cycles of the plasmapheresis should be continued until delivery. In HUS it may not be very effective; the management of treatment is supportive care, renal dialysis, and red cell transfusion. Platelet transfusion should be avoided as it may precipitate or exacerbate the disease [27].

11.4 Consumptive Coagulopathy

Disseminated intravascular coagulation (DIC) is characterized by systemic activation of blood coagulation, which results in generation and deposition of fibrin, leading to microvascular thrombi in various organs that contribute to multiple organ dysfunction syndrome [28]. This massive activation of coagulation usually results in depletion of coagulation factors and platelets and leads to a bleeding diathesis. DIC is generally secondary to an underlying disorder: abruptio placentae, severe preeclampsia/eclampsia, or HELLP syndrome, amniotic fluid embolism, acute fatty liver of pregnancy, dead fetus syndrome, septic abortions, massive hemorrhage due to placenta previa, uterine rupture, placenta accreta, or postpartum uterine atony [29].

The laboratory findings of DIC are prolongation of PT, aPTT, and thrombin times, thrombocytopenia, elevated fibrin degradation products, and low fibrinogen concentration [30]. Early in the course of the syndrome, sometimes normal levels of PTT and PT can be seen. Fibrinogen levels are low, usually less than 200 mg/dL, but it is a late finding. D-dimer is the most commonly used parameter to assess fibrin-related degradation products and often 2000 ng/mL in cases of coagulopathy. Hemoglobinuria may show the evidence of microangiopathic hemolysis [27].

Removal of the underlying cause, providing supportive care, and replacement of blood products are the goals of the treatment. Delivery of the fetus is often required. In general, platelet concentrate is transfused to patients with a platelet count of less than 50×10^9/L who are actively bleeding. A much lower threshold ($<30 \times 10^9$/L) may be used if there is no active bleeding. In the presence of active hemorrhage and prolonged PT and aPTT, transfusion of FFP (10–20 mL/kg) can be useful. In some conditions such as fluid overload, FFP cannot be used so that prothrombin complex concentrate (PCC) (25–30 U/kg) may be considered. Cryoprecipitate or virally inactivated fibrinogen concentrate are administered in low fibrinogen levels. Two cryoprecipitate pools (ten donor units) or 3–5 g of fibrinogen concentrate is expected to raise plasma fibrinogen level by approximately 1 g/L. Heparin is generally not recommended except in cases of retained dead fetus.

In recent years recombinant factor VIIa (rFVIIa) has been used in massive obstetric hemorrhage. But it is still not licensed for use in postpartum hemorrhage and pregnancy. However, its dose in refractory massive obstetric hemorrhage is ranging from 15 to 120 µg/kg. Patients with less severe coagulopathy (platelet count >100 × 10⁹/L) are more likely to respond to rFVIIa. Also rFVIIa has been associated with thromboembolic complications in some cases [31]. Recombinant activated protein C (raPC) has been successfully used in sepsis-related obstetric consumptive coagulopathy at a dose of 24 µg/kg/h in a 96 h infusion [32].

11.5 Factor VIII Inhibitors

Acquired hemophilia A (AHA), is caused by spontaneous development of autoantibodies directed against coagulation FVIII. The incidence is approximately 1.5 cases/million/year [33]. Laboratory findings are normal bleeding time, PT, and platelet count, prolonged aPTT not corrected by incubating the patient's plasma with equal volumes of normal plasma, and reduced factor VIII levels. FVIII levels must be increased; therefore, DDAVP and/or FVIII concentrate can be used in cases of mild bleeding. But rFVIIa and/or activated prothrombin complex concentrates are more effective in severe acute hemorrhage. For the eradication of inhibitors, methylprednisolone at a dose of 1 mg/kg/day, or an equivalent dose of prednisone, has been used successfully [34].

11.6 Congenital Coagulopathies

Platelet function disorders include Bernard-Soulier syndrome (BSS) and Glanzmann thrombasthenia (GT). Hemophilias A and B together with von Willebrand Disease (VWD), a defect of primary hemostasis, include 95% of all the inherited deficiencies of coagulation factors, whereas rare bleeding disorders (inherited fibrinogen disorders, FII, FV, FV+FVIII, FVII, FX, FXI, and FXIII) represent the remaining 3–5% [35].

11.6.1 Congenital Platelet Disorders

They are uncommon diseases and caused by a reduction in the number of platelets (thrombocytopenia) or by platelet function defects (thrombocytopathies). Congenital thrombocytopathies can be classified according to platelet function into adhesion, activation, secretion, and aggregation defects [36].

11.6.1.1 Platelet Adhesion Disorders: Bernard-Soulier Syndrome

Clinical manifestations are purpura, epistaxis, menorrhagia, and gingival and gastrointestinal bleeding. Thrombocytopenia, large platelets, prolonged bleeding time, and poor platelet aggregation in vitro to ristocetin are the laboratory findings. Treatment is generally supportive and requires no medications. Bleeding episodes may require tranexamic acid, desmopressin (DDAVP), rFVIIa, and platelet transfusion. Antifibrinolytic therapy with tranexamic acid or rFVIIa can be considered in labor and uncomplicated delivery [37].

11.6.1.2 Platelet Aggregation Disorders: Glanzmann's Thrombasthenia (GT)

The laboratory findings include a normal platelet count, PT, and aPTT and prolonged bleeding time [38]. Tranexamic acid and rFVIIa are effective in the treatment. For mild to moderate bleeding episodes, local measures and/or anti-fibrinolytic drugs (tranexamic acid and epsilon aminocaproic acid) may resolve bleeding. These agents, used alone or as adjunctive therapy with rFVIIa, have proven to be useful and safe agents in treatment. Platelet transfusion allows the partial correction of the functional defect in patients with GT and is considered standard therapy for patients when local measures and/or antifibrinolytics fail to control bleeding [39].

11.6.2 Defect of Primary Hemosatsis

11.6.2.1 Von Willebrand Disease

von Willebrand Disease (VWD) is the most common bleeding disorder in the general population (%1). VWF adheres to injured tissues and causes platelet adherence at the injury site. Also it binds and stabilizes the procoagulant protein factor VIII, which degrades rapidly when not attached to VWF. It results from either a deficiency or a functional defect in VWF. Three types of VWD have been described. VWD type1 is the most common one (70–80%) and characterized by decreased but functionally normal levels of VWF. Patients with type 2 VWD have a qualitative defect in VWF with the incidence of 10–20%. VWD type 2 is further divided into four variants (2A, 2B, 2N, 2M) based on characteristics of dysfunctional VWF. Although recent evidence indicates the existence of at least three more subtypes (C, D, E). These categories correspond to distinct molecular mechanisms, with corresponding clinical features and therapeutic recommendations. The least frequent of three forms, type 3 VWD, is characterized by a quantitative defect of VWF with resultant secondary deficiency of factor VIII [27].

In the treatment of VWD DDAVP has been used. It increases plasma levels of VWF and factor VIII transiently [40]. Treatment is more indicated to raise factor VIII level and VWF above 50%. DDAVP should be administered prophylactically to women with low VWF levels and either type 1 disease or a known response to DDAVP approximately 1 h before anticipated delivery. Patients with type 2 and 3 VWD usually require VWF concentrate. Patients who are unresponsive to DDAVP treatment or those with continued bleeding usually require cryopresipitate or VWF concentrate. DDAVP should be avoided in type 2B VWD in order not to exacerbate thrombocytopenia. FVIII level and VWF activity should be greater than 50% for 3 days following vaginal delivery and 5–7 days following cesarean delivery [37]. All patients must be evaluated individually on deciding anesthesia type [41]. There is no consensus among anesthesiologists about the anesthetic and hematologic management of patients with VWD. Several authors have reported the successful use of neuraxial techniques in patients with VWD [42]. In type 1 VWD, when FVIII and VWF activities have spontaneously corrected, epidural anesthesia is likely to be safe [43]. For type 2 or type 3 VWD, alternative techniques can be used. After delivery the epidural catheter should be removed as soon as possible because factor concentrations decrease rapidly after delivery, and normal factor concentrations should be obtained before removal [44].

11.6.2.2 Hemophilias

Hemophilias A and B are associated with reduced or absent coagulation FVIII and FIX, respectively. Severity of the clinical symptoms is directly related to plasma concentrations of FVIII/FIX. Values lower than 1% of normal have associated with severe hemophilia and the most frequent bleedings. The levels of Factor VIII tend to rise during normal pregnancy. So carriers of hemophilia A usually do not require prophylaxis or treatment at the time of delivery. Levels less than 40–50 IU/dL at the time of delivery or other invasive procedure or the setting of acute bleeding should prompt treatment of hemophilia A carriers. DDAVP can be used for these women [44].

Epidural anesthesia may be used in hemophilias if coagulation defects have been corrected and the relevant factor level is above 50% or has been raised to more than 50% [44].

Postpartum period is risky for the carriers of hemophilia because FVIII levels may decrease rapidly after delivery. On the other hand, FIX levels do not increase during pregnancy so patients with Hemophilia B carriers are more likely to experience postpartum hemorrhage. Hemophilia B carriers do not respond to DDAVP and should receive prophylactic FIX concentrate for factor levels less than 40–50 IU/dL or in the setting of acute bleeding. Supportive therapy should be continued for at least 3 days after vaginal delivery and for at least 5 days after cesarean delivery [44].

11.6.3 Other Factor Deficiencies

Factor II (prothrombin) and Factor V deficiencies are rare inherited bleeding disorders. They are associated with postpartum hemorrhage [45].

Factor VII deficiency is an autosomal recessive condition that produces severe deficiency in the homozygote and moderate deficiency without a bleeding tendency in the heterozygote individuals. It is the most common cause of the rare inherited coagulation disorders. Clinical symptoms are spontaneous epistaxis, genitourinary and gastrointestinal hemorrhages, hemarthrosis, and deep subcutaneous bleeding, but rarely it can result in fatal bleeding. In laboratory findings there is a prolonged PT and a normal aPTT and fibrinogen level [37].

Women with severe deficiency or positive bleeding history are more likely to be at risk of postpartum hemorrhage and require prophylactic requirement [46]. The first choice for congenital FVII deficiency is rFVIIa. The other options are plasma-derived FVII concentrates, plasma, prothrombin complex concentrates, and antifibrinolytics [45].

Factor X deficiency is an autosomal recessive disease. FX levels increase during pregnancy, but women with severe deficiency or history of bleeding may benefit from treatment. FFP or prothrombin complex concentrates are used for the treatment. The decision for the mode of delivery should be individualized [45].

Factor XI deficiency (HEMOPHILIA C) is an autosomally inherited disorder with an incidence of 1 in 1 million. FXI deficiency is associated with variable bleeding tendency and does not correlate well with FXI levels. FXI level, personal/family bleeding history, and the mode of delivery must be taken into account. Levels greater than 20% with no history of significant bleeding do not require specific therapy for delivery, but tranexamic acid can be considered. In patients with severe FXI disease, FXI concentrates (15 U/kg) or fresh frozen plasma (10–20 mL/kg) should be considered [47]. When aPTT is normalized in these patients, the factor XI level usually reaches 25–30%, which is sufficient for hemostasis [48].

In some cases successful neuraxial anesthesia has been used. It may be used in patients with partial FXI deficiency and following FFP or FXI transfusion in patients with severe deficiency. However current evidence on the choice of anesthesia technique is still insufficient [48].

Factor XIII deficiency is an autosomal recessive disorder. Delayed and impaired wound healing with bleeding occurring 24–36 h after surgery and trauma, soft tissue bleedings, and recurrent pregnancy loss are associated with this disorder. In laboratory findings the PT, PTT, and bleeding time are normal. Diagnosis is made with abnormal clot solubility test. FXIII levels fall during pregnancy, and most women need monthly infusions of FXIII concentrate [49].

11.6.3.1 Inherited Abnormalities of Fibrinogen

These are quantitative (afibrinogenemia and hypofibrinogenemia) or qualitative deficiencies (dysfibrinogenemia) of fibrinogen [39]. Although replacement therapy may be required in women with hypofibrinogenemia depending on the fibrinogen level and the bleeding, it should be begun immediately in afibrinogenemia. To maintain levels of fibrinogen greater than 100–150 mg/dL, plasma-derived fibrinogen concentrate and cryoprecipitate have been used. Dysfibrinogenemia is a functional disorder. The most sensitive test for this disorder is prolonged thrombin time [27].

11.6.4 Labor, Delivery, and Therapeutic Management in Congenital Coagulopathies

These patients are at increased risk of bleeding complications during and after delivery. At the beginning of labor, maternal full blood count and coagulation screening should be performed. Factor levels are generally not measurable in the acute setting. Planning for delivery should be done on the basis of the third trimester [50].

Neuraxial techniques are controversial in women with congenital disorders. However, if the coagulation status is in the normal range after replacement therapy, there is no contraindication to a regional anesthesia. It is particularly important to check factor levels prior removal of the epidural catheter because the pregnancy-induced increase in factor levels may be quickly reversed after birth [45].

11.7   Anticoagulant Therapy During Pregnancy

Anticoagulants help preventing blood clot formation in the vessels. Their indications in pregnancy and/or in the puerperium period are found in women who are at high risk for deep vein thrombosis and women with prosthetic heart valves, atrial fibrillation, cerebral venous sinus thrombosis, previous miscarriages, left ventricular dysfunction.

Low molecular weight heparins (LMWHs), unfractionated heparin (UFH), vitamin K antagonists, and direct thrombin and factor Xa inhibitors are the preferred agents for anticoagulant therapy. The American Society of Regional Anaesthesia and Pain Medicine (ASRA) and the European Society of Anaesthesiologists (ESA) published similar consensus guidelines in 2010 [51, 52]. They both recommended that neuraxial anesthesia in patients using prophylactic UFH up to 5000 units twice daily is safe and no further testing is required before neuraxial anesthesia techniques. Doses of over 5000 units twice a day require documentation of a normal PTT before placement. A platelet count should be checked to exclude heparin-induced thrombocytopenia after a 4-day course of heparin therapy [50].

Neuraxial anesthesia should be withheld for either 12 or 24 h from the last injection of LMWH depending on whether the patient is receiving prophylactic or therapeutic doses of LMWH, respectively. If the patient has an epidural catheter placed, LMWH administration should be delayed for 4 h after catheter removal [50].

If a pregnant woman is taking the newer oral anticoagulants, such as dabigatran or rivaroxaban, neuraxial placement should be delayed by 5 and 3 days, respectively [43].

> **Key Learning Points**
> - The management of the coagulation defects in pregnant patients requires multidisciplinary approach including anesthesiologist, hematologist, and obstetricians.
> - Women whom have known or suspected disorder of coagulation during pregnancy should be evaluated at antepartum period.
> - Women whose first manifestation of coagulation disturbance is obstetric hemorrhage should receive standard treatment for hemorrhage and subsequently should be evaluated for disorders of coagulation.

References

1. Brenner B. Haemostatic changes in pregnancy. Thromb Res. 2004;114:409–14.
2. James AH. Pregnancy and thrombotic risk. Crit Care Med. 2010;38:57–63.
3. Abbassi-Ghanavati M, Greer LG, Cunningham FG. Pregnancy and laboratory studies: a reference table for clinicians. Obstet Gynecol. 2009;114:1326–31.
4. Hellgren M, Blomback M. Studies on blood coagulation and fibrinolysis in pregnancy, during delivery and in the puerperium. I. Normal condition. Gynecol Obstet Investig. 1981;12:141–54.
5. Stirling Y, Woolf L, North WR, Seghatchian MJ, Meade TW. Haemostasis in normal pregnancy. Thromb Haemost. 1984;52:176–82.
6. Uchikova EH, Ledjev II. Changes in haemostasis during normal pregnancy. Eur J Obstet Gynecol Reprod Biol. 2005;119:185–8.
7. Dalaker K. Clotting factor VII during pregnancy, delivery and puerperium. Br J Obstet Gynaecol. 1986;93:17–21.
8. McCrae KR. Thrombocytopenia in pregnancy: differential diagnosis, pathogenesis and management. Blood Rev. 2003;17:7–14.
9. Tanaka M, Balki M, McLeod A, Carvalho JC. Regional anesthesia and non-preeclamptic thrombocytopenia: time to re-think the safe platelet count. Rev Bras Anestesiol. 2009;59:142–53.
10. Kam PC, Thompson SA, Liew AC. Thrombocytopenia in the parturient. Anaesthesia. 2004;59:255–64.
11. Chang M, Nakagawa PA, Williams SA, Schwartz MR, Imfeld KL, Buzby JS, et al. Immune thrombocytopenic purpura (ITP) plasma and purified ITP monoclonal autoantibodies inhibit megakaryocytopoiesis in vitro. Blood. 2003;102:887–95.
12. Webert KE, Mittal R, Sigouin C, Heddle NM, Kelton JG. A retrospective 11-year analysis of obstetric patients with idiopathic thrombocytopenic purpura. Blood. 2003;102:4306–11.
13. Bussel JB, Pham LC. Intravenous treatment with gamma globulin in adults with immune thrombocytopenic purpura: review of the literature. Vox Sang. 1987;52:206–11.
14. Galli M, Finazzi G, Barbui T. Thrombocytopenia in the antiphospholipid syndrome: pathophysiology, clinical relevance and treatment. Ann Med Interne. 1996;47:24–7.
15. Miyakis S, Lockshin MD, Atsumi T, Branch DW, Brey RL, Cervera R, et al. International consensus statement on an update of the classification criteria for definite antiphospholipid syndrome (APS). J Thromb Haemost. 2006;4:295–306.
16. Royal College of Obstetricians and Gynaecologists. Guidelines. Reducing the risk of thrombosis and embolism during pregnancy and the puerperium. Guidelines No 37a, London: RCOG; 2009.
17. Chakravarty EF, Nelson L, Krishnan E. Obstetric hospitalizations in the United States for women with systemic lupus erythematosus and rheumatoid arthritis. Arthritis Rheum. 2006;54:899–907.
18. Silva CA, Hilario MO, Febronio MV, Oliveira SK, Almeida RG, Fonseca AR, et al. Pregnancy outcome in juvenile systemic lupus erythematosus: a Brazilian Multicenter Cohort Study. J Rheumatol. 2008;35:1414–8.
19. Litttleton N. Thrombocytopenia in HIV. CME. 2007;25:272–5.
20. Aster RH, Bougie DW. Drug-induced immune thrombocytopenia. N Engl J Med. 2007;357:580–7.
21. Greinacher A. Clinical practice. Heparin-induced thrombocytopenia. N Engl J Med. 2015;373:252–61.
22. Ciurzynski M, Jankowski K, Pietrzak B, Mazanowska N, Rzewuska E, Kowalik R, et al. Use of fondaparinux in a pregnant woman with pulmonary embolism and heparin-induced thrombocytopenia. Med Sci Monit. 2011;17:56–9.
23. Greinacher A, Eckhardt T, Mussmann J, Mueller-Eckhardt C. Pregnancy complicated by heparin associated thrombocytopenia: management by a prospectively in vitro selected heparinoid (Org 10172). Thromb Res. 1993;71:123–6.
24. Gernsheimer T, James AH, Stasi R. How I treat thrombocytopenia in pregnancy. Blood. 2013;121:38–47.

25. George JN. Clinical practice. Thrombotic thrombocytopenic purpura. N Engl J Med. 2006;354:1927–35.
26. Esplin MS, Branch DW. Diagnosis and management of thrombotic microangiopathies during pregnancy. Clin Obstet Gynecol. 1999;42:360–8.
27. Silver RM, Major H. Maternal coagulation disorders and postpartum hemorrhage. Clin Obstet Gynecol. 2010;53:252–64.
28. Thachil J. Disseminated intravascular coagulation-new pathophysiological concepts and impact on management. Expert Rev Hematol. 2016;9:803–14.
29. Thachil J, Toh CH. Disseminated intravascular coagulation in obstetric disorders and its acute haematological management. Blood Rev. 2009;23:167.
30. Montagnana M, Franchi M, Danese E, Gotsch F, Guidi GC. Disseminated intravascular coagulation in obstetric and gynecologic disorders. Semin Thromb Hemost. 2010;36:404–18.
31. Haynes J, Laffan M, Plaat F. Use of recombinant activated factor VII in massive obstetric haemorrhage. Int J Obstet Anaesth. 2007;16:40–9.
32. Maclean A, Almeida Z, Lopez P. Complications of acute fatty liver of pregnancy treated with activated protein C. Arch Gynecol Obstet. 2005;273:119–21.
33. Collins PW, Hirsch S, Baglin TP, Dolan G, Hanley J, Makris M, Keeling DM, Liesner R, Brown SA, Hay CR, UK Haemophilia Centre Doctor's Organisation. Acquired haemophilia a in the United Kingdom: a 2-year national surveillance study by the United Kingdom Haemophilia Centre Doctor's Organisation. Blood. 2007;109:1870–7.
34. Boggio LN, Green D. Acquired hemophilia. Rev Clin Exp Hematol. 2001;5:389–404.
35. Peyvandi F, Bidlingmaier C, Garagiola I. Management of pregnancy and delivery in women with inherited bleeding disorders. Semin Fetal Neonatal Med. 2011;16:311–7.
36. D'Andrea G, Chetta M, Margaglione M. Inherited platelet disorders: thrombocytopenias and thrombocytopathies. Blood Transfus. 2009;7:278–92.
37. Ganchev RV, Ludlam CA. Acquired and congenital hemostatic disorders in pregnancy and the puerperium. In: Arulkumaran S, Karoshi M, Keigh L, Lalonde A, B-Lynch C, editors. A comprehensive textbook of postpartum hemorrhage: an essential clinical reference for effective management. 2nd ed. London: Sapiens Publications; 2012. p. 199–217.
38. Fiore M, Nurden AT, Nurden P, Seligsohn U. Clinical utility gene card for: Glanzmann thrombasthenia. Eur J Hum Genet. 2012;20:1102.
39. Nurden AT, Pillois X, Wilcox DA. Glanzmann thrombasthenia: state of the art and future directions. Semin Thromb Hemost. 2013;39:642–55.
40. Kujovich JL. von Willebrand disease and pregnancy. J Thromb Haemost. 2005;3:246–53.
41. Choi S, Brull R. Neuraxial techniques in obstetric and nonobstetric patients with common bleeding diatheses. Anesth Analg. 2009;109:648–60.
42. Federici AB. Highly purified VWF/FVIII concentrates in the treatment and prophylaxis of von Willebrand disease: the PRO.WILL study. Haemophilia. 2007;13:15–24.
43. Butwick AJ, Carvalho B. Neuraxial anesthesia for cesarean delivery in a parturient with type 1 von Willebrand disease and scoliosis. J Clin Anesth. 2007;19:230–3.
44. Lee CA, Chi C, Pavord SR, Bolton-Maggs PH, Pollard D, Hinchcliffe-Wood A, Kadir RA, UK Haemophilia Centre Doctors' Organization. The obstetric and gynaecological management of women with inherited bleeding disorders–review with guidelines produced by a taskforce of UK Haemophilia Centre Doctors' Organization. Haemophilia. 2006;12:301–36.
45. Kadir R, Chi C, Bolton-Maggs P. Pregnancy and rare bleeding disorders. Haemophilia. 2009;15:990–1005.
46. Eskandari N, Feldman N, Greenspoon JS. Factor VII deficiency in pregnancy treated with recombinant factor VIIa. Obstet Gynecol. 2002;99:935–7.
47. Singh A, Harnett MJ, Connors JM, Camann WR. Factor XI deficiency and obstetrical anesthesia. Anesth Analg. 2009;108:1882–5.
48. Bhoi D, Sreekumar EJ, Anand RK, Baidya DK, Chhabra A. Anaesthesia management of caesarean section in a patient with severe factor XI deficiency. J Obstet Anaesth Crit Care. 2013;3:37–9.

49. Asahina T, Kobayashi T, Takeuchi K, Kanayama N. Congenital blood coagulation factor XIII deficiency and successful deliveries: a review of the literature. Obstet Gynecol Surv. 2007;62:255–60.
50. Katz D, Beilin Y. Disorders of coagulation in pregnancy. Br J Anaesth. 2015;15:ii75–88.
51. Horlocker TT, Wedel DJ, Rowlingson JC, Enneking FK. Executive summary: regional anesthesia in the patient receiving antithrombotic or thrombolytic therapy: American Society of Regional Anesthesia and Pain Medicine Evidence-Based Guidelines (Third Edition). Reg Anesth Pain Med. 2010;35:102–5.
52. Gogarten W, Vandermeulen E, Van Aken H, Kozek S, Llau JV, Samama CM. Regional anaesthesia and antithrombotic agents: recommendations of the European Society of Anaesthesiology. Eur J Anaesthesiol. 2010;27:999–1015.

Pregnant Patients on Anticoagulants

12

Sunanda Gupta and Anju Grewal

12.1 Introduction

Anticoagulation is prescribed for a variety of obstetric and medical conditions in antenatal period [1, 2]. However, anticoagulation poses an increased risk of spinal epidural hematoma (SEH) following neuraxial blocks (NB), with consequent permanent neurologic deficits [1–3]. Anesthesia provider should proceed after evaluating the need for initial anticoagulation versus risks of withholding anticoagulation with the benefits of NB performance [1–4].

12.2 Why Do Pregnant Patients Need Anticoagulation?

Alterations in procoagulant, anticoagulant, and fibrinolytic system during pregnancy result in a hypercoagulable state, which is an adaptation to the expected hemostatic challenge during delivery [5]. However, these physiologic changes also increase the incidence of venous thromboembolism (VTE), leading to an increased use of thromboprophylaxis or high-dose anticoagulation.

In addition, women with mechanical prosthetic heart valves need long-term anticoagulation to prevent valve thrombosis and systemic embolization. The dilemma of balancing the benefits of an ideal anticoagulation using warfarin with risks of adverse fetal outcome is overcome by switching over to high-dose unfractionated heparin (UFH) or low-molecular-weight heparin (LMWH) anticoagulation [1, 2, 6].

S. Gupta (✉)
Department of Anaesthesiology and Critical Care, Geetanjali Medical College and Hospital, Udaipur, Rajasthan, India

A. Grewal
Department of Anaesthesiology, Dayanand Medical College and Hospital, Ludhiana, Punjab, India

© Springer International Publishing AG, part of Springer Nature 2018
B. Gunaydin, S. Ismail (eds.), *Obstetric Anesthesia for Co-morbid Conditions*,
https://doi.org/10.1007/978-3-319-93163-0_12

Recurrent early pregnancy losses, placental abruption, and inherited or acquired thrombophilias are also candidates for thromboprophylaxis [1, 2].

12.3 What Are the Challenges Posed by Anticoagulated Parturients?

Anticoagulation has been reported to be associated with spontaneous SEH [2, 7]. The major fears of adding instrumentation by use of neuraxial techniques to antico-agulated parturients are related to the distressing neurological complications of SEH especially paraplegia. Fortunately the incidence of reported major complica-tions following neuraxial anesthesia in obstetric population is extremely low vary-ing from 0.5:100,000 to 1:200,000–1:250,000, compared to 1:3600 SEH incidence in elderly female orthopedic population [1–3, 8–10]. This low incidence in obstet-rics has been validated in the report from Multicenter Perioperative Outcomes Group Research Consortium (MPOG) and in a recent systematic review which did not identify even a single case of SEH after neuraxial block in obstetric patients receiving UFH and LWMH [11, 12], which has been ascribed to the hypercoagula-ble state, along with a more compliant epidural or foraminal space in these young parturients.

Neuraxial anesthesia and/or analgesic techniques, viz., spinal, epidural, and combined spinal epidural, are the gold standard for optimal labor pain relief and providing anesthesia for cesarean delivery (CD), mainly because general anesthesia (GA) has been associated with significant risks both to the mother and fetus [1, 4].

However, labor and delivery usually have unpredictable timings, which can make decision to time the insertion of NB difficult. Furthermore, the physiological changes of pregnancy affect the pharmacokinetics (PK) and pharmacodynamics (PD) of anticoagulant drugs necessitating use of higher doses at term, albeit with lower peak plasma concentration, lower anti-Xa activity, and rapid renal clearance [1, 4, 13] (Table 12.1). This adds to the dilemma in adopting safe time lines for NB or catheter insertion/removal (CR) from current guidelines, which neither are pregnancy-specific nor address the varying LMWH dosing regimens used by obste-tricians [1, 4].

12.4 Are There Any Pregnancy-Specific Guidelines?

Recently the Society for Obstetric Anesthesia and Perinatology (SOAP) combined with the American Society of Regional Anesthesia (ASRA) and hematology issued a consensus statement to bridge this gap and challenges based on a thorough sys-tematic and general review of relevant literature and an exhaustive modified Delphi process [4]. Guidelines with regard to various time lines and PK-PD data from the ASRA 2010 and 2015 update have been compiled in Table 12.2 [1–4, 14–20].

As a general rule, Rosencher et al. [17] proposed a management strategy that can be applied to majority of anticoagulants especially NOACs. NB and subsequent CR

Table 12.1 Impact on pharmacokinetics and pharmacodynamics of anticoagulants in the obstetric population

Increased volume of distribution (Vd) for water-soluble drugs secondary to an increased plasma volume	Increased binding to nonspecific heparin-neutralizing proteins Increase in free fraction of protein-bound drugs due to decrease in serum albumin	Increased levels of fibrinogen and other coagulation factors especially factor VIII	Increase in renal blood flow and glomerular filtration rate
Significantly lower peak plasma concentration of UFH and LMWH and lower anti-Xa activity		aPTT response to UFH is decreased Anti-Xa activity used to regulate dose of LMWH and also a guide for emergency neuraxial block insertion (values less than 0.01 IU/mL deemed reassuring)	Rapid clearance of drugs excreted by renal route
These changes result in heparin resistance and a need for increasing dose as pregnancy progresses with peak effects in the third trimester (36 weeks of gestation), but resolution of changes starts to occur by the second week postpartum. Both physiological procoagulant state of pregnancy and response to anticoagulants make interpretation of coagulation tests challenging [1, 4, 13]			

should only be performed at least two elimination half-lives after the last dose of anticoagulant drug. The next dose of that anticoagulant should only be administered after a time interval which is obtained by subtracting the time necessary for that specific anticoagulant to reach maximum plasma levels from the time necessary to produce a stable blood clot (i.e., 8 h) [3, 21].

The salient features of the recent SOAP and updated ASRA guidelines are as follows [4, 14, 15, 20]:

Antepartum Recommendations
1. A multidisciplinary team comprising of an experienced hematologist, obstetrician, and obstetric anesthesiologist should engage in shared informed decision-making with the anticoagulated parturient.
2. An antepartum anesthesia consultation should be mandatory both for in and out patients especially at 36 weeks of gestation or in patients with concomitant medical/obstetric morbidity. It is critical that the last dose with exact timing be conveyed promptly to the obstetric anesthesia provider in parturients with imminent or high-risk delivery.
3. Consider switch from LMWH to UFH low-dose 5000 U/day SQ twice daily at 36 weeks of gestation in combination with mechanical thromboprophylaxis in women with additional comorbidities like obesity with difficult airway or in women with high risk of emergent operative high-risk mode of delivery or preterm labor.

Table 12.2 Anticoagulant and antithrombotic drugs: mechanism of action, PK-PD data, and time lines for NB/CR as per updated ASRA and ESRA guidelines

Drug	Mode of action	Onset of action	Time and peak effect	Elimination half-life	Acceptable time after drug for block performance	Acceptable time after block performance or catheter removal for next drug dose	Administration of drug while spinal or epidural catheter in place
Heparins							
UFH SQ prophylaxis low-dose / UFH SQ treatment (intermediate- or high-dose UFH)	Bind ATIII	Within 2 h (SQ); immediate (IV)	<30 min	1–2 h	>4–6 h or normal APTTR: low-dose UFH; ≥12 h and normal APTTR: intermediate-dose UFH; ≥24 h and normal APTTR: high-dose UFH	≥1 h	Caution: only use indwelling catheters with low-dose UFH. Hold NSAIDs including aspirin except acetaminophen until CR if receiving UFH/LMWH
UFH IV treatment	Bind ATIII		<5 min	1–2 h	4–6 h or normal APTTR	≥1 h (4 h)	Caution
LMWH SQ prophylaxis	Bind ATIII	±3–4 h	3–4 h	3–7 h	≥12 h	≥12 h after NB and ≥4 h after CR. CR can be done ≥12 h after LMWH dose with subsequent LMWH dosing to be given ≥4 h after CR	Caution
LMWH SQ treatment Intermediate and high dose	Bind ATIII		3–4 h	3–7 h	≥24 h	12–24 h and ≥24 h, respectively, after NB and ≥4 h after CR for next drug dose	Not recommended

Heparin alternatives

Argatroban	Direct thrombin inhibitors	1–3 h (with IV infusion)	<30 min	30–35 min	4 h or normal APTTR	6 h	Not recommended
Fondaparinux prophylaxis	Selective inhibition of factor Xa	Within 2 h	1–2 h	17–20 h	36–42 h (Consider anti-Xa levels) (36 h or 5 half-lives, if interventional pain procedure is planned)	6–12 h	Not recommended
Fondaparinux treatment			1–2 h	17–20 h	Avoid NB (consider anti-Xa levels)	12 h after CR Indwelling epidural catheter not recommended	Not recommended

Antiplatelet drugs

NSAIDs			1–12 h	1–12 h	No additional precautions	No additional precautions	No additional precautions
Aspirin	Irreversible inhibition of COX-1	Rapid (with 160 mg dose)	12–24 h	Not relevant irreversible effect	No additional precautions	No additional precautions	No additional precautions
Clopidogrel	Inhibit ADP-induced platelet aggregation	Within 5 h	12–24 h	Not relevant irreversible effect	7 days	6 h	Not recommended
Prasugrel	Inhibitor of platelet activation and aggregation through the irreversible binding of its active metabolite to the P2Y12 class of ADP receptors on platelets		15–30 min	Not relevant irreversible effect	7–10 days	6 h	Not recommended

(continued)

Table 12.2 (continued)

Drug	Mode of action	Onset of action	Time and peak effect	Elimination half-life	Acceptable time after drug for block performance	Acceptable time after block performance or catheter removal for next drug dose	Administration of drug while spinal or epidural catheter in place
Ticagrelor	Interact with the platelet $P2Y_{12}$ ADP receptor to prevent signal transduction and platelet activation		2 h	8–12 h	5–7 days	6 h	Not recommended
Tirofiban	Inhibition of fibrinogen binding to GPIIb/IIIa receptors	Maximal effect within 5 min	<5 min	4–8 h	8 h	6 h	Not recommended
Eptifibatide	Inhibition of fibrinogen binding to GPIIb/IIIa receptors	Within 15 min	<5 min	4–8 h	8 h	6 h	Not recommended
Abciximab	Inhibition of fibrinogen binding to GPIIb/IIIa receptors	Maximal effect 2 h after IV bolus	<5 min	24–48 h	48 h	6 h	Not recommended
Dipyridamole			75 min	10 h	No additional precautions		No additional precautions
Oral anticoagulants							
Warfarin	Inhibit γ-carboxylation of factors II, VII, IX, and X; Vitamin K antagonist	Within 90 min	3–5 days	4–5 days	INR ≤ 1.4	After catheter removal	Not recommended

Drug	Class					
Rivaroxaban prophylaxis (CrCl > 30 ml min⁻¹)	Factor Xa inhibitor		3 h	7–9 h	18 h updated ASRA: 3 days	6 h	Not recommended
Rivaroxaban treatment (CrCl > 30 ml min⁻¹)		3 h	7–11 h	48 h 2015 update of ASRA suggests discontinuation for 3 days before puncture/catheter removal or manipulation	6 h	Not recommended
Dabigatran prophylaxis or treatment	Direct thrombin inhibitor					
(CrCl > 80 ml min⁻¹)		0.5–2.0 h	12–17 h	48 h	6 h	Not recommended
(CrCl 50–80 ml min⁻¹)		0.5–2.0 h	15 h	72 h	6 h	Not recommended
(CrCl 30–50 ml min⁻¹)		0.5–2.0 h	18 h	96 h 2015 update of ASRA suggests discontinuation for 5 days before puncture/catheter removal or manipulation	6 h	Not recommended
Apixaban prophylaxis	Factor Xa inhibitor	3–4 h	12 h	24–48 h 2015 update of ASRA suggests discontinuation for 3 days before puncture/catheter removal or manipulation	6 h	Not recommended
Thrombolytic drugs						
Alteplase, anistreplase, reteplase, streptokinase		<5 min	4–24 min	10 days	10 days	Not recommended

Data used to fill this table are derived from ASRA and ESRA guidelines 2010 and 2015 update, SOAP guidelines 2017, and other data sources [1–5, 14, 15, 17–21]. These recommendations relate primarily to neuraxial blocks and to patients with normal renal function except where indicated

UFH unfractionated heparin, *SQ* subcutaneous, *APTTR* activated partial thromboplastin time ratio, *IV* intravenous, *LMWH* low molecular weight heparin, *NSAIDs* nonsteroidal anti-inflammatory drugs, *INR* international normalized ratio, *CrCl* creatinine clearance

4. If parturient is on LMWH beyond 36 weeks of gestation, anticipate timing for holding the appropriate dose timely by planning induction of labor [22, 23].
5. LMWH or UFH should be discontinued at least 36 h before planned induction of labor or CD, especially for patients diagnosed with VTE during current pregnancy.
6. Intravenous UFH is recommended during labor for very-high-risk parturients with recurrent thromboembolism (e.g., pulmonary embolism within 4 weeks of delivery etc.). Intravenous UFH should be discontinued 4–6 h before anticipated delivery.
7. In all women on UFH > 4 days, platelet count should be checked prior to NB to rule out heparin-induced thrombocytopenia (HIT).
8. Oral NOACs should be switched to LMWH or UFH at ≤36 weeks of gestation.

Intrapartum Recommendations
9. SOAP has developed decision aids to help during urgent and emergent unplanned delivery situations based on the latest ASRA guidelines, PK of anticoagulants (UFH & LMWH), while considering the risks of general anesthesia and concerns for maternal-fetal well-being (Figs. 12.1 and 12.2).
10. The highlight of this decision aid is to consider risks of GA as unacceptable to less probable risk of SEH from NB in parturients receiving low- and intermediate-dose UFH and LMWH.

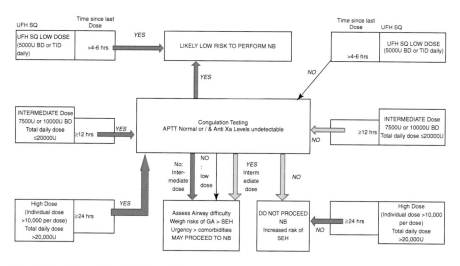

Fig. 12.1 Adapted from decision aid for urgent/emergent neuraxial procedures in obstetric patient with normal renal functions, body weight <40 kg, and receiving UFH [4]

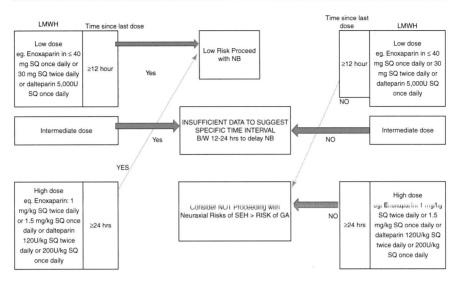

Fig. 12.2 Adapted from decision aid for urgent/emergent neuraxial procedures in obstetric patient with normal renal functions, body weight <40 kg, and receiving LMWH [4]

11. Pre-procedure huddles and multidisciplinary rounds emphasizing on the mode, timing, and dose of anticoagulants and plans for reinstating anticoagulation should be a norm.

12. The decision in elective obstetric procedures for ensuring safe time intervals between last anticoagulant dose and performance of NB/CR is based on the magnitude of last and total daily dose being received by the parturient (Table 12.2).

13. Interindividual variability is wider and therapeutic index narrower for UFH at intermediate and higher doses. Hence, combining time intervals and coagulation status assessment are recommended prior to neuraxial anesthesia.

14. Timings for elective discontinuation after last dose for low-dose, intermediate-dose, and high-dose UFH are 4–6 h, 12 h, and 24 h, respectively, along with coagulation testing.

15. Intravenous infusions of heparin can be stopped 4–6 h prior to NB. However, assessment of coagulation status should be done before placing the NB.

16. Protamine can be considered where UFH needs to be urgently reversed.

17. Indwelling catheters can be maintained with low-dose UFH.

18. CR should occur ≥4–6 h after a dose of subcutaneous (SQ) and IV UFH, and subsequent anticoagulation reinitiation of UFH dosing should occur ≥1 h after CR/NB.

19. Guidelines for LMWH are based on both coagulation assessment and quantum of dose. Thus time intervals for holding low-dose, intermediate-dose, and high-dose LMWH are $\geq$12 h, 12–24 h, and $\geq$24 h, respectively prior to NB performance.
20. There are insufficient data to recommend a specific interval between 12 and 24 h in case of intermediate-dose LMWH.
21. Wait for $\geq$12 h after NB and $\geq$4 h after CR before initiating LMWH low-dose thromboprophylaxis. Catheters can be maintained with low-dose LMWH, and CR can occur $\geq$12 h after a LMWH dose with subsequent dosing at $\geq$4 h after CR.
22. In case of higher-dose LMWH, consider waiting $\geq$24 h after NB and $\geq$4 h after CR prior to restarting LMWH.
23. Bridging with UFH 5000U SQ BD/TID daily can be considered for patients needing early post-CD thromboprophylaxis, patients with risk of PPH after CD, planned postpartum surgical procedure, and in cases where an indwelling postpartum catheter needs removal.
24. Aspirin and other NSAIDs except acetaminophen should be withheld until CR if receiving thromboprophylaxis with either UFH/LMWH SQ.
25. It is advisable to use dilute solutions/lower concentrations of local anesthetics to help early detection of early symptoms of SEH.

12.5 Can We Optimize Neurologic Outcomes if SEH Does Occur?

We must focus not only on the prevention but also on rapid diagnosis and treatment of SEH to optimize neurologic outcome. Risk of permanent neurologic deficit is increased if early surgical decompression gets delayed beyond 8–12 h from onset of neurologic symptoms. Protocols must be in place for urgent magnetic resonance imaging and hematoma evacuation (<6–8 h of symptom onset) if there is a change in neurologic status. Alerting symptoms for a neurologic deficit include an effect of neuraxial block persisting for more than the expected duration, local or back pain/tenderness, persistent numbness or motor weakness of lower limbs, and anal sphincter dysfunction. Hence vigilant monitoring is critical. It is also essential to have vigilance for longer time intervals beyond 24 h when NOAC or high-dose anticoagulants are on board [3, 11, 24].

These guidelines and algorithms should be used as a general guide to tailor management using multidisciplinary team along with shared decisions while assessing risks versus benefits for each individual parturient [4]. Rigorous reporting of complications especially incidence of SEH after NB in pregnant women can better update future guidelines for this special group of patients.

Key Learning Points

- A well-knit proactive relationship must evolve between the obstetric anesthesiologist, the obstetrician, hematologist, and parturient to ensure good closed-loop communication for safer neurologic outcomes.
- When possible, an induction or elective CD should be planned and an anesthesia consultation be obtained to plan an appropriate window of "off anticoagulation" while comprehending the PK-PD characteristics of the drug being used for anticoagulation.
- NB and subsequent CR should only be performed at least two elimination half-lives after the last dose of anticoagulant drug. NOAC may need to be withheld for at least five times the elimination half-lives. The next dose of that anticoagulant should only be administered after a time interval which is obtained by subtracting the time necessary for that specific anticoagulant to reach maximum plasma levels from the time necessary to produce a stable blood clot (i.e., 8 h).
- The updates ASRA and SOAP recognize that the risks of SEH in pregnant women may indeed be lower than the risks of subjecting pregnant women to general anesthesia.
- Hence in urgent or emergent scenarios, placement of NB without delay by an experienced provider may be appropriate especially if intermediate or low doses of anticoagulants are being administered and the parturients fall short of times since last dose with undetectable factor Xa activity.
- Anticoagulants on high dose and not meeting criteria for safe time lines should preferably be weighed carefully for risks of GA versus SEH with the shared decision in favor of maternal and fetal safety.
- Vigilant monitoring for longer periods is critical to detect early neurological symptoms with protocols for early surgical decompression preferably within 8–12 h for favorable neurologic outcomes.
- Indwelling catheters should be reserved only for low- or intermediate-dosing regimens and preferably should not be used for parturients on high-dose anticoagulation or on therapeutic NOACs presenting outside the safe time lines since last dose.

References

1. Butwick AJ, Carvalho B. Neuraxial anesthesia in obstetric patients receiving anticoagulants and antithrombotic drugs. Int J Obstet Anesth. 2010;19:193–201.
2. Butwick AJ, Carvalho B. Anticoagulant and antithrombotic drugs in pregnancy: what are the anesthetic implications for labor and cesarean delivery? J Perinatol. 2011;31:73–84.
3. Vandermeulen E. Regional anaesthesia and anticoagulation. Best Pract Res Clin Anaesthesiol. 2010;24:121–31.

4. Leffert L, Butwick A, Carvalho B, et al. The Soicety for Obstetric Anesthesia and Perinatalogy concensus statement on the anesthetic management of pregnant and postpartum women receiving thromboprophylaxis or higher dose anticoagulants. Anesth Analg. 2017;126:928–44. https://doi.org/10.1213/ANE0000000000002530.
5. Gonzalez-Fiol A, Eisenberger A. Anesthesia implications of coagulation and anticoagulation during pregnancy. Semin Perinatol. 2014;38:370–7.
6. Nishimura RA, Warnes CA. Anticoagulation during pregnancy in women with prosthetic valves: evidence, guidelines and unanswered questions. Heart. 2015;0:1–6. https://doi.org/10.1136/heartjnl-2014-306500.
7. Forsnes E, Occhino A, Acosta R. Spontaneousspinal epidural hematoma in pregnancy associated with using low molecular weight heparin. Obstet Gynecol. 2009;113:532–3.
8. D'Angelo R, Smiley RM, Riley ET, Segal S. Serious complications related to obstetric anesthesia: the serious complication repository project of the Society for Obstetric Anesthesia and Perinatology. Anesthesiology. 2014;120:1505–12.
9. Moen V, Dahlgren N, Irestedt L. Severe neurological complications after central neuraxial blockades in Sweden 1990–1999. Anesthesiology. 2004;101:950–9.
10. Popping DM, Zahn PK, Van Aken HK, Dasch B, Boche R, Pogatzki-Zahn EM. Effectiveness and safety of postoperative pain management: a survey of 18 925 consecutive patients between 1998 and 2006 (2nd revision): a database analysis of prospectively raised data. Br J Anaesth. 2008;101:832–40.
11. Bateman BT, Mhyre JM, Ehrenfeld J, et al. The risk and outcomes of epidural hematomas after perioperative and obstetric epidural catheterization: a report from the Multicenter Perioperative Outcomes Group Research Consortium. Anesth Analg. 2013;116:1380–5.
12. Leffert LR, Dubois HM, Butwick AJ, Carvalho B, Houle TT, Landau R. Neuraxial anesthesia in obstetric patients receiving thromboprophylaxis with unfractionated or low-molecular-weight heparin: a systematic review of spinal epidural hematoma. Anesth Analg. 2017;125(1):223–31. https://doi.org/10.1213/ANE.0000000000002173.
13. Ansari J, Carvalho B, Shafer SL, Flood P. Pharmacokinetics and pharmacodynamics of drugs commonly used in pregnancy and parturition. Anesth Analg. 2016;122:786–804.
14. Horlocker TT, Wedel DJ, Rowlingson JC, Kayser Enneking F, Kopp SL, Benzon HT, et al. Regional anesthesia in the patient receiving antithromboticor thrombolytic therapy. American Society of Regional Anesthesia and Pain Medicine Evidence-Based Guidelines (Third Edition). Reg Anesth Pain Med. 2010;35(1):64–101.
15. Gogarten W, Vandermeulen E, Van Aken H, Kozek S, Llau JV, Samama CM. Regional anaesthesia and antithrombotic agents: recommendations of the European Society of Anaesthesiology. Eur J Anaesthesiol. 2010;27:999–1015.
16. Bates SM, Greer IA, Pabinger I, Sofaer S, Hirsh J. Venous thromboembolism, thrombophilia, antithrombotic therapy, and pregnancy: American College of Chest Physicians evidence-based clinical practice guidelines (8th edition). Chest. 2008;133:844S–86S.
17. Rosencher N, Bonnet MP, Sessler DI. Anaesthesia and antithrombotic agents. Anaesthesia. 2007;62:1154–60.
18. Horlocker TT. Regional anaesthesia in the patient receiving antithrombotic and antiplatelet therapy. Br J Anaesth. 2011;107(51):i96–i106.
19. Green L, Machin SJ. Managing anticoagulated patients during neuraxial anaesthesia. Br J Haematol. 2010;149:195–208.
20. Oprea AD, Noto CJ, Halaszynski TM. Risk stratification, perioperative and periprocedural management of the patient receiving anticoagulant therapy. J Clin Anesth. 2016;34:586–99.
21. Harrop-Griffiths W, Cook T, Gill H, Hill D, Ingram M, Makris M, Malhotra S, Nicholls B, Popat M, Swales H, Wood P. Regional anaesthesia and patients with abnormalities of coagulation. Anaesthesia. 2013;68:966–72. https://doi.org/10.1111/anae.12359.

22. Butwick A, Hass C, Wong J, Lyell D, El-Sayed Y. Anticoagulant prescribing practices and anesthetic intervention among anticoagulated pregnant patients: a retrospective study. Int J Obstet Anesth. 2014;23:238–45.
23. American College of Obstetricians and Gynecologists Womens Healthcare Physicians. ACOG practice bulletin No. 138: inherited thrombophilias in pregnancy. Obstet Gynecol. 2013;122:706–16.
24. Benzon HT, Avram MJ, Green D, Bonow RO. Newer anticoagulants and regional anesthesia. Br J Anaesth. 2013;11(S1):i96–i113. https://doi.org/10.1093/bja/aet401.

Anesthesia for Pregnant Patient with Cardiac Disease

13

Demet Coskun and Ahmet Mahli

13.1 Introduction

Approximately 15% of pregnancy-related mortality is caused by heart disease indirectly which is also among the main causes of maternal mortality. The preexistence of cardiac disease may have favorable results as long as the patient is able to cope with the physiological demands of pregnancy. When those demands are not met, complications may occur. Therefore, in order to enhance care of such patients, the regular changes in physiology during pregnancy should be taken into consideration [1, 2].

Currently, the prevalence of cardiac disease during pregnancy ranges between 0.4 and 4.1%. Today, with the improvement in congenital heart surgery, more patients are likely to live up to the childbearing age, and thus congenital heart disease has replaced rheumatic heart disease and become the major cause of cardiac disease during pregnancy. Before conception, women with cardiac diseases should receive counseling as this is not only intended for detailed history taking and evaluation including some invasive procedures such as cardiac catheterization with fluoroscopy, when needed, but also improves both maternal and fetal outcome since it is possible to repair correctable lesions prior to conception [3, 4].

The severity of cardiac disease has a direct effect on the overall maternal and fetal morbidity and mortality. According to the New York Heart Association

D. Coskun (✉)
Gazi University School of Medicine, Department of Anesthesiology
and Reanimation, Ankara, Turkey
e-mail: dcoskun@gazi.edu.tr

A. Mahli
Yuksek Ihtisas University School of Medicine, Department of Anesthesiology
and Reanimation, Ankara, Turkey
e-mail: amahli@gazi.edu.tr

© Springer International Publishing AG, part of Springer Nature 2018
B. Gunaydin, S. Ismail (eds.), *Obstetric Anesthesia for Co-morbid Conditions*,
https://doi.org/10.1007/978-3-319-93163-0_13

Table 13.1 The New York Heart Association functional capacity and objective assessment

Functional capacity	Objective assessment
Class I. Patients with cardiac disease but without resulting limitation of physical activity. Ordinary physical activity does not cause undue fatigue, palpitation, dyspnea, or anginal pain	A. No objective evidence of cardiovascular disease
Class II. Patients with cardiac disease resulting in slight limitation of physical activity. They are comfortable at rest. Ordinary physical activity results in fatigue, palpitation, dyspnea, or anginal pain	B. Objective evidence of minimal cardiovascular disease
Class III. Patients with cardiac disease resulting in marked limitation of physical activity. They are comfortable at rest. Less than ordinary activity causes fatigue, palpitation, dyspnea, or anginal pain	C. Objective evidence of moderately severe cardiovascular disease
Class IV. Patients with cardiac disease resulting in inability to carry on any physical activity without discomfort. Symptoms of heart failure or the anginal syndrome may be present even at rest. If any physical activity is undertaken, discomfort is increased	D. Objective evidence of severe cardiovascular disease

(NYHA), maternal mortality varies between 0.4% class I–II disease and 6.8% class III–IV disease (Table 13.1) [5].

When a pregnant woman is unable to meet the extra demands that are the results of the physiological changes of pregnancy and parturition, cardiac decompensation becomes the major concern. The physiological changes that develop during pregnancy are as follows [6]:

1. Intravascular volume which peaks by early- to mid-third trimester increases by 50%.
2. There is a progressive decrease in systemic vascular resistance (SVR) throughout pregnancy. In spite of 30–40% increase in cardiac output (CO), mean arterial pressure remains at normal values. Further, the heart rate increases by 15%.
3. During labor, significant fluctuations in CO occur along with tachycardia, and during each uterine contraction, about 500 mL of blood is added to the circulation.
4. Pregnancy-related hypercoagulability occurs.
5. Functional residual capacity is reduced.

A team consisting of representatives from obstetrics and perinatology, anesthesiology, neonatology, cardiology, cardiothoracic surgery, intensive care, nursing, and social support service should be involved in the management of a pregnant woman with heart disease [7].

First of all, the pharmacology and teratogenic effects of the drugs that are generally administered in anesthesia management of pregnant women should be considered, and hypotension either due to drugs or anesthesia itself (general or regional anesthesia) should be treated. Additionally, the importance of perioperative fetal monitoring during anesthesia in pregnant women should be taken into account.

13.2 Pharmacology

Administration of drugs must be titrated appropriately according to the changes in pharmacokinetic and pharmacodynamic profiles during pregnancy. Secondary to pregnancy-induced increase in blood volume, the volume of distribution is increased. Increased α-1-glycoprotein concentration is observed along with the physiologic hypoalbuminemia of pregnancy. The free or unbound fraction of drugs is changed, and the doses of drugs such as local anesthetic agents are reduced because of altered plasma protein binding. Still, individual pharmacokinetic and pharmacodynamic alterations are heterogeneous, which indicates different pregnancy-related changes in each metabolizing organ system [8].

13.3 Teratogenicity

The observation of any critical change in the function or form of a child secondary to prenatal treatment is teratogenicity. The greatest risk to fetuses is posed by perioperative incidents that lead to severe maternal hypotension or hypoxemia. It has also been shown that derangements in carbohydrate metabolism and hyperthermia are teratogenic, but hypothermia is associated with no adverse fetal outcome [9].

Lipid-soluble drugs and drugs that have low molecular weight move across the trophoblast, which acts as a lipid membrane, easily by passive diffusion. On condition that sufficient exposure takes place at a sensitive developmental stage, any agent can be teratogenic in animals. The dose of any drug and the gestational age at which it is administered determine its impact. While a small dose of a given drug may be destructive to the early embryo, a large dose of the same drug may not have any effects on a fetus at an advanced stage of development. Drug exposure during the period of organogenesis (days 31–71) caused many iatrogenic structural abnormalities. It has been shown that drug exposure during late pregnancy resulted in functional abnormalities [8].

No increase in congenital anomalies among the offspring of women who underwent surgery during pregnancy has been observed in the large survey studies. However, an increase in the risk for abortions, growth restriction, and increased frequency of low-birth-weight and very low-birth-weight neonates was observed, and their reasons were attributed to the requirement for surgery, not to anesthesia [10].

13.4 Hypotension

A major risk to fetuses is posed by hypotension caused by hypovolemia, anesthetic drugs, central neuraxial blockade, or aortocaval compression. Since the uteroplacental circulation is not subject to autoregulation, perfusion is totally dependent on the maintenance of adequate maternal systemic blood pressure. In order to ameliorate hypotension, the use of intravenous (IV) fluid boluses is possible, but care is required as patients are predisposed to pulmonary edema with the concomitant administration of tocolytics and increased capillary permeability [8].

Ephedrine is extensively used for the treatment of maternal hypotension refractory to IV fluid administration. Ephedrine is an indirect-acting sympathomimetic agent that releases noradrenaline from postganglionic sympathetic nerve endings. For this reason, ephedrine has a comparatively slow onset and long duration of action. Furthermore, tachyphylaxis, which is caused in part by depletion of noradrenaline from presynaptic nerve endings and prolonged blockade of receptors, is prevalent. For that reason titration of ephedrine doses is difficult. The alpha agonists phenylephrine and metaraminol are more effective in the maintenance of maternal blood pressure, preventing fetal acidosis [11, 12].

13.5   Fetal Monitoring

Continuous fetal heart rate (FHR) monitoring is appropriate from 18 weeks' gestation. Since maternal hemodynamic stability alone is not an ample indicator of fetal well-being, fetal monitoring is a must as long as it is technically possible. Another practical indicator of fetal well-being is FHR variability, and it can be monitored from 25 to 27 weeks' gestation onward. As anesthetic agents reduce both baseline FHR and FHR variability, readings must be interpreted by taking the context of administered drugs into consideration. The human fetus may be responsive to several environmental stimuli such as noise, pressure, pain, and cold temperature. Noxious stimuli cause an autonomic response as well as a rise in stress hormones. Persistent fetal bradycardia is generally an indication of true fetal distress and requires immediate therapeutic measures. It should be noted that when administered with glycopyrrolate, neostigmine causes fetal bradycardia due to the reduced placental transfer of the former compound [9].

Intraoperative FHR monitoring is valuable in detecting early compromise, which then allows the optimization of maternal hemodynamics and oxygenation with appropriate fluid therapy, vasopressors, blood product administration, hyperventilation, or position adjustment. During laparoscopic surgery, changes in the FHR may be an indication of the requirement for temporary deflation of the pneumoperitoneum [13].

13.6   General Principles of Anesthetic Management

During pregnancy, due to any potential compromise to the fetus, surgery of any type is usually avoided. The management of the pregnant patient with heart disease often involves medical therapy including long periods of bed rest, if required. In the presence of a surgical lesion, every attempt is made in order to postpone the definitive procedure until after delivery of the infant. But still, there are patients who decompensate so severely from the cardiovascular stress imposed by pregnancy that their chance of survival is very low if surgical correction is not performed. Such patients mostly suffer from rheumatic valvular disease and, more often, mitral stenosis [1].

In pregnant patients, cardiac surgery for decompensated valve disease, coronary artery bypass grafting, atrial myxoma, and aortic dissection has been performed safely without fetal loss. The optimization of fetal outcome is possible by intervention prior to the development of NYHA class IV disease and by the use of normothermic, high-flow, and high-pressure extracorporeal circulation. Maintenance of uteroplacental perfusion is the main goal in the management of anesthesia of high-risk parturient patients, where the role of a multidisciplinary team is crucial [9, 14].

Most of the women with cardiac disease remaining asymptomatic throughout entire pregnancy tolerate labor and delivery well. Surgery on patients in functional NYHA class III–IV categories with surgically correctable lesions should be performed either before pregnancy or during the second trimester of pregnancy before labor and delivery [15].

The four main goals of anesthetic management during labor and delivery in pregnant women with heart disease are to provide analgesia and hemodynamic monitoring, optimize cardiovascular and respiratory functions with the manipulation of various hemodynamic factors, customize anesthetic technique for maternal and fetal well-being, and perform resuscitation including airway and ventilatory management if necessary. In accordance with Moore's concept, five hemodynamic factors comprise preload, pulmonary vascular resistance (PVR), SVR, heart rate, and myocardial contractility, and they are related to patient's cardiac disease (Table 13.2) [16]. The anesthetist can control these factors, and they can be adjusted by manipulation of the anesthetic technique or the employment of specific drugs.

The minimum mandatory monitoring required in all cardiac patients undergoing labor and delivery is noninvasive blood pressure, electrocardiogram (for detecting arrhythmias) and heart rate, pulse oximetry, and respiratory rate. Signs of persistent

Table 13.2 Hemodynamic parameters controllable by the anesthetist

Parameter	Increase	Decrease
Preload	Fluid therapy, capacitance vessel constriction—phenylephrine, mephentermine	Phlebotomy, bleeding, capacitance vessel dilation –nitroglycerine, trimethaphan, ventilation, large tidal volume, PEEP
PVR	Increased $PaCO_2$, hypoventilation, decreased PaO_2, acidosis	Decreased $PaCO_2$, hyperventilation, increased PaO_2, alkalosis
SVR	Arteriolar constriction—phenylephrine, mephentermine Anesthetics—ketamine, nitrous oxide	Arteriolar dilation—nitroprusside isoproterenol Anesthetics—droperidol, propofol, isoflurane, sevoflurane Relaxants—D-tubocurarine
HR	Anticholinergics—atropine Relaxants—pancuronium, gallamine	Esmolol, metoprolol, digoxin Relaxants—vecuronium Anesthetics—halothane, fentanyl
Contractility	Inotropes—adrenaline, dopamine, dobutamine, isoproterenol Calcium Digoxin, amrinone, milrinone	β-blockers—esmolol, metoprolol Anesthetics—halothane, propofol, sevoflurane

PVR pulmonary vascular resistance, *SVR* systemic vascular resistance, *HR* heart rate, *PEEP* positive end-expiratory pressure respiratory distress, four hourly temperature, and input–output fluid balance are also followed. With regard to parturients in functional classes III and IV, some additional invasive monitoring such as intra-arterial pressure, pulmonary artery (PA) pressure, pulmonary capillary wedge pressure (PCWP), and arterial blood gas analysis may be necessary. If the condition of parturient worsens and simultaneous cardiac surgery needs to be planned, perioperative transesophageal echocardiography (TEE) may be required [4, 17].

In patients with a history of thromboembolism or those with valvular heart disease or prosthetic heart valves, anticoagulant therapy is used in pregnancy as long-term thrombolysis or prophylaxis, respectively. However, oral anticoagulant therapy during pregnancy is contraindicated. As heparin is a large molecule that does not cross the placenta, it is the drug of choice in pregnancy. As low molecular weight heparin has a long half-life which allows once-a-day dosing and is more bioavailable after subcutaneous injection and does not enter the fetal circulation, it is used widely. Other treatments such as streptokinase and urokinase are relatively contraindicated in pregnancy [18, 19].

Cardiac diseases that are present in pregnancy can be classified as follows [2]:

1. Valvular heart disease
2. Congenital heart disease
3. Cardiac dysrhythmias and conduction defects during pregnancy
4. Others

In this chapter, mainly the heart diseases in pregnancy that are important in terms of anesthesia management will be reviewed.

13.7 Valvular Heart Diseases

13.7.1 Mitral Stenosis

Mitral stenosis causes 90% of rheumatic heart disease in pregnancy, and 25% of the patients develop symptoms for the first time during late pregnancy. As pregnancy advances, relative obstruction across the valve increases due to the greater blood volume, heart rate, and CO. Pulmonary venous congestion occurs due to increased obstruction, and it may result in pulmonary edema. The most common pathology related to acute pulmonary edema in pregnancy is pure mitral stenosis, and it is followed by aortic valve disease and/or primary myocardial disease. Thrombi within the enlarged left atrium (LA) characterize a major therapeutic challenge due to the risks and side effects of anticoagulation [20, 21].

In order to avoid changes in monitored hemodynamic parameters, lumbar epidural anesthesia is the best choice regarding anesthesia for labor and vaginal delivery. After the development of reflex tachycardia, a sudden decrease in SVR may not be tolerated well. Even though it is possible to use other analgesic modalities, epidural analgesia does not only allow for careful titration to the desired result but also minimizes undesirable changes. The addition of opioids, such as fentanyl, to the dilute local anesthetic mixture improves the quality of analgesia yet does not add to the sympathetic blockade. For the critically ill patient, opioids alone may be administered through the epidural or intrathecal route. In cases where epidural anesthesia has not been employed, a low spinal anesthesia may be administered to make a controlled second stage and delivery possible. Another rational and a rarely selected option is caudal anesthesia. For some patients sufficient, though not ideal, pain relief can be provided by pudendal nerve block [22, 23].

The reason for the preference of epidural anesthesia over spinal anesthesia is because the former results in slower onset of blockade leading to more controllable hemodynamic alterations. With epidural anesthesia, such patients may be prone to hypotension, secondary to a combination of venous pooling and prior beta-adrenergic blockade and diuretic therapy. Because it may result in tachycardia, the usual vasopressor choice of ephedrine should be avoided. Instead, judicious use of metaraminol or low-dose (20–40 mcg) phenylephrine helps maternal blood pressure to be restored with little or no unwanted effect on uteroplacental perfusion [24].

General anesthesia should be carefully induced without using drugs that commonly cause tachycardia. The use of a high-dose narcotic-based technique may be required because of the need to blunt the hemodynamic response to endotracheal intubation depending on the severity of the disease. Thus, myocardial depression and the decreases in SVR that may occur with commonly employed short-acting barbiturates are also avoided. The maintenance of anesthesia is accomplished with narcotics, muscle relaxants, nitrous oxide, and oxygen [25].

The major anesthetic concerns for mitral stenosis include prevention of rapid ventricular rates to maintain sinus rhythm and prevention of increases in central blood volume. However, maintaining optimal LA preload; avoiding large, rapid falls in SVR; and also avoiding hypoxemia and/or hypoventilation, both of which may increase PA pressures and cause right ventricle (RV) failure.

13.7.2 Mitral Insufficiency

The second most prevalent valvular lesion in pregnancy is mitral valve insufficiency and regurgitation. Chronic left ventricular volume overload and work are usually well tolerated, and their symptoms develop comparatively late in life after child-bearing age. Therefore, most patients who have mitral regurgitation tolerate pregnancy well. An increased risk of atrial fibrillation during pregnancy, bacterial endocarditis requiring antibiotic prophylaxis, systemic embolization, and pulmonary congestion during pregnancy is among the complications. With a presence of 10–17% in pregnancies, congenital mitral valve prolapse is much more prevalent during pregnancy than mitral regurgitation. It is tolerated well and a typically benign form of mitral regurgitation, and thus, therapeutic interventions are rarely required [3, 26].

It is possible to provide safe anesthetic management of labor and delivery using any of the available techniques, including lumbar epidural anesthesia. Providing adequate analgesia and anesthesia, peripheral vasoconstriction will be minimized, and thus the increase in left ventricle (LV) afterload related to labor pain will be attenuated, and thereby the forward flow of blood will be augmented. In this regard, sympathetic blockade-induced decrease in SVR is advantageous. It should be noted that as venous capacitance increases, in order to maintain LV filling volume, one must be ready to augment preload carefully with IV fluid infusion [1].

13.7.3 Aortic Insufficiency

Aortic insufficiency may be either congenital or acquired. If congenital, it is generally associated with other lesions, whereas if acquired, it may be secondary to rheumatic heart disease or endocarditis in association with aortic root dissection. The development of the symptoms that follow rheumatic fever usually occurs during the fourth or fifth decade of life. Thus, most women having this as dominant lesion have event-free pregnancies. The basic pathophysiology is of chronic volume overloading of the left ventricle which results in hypertrophy and dilation associated with increased compliance. As a result of hypertrophy, requirements for myocardial oxygen are higher than normal, yet a decrease in diastolic pressure and an increased left ventricular end-diastolic pressure may reduce perfusion pressure and thus oxygen supply. Since the anesthetic concerns are similar to those in question for patients with mitral regurgitation, epidural anesthesia for labor and delivery is desirable to prevent increases in peripheral vasoconstriction. Epidural anesthesia with reasonable avoidance of direct myocardial depressants is more suitable than general anesthesia in providing surgical anesthesia [1, 27].

Thus, anesthetic considerations focus on minimizing pain, thereby prevention of increases in SVR is induced by circulating catecholamines, avoiding bradycardia as it increases regurgitant flow time and also avoiding myocardial depressants as they may aggravate failure.

13.7.4 Aortic Stenosis

In women of childbearing age, aortic stenosis is very rare, and it is associated with high fetal and maternal mortality in the presence of moderate to severe form. In pregnant patients with aortic stenosis, as a consequence of more blood volume and less SVR, transvalvular gradients increase progressively during pregnancy. Such increases can cause syncope, angina, and reduced perfusion to the placenta and fetus. In parturients with severe aortic stenosis, carefully titrated epidural anesthesia or combined spinal epidural anesthesia for labor and delivery is supported. Based on the concern that induction of general anesthesia and tracheal intubation may result in hypertension and tachycardia, and thus a decrease in CO and coronary blood flow, these reports argue against general anesthesia for women with severe aortic stenosis. In some cases, the CO might be low as a result of a high SVR that is related to pain and anxiety. A gradual reduction in SVR associated with induction of epidural anesthesia provides an improvement in CO when a fixed stroke volume is present, with the assumption that the filling pressures are sufficient [28, 29].

When a general anesthetic technique is used, an opioid-based anesthetic is applicable when LV function is compromised. Nonetheless, that the slow induction period associated with general anesthetic technique increases the risk of pulmonary aspiration is a concern. As long as the risks and benefits are acknowledged, drugs are titrated carefully, and invasive monitoring is used as a guide to appropriate therapy in the event of adverse hemodynamic changes, any anesthetic technique that is well-managed is appropriate [30].

Employment of labor analgesia with epidural anesthesia is still a controversial issue as these patients may not be able to tolerate the decreases in preload and afterload that may accompany epidural analgesia associated with sympathetic blockade. Other suitable choices are intrathecal or epidural opioids, whether alone or in combination with an epidural segmental anesthetic. Spinal opioids do not have any cardiovascular effects. In particular, with the use of this technique, myocardial contractility remains unaltered, preload is preserved, and, most important of all, SVR is unchanged. It is considered that local anesthetics and opioids act synergistically, allowing a decrease in the concentration of both drugs when used together. Of note, tachycardia associated with labor pain can be prevented by effective analgesia [20, 31].

The following goals are encompassed by anesthetic management that includes avoiding tachycardia and bradycardia, maintaining adequate preload so that the LV may produce a sufficient CO across the stenotic valve.

13.7.5 Mixed Valvular Lesions

In case of mixed valvular lesions, the dilemma is to treat which lesion first. As a general rule, the management of the dominant lesions should be the target of therapy. For example, in a woman presenting with moderate-to-severe mitral regurgitation and mild mitral stenosis, management should be first directed to the treatment of the regurgitant lesion even though this conflicts with the usual management of the mitral stenosis [2].

13.8 Congenital Heart Disease

13.8.1 Congenital Heart Disease Without Shunt

13.8.1.1 Coarctation of the Aorta

Narrowing of the aorta at or near the insertion of ductus arteriosus characterizes coarctation of the aorta. Hereby, the principal concern is maternal hypertension, specifically in the upper body. An arm-to-leg systolic blood pressure gradient of less than 20 mmHg is with a satisfactory outcome during pregnancy. In a pregnant woman with an uncorrected coarctation or a residual decrease in aorta diameter, a high risk for left ventricular failure and/or aortic rupture or dissection is in question. As a result of the decreased uterine perfusion distal to the aorta lesion, fetal mortality rate may reach up to 20% in such pregnancies. In order to decrease the risk of aortic dissection and/or rupture, it is critical to control maternal hypertension by beta blockers as indicated. Although risk of fetal growth retardation is increased with the administration of beta blockers during pregnancy, maternal safety is the priority. For cesarean delivery, although epidural anesthesia has also been used because of its slow onset, general anesthesia is most commonly preferred [32, 33].

Physiologically, a fixed obstruction to aortic outflow with distal hypoperfusion is represented by an uncorrected coarctation of the aorta. It is recommended that in order to avoid compromising the placental blood flow, a maternal lower-limb systolic blood pressure at more than 100 mmHg should be maintained. During anesthesia, FHR monitoring should be performed continuously so as to detect any compromise in the placental circulation. Fetal bradycardia can also be an indication of placental hypoperfusion but only after a time lag. Due to their mild positive chronotropic effects, ephedrine and dopamine are vasopressors of choice [34].

Anesthetic goals include invasive hemodynamic monitoring, maintaining normal to slightly elevated SVR and heart rate, and maintaining adequate intravascular volume and venous return as well.

13.8.2 Congenital Heart Disease with Shunt

Congenital heart diseases with intracardiac shunts are divided into two main categories, as acyanotic and cyanotic lesions. The optimal cardiovascular parameters that are required in parturients with intracardiac shunts during induction and maintenance of anesthesia are shown in Table 13.3 [35].

Table 13.3 Optimal cardiovascular parameters for parturients with shunt

Cardiovascular parameter	Right-to-left shunt (cyanotic)	Left-to-right shunt (acyanotic)
HR	N	N
Heart rhythm	Sinus	Sinus
Preload	Maintain	Maintain
Contractility	N	N to ↑
Afterload (SVR)	↑	↓
PVR	↓	↑
Anesthetic considerations	Avoid large fall in SVR at induction/abrupt sympathectomy by central neuraxial blocks	Avoid pulmonary artery vasodilators and myocardial depressants
	Use oxytocin cautiously	Avoid increases in SVR from cold, anxiety, or pain
	Avoid increases in PVR from hypoxia, acidemia, hypoventilation, or excessive positive pressure ventilation	Avoid the use of ergometrine
	Avoid prostaglandin F2-alfa	

↑ increase, ↓ decrease, *N* normal, *PVR* pulmonary vascular resistance, *SVR* systemic vascular resistance, *HR* heart rate

13.8.2.1   Acyanotic Heart Lesions (Left-to-Right Shunts)

The most common acyanotic heart lesion is atrial septal defect (ASD) which can be easily missed during screening. Women with left-to-right shunts, without pulmonary hypertension, can generally tolerate pregnancy well because of the associated physiologic decrease in SVR even when pulmonary blood flow is increased. However, there is an increase in the risk of LV failure during pregnancy. Increases in atrial volume lead to biatrial enlargement, and therefore, supraventricular dysrhythmias are common. Increased plasma volume and cardiac output related to pregnancy serve to accentuate the left-to-right shunt, right ventricular volume work, and pulmonary blood flow, with the possibility of pulmonary hypertension development and left and right ventricular failure. Peripartum management focuses on avoiding vascular resistance changes which may possibly increase the degree of shunt. Increases in SVR or decreases in PVR may not be tolerated well. In spite of the usefulness of all of the common methods of providing labor analgesia, lumbar epidural analgesia for labor and vaginal delivery or cesarean delivery decreases the risks of increased SVR. Provided that increases in SVR are avoided and sinus rhythm is maintained, general anesthesia for cesarean delivery is also tolerated well [2, 27].

In 7% of adults with congenital heart disease, ventricular septal defect (VSD) develops. Patients with uncorrected lesions do well during pregnancy when pulmonary hypertension is not present. In patients with large VSDs and coexisting pulmonary hypertension, the percentage of which is small, maternal mortality ranges between 7 and 40%. The major ensuing complication is severe right ventricular failure with shunt reversal (Eisenmenger syndrome). A rise in plasma volume, cardiac output, and heart rate during pregnancy may increase left-to-right shunt and may deteriorate pulmonary hypertension to a further degree [33, 36].

For the optimal achievement of anesthesia for labor and vaginal delivery, segmental epidural anesthesia consisting of local anesthetics, opioids, or their combination is employed; in this way, painful stimuli can be controlled, and thus the changes in heart rate and SVR are minimized. It is possible to accomplish anesthesia for cesarean delivery either with slow titration of an epidural anesthetic agent to allow time for correction of pressure changes or with a general anesthetic agent combining opioid and inhalation technique in order to depress the adrenergic response to endotracheal intubation and minimize myocardial depression [33].

Almost 15% of all cases of congenital heart disease are caused by patent ductus arteriosus (PDA); today most patients with a large PDA (>1 cm) receive early surgical intervention. Patients with a small PDA typically have normal pregnancies, but maternal mortality may reach 5–6% from ventricular failure in pregnant women with superimposed pulmonary hypertension. It is possible to associate the progressive decrease in SVR development throughout pregnancy with shunt reversal and peripheral cyanosis. Avoidance of increases in SVR and hypervolemia is among the anesthetic considerations. Contrarily, acute decreases in SVR may lead to reversal of shunt in patients with preexisting pulmonary hypertension and right ventricular compromise. Again, depending on the severity of the disease, all modalities may be used. Pain-associated increase in SVR is decreased with continuous lumbar epidural analgesia for labor and delivery. For cesarean delivery, epidural or general anesthesia is appropriate as long as the increases in SVR related to endotracheal intubation and surgical stimulation are adequately handled [36].

After all, small ASD or VSD or PDA with modest left-to-right shunt is often well tolerated during pregnancy. Early epidural analgesia is desirable in order to avoid pain and the resulting increase in SVR and therefore potential left-to-right shunt. Since a rapid decrease in SVR is likely to result in reversal of shunt flow and hypoxemia, slowly titrated epidural anesthesia is preferred [33, 34].

Anesthetic goals include avoidance of accidental injection of air intravenously, avoidance of decrease in SVR, and also prevention of hypoxia, hypercapnia, and acidosis. Intrapartum monitoring of mother with TEE is beneficial.

13.8.2.2   Cyanotic Heart Lesions (Right-to-Left Shunts)

A congenital heart lesion characterized by right-to-left shunt is related to recirculation of desaturated blood. In case of unsaturated hemoglobin level more than 5 g/dL, peripheral cyanosis is present. Hematocrit level has a direct influence on the degree of cyanosis. While an anemic parturient with poor oxygen saturation may not manifest cyanosis, a woman with polycythemia may appear cyanotic even at higher oxygen saturations [37].

The commonest congenital heart disease with right-to-left shunt is tetralogy of Fallot (TOF). It causes 5% of cases of congenital heart disease in pregnancy. It involves four components: a VSD, infundibular or right ventricular outflow tract obstruction, overriding of the aorta sitting over the VSD, and right ventricular hypertrophy. Pregnant women with tetralogy usually had undergone corrective surgery such as the closure of VSD and widening of pulmonary outflow tract in childhood. In some pregnant women, a small residual VSD may still be present, or progressive hypertrophy of pulmonary outflow tract may occur slowly over decades [33].

Patients who have corrected tetralogy, even if it has been asymptomatic for many years, should undergo echocardiography both before and during early pregnancy. Due to surgical injury to cardiac conduction system, such patients may manifest atrial and ventricular arrhythmias. As IV air bubble infusion may result in systemic embolization, meticulous attention should be given to avoid it. In uncorrected TOF or corrected TOF with residual disease, anesthetic management targets to avoid decrease in SVR, which increases right-to-left shunt. The maintenance of intravascular volume and venous return is important. In early labor, administration of epidural anesthesia is recommended in order to avoid pain and consequent right ventricular outflow tract spasm and increase in right-to-left shunt. For cesarean delivery, the onset of regional block should be slow, and as a sudden decrease in SVR may cause increase in right-to-left shunt, single-shot spinal is not a good choice [34, 36].

In TOF, and similar lesions with obstructed pulmonary outflow tracts, a pure α-agonist such as phenylephrine is the best option for the treatment of a reduction in SVR and blood pressure. In the case of an obstruction of the RV outflow tract, catecholamine release from inadequate pain relief and light general anesthesia and/ or catecholamine release related to exogenous factors like stress or anxiety should be avoided. Inhalation anesthetics such as halothane and sevoflurane and short-acting beta blockers can relieve infundibular obstruction. Hypovolemia, hypercarbia, acidosis, rise in PVR, and fall in SVR are not tolerated [27, 35].

Anesthetic goals include avoidance of decrease in SVR and maintenance of adequate intravascular volume and venous return, placing epidural catheter for analgesia early in labor. Besides, intrapartum monitoring of mother with TEE is beneficial.

13.8.2.3 Eisenmenger Syndrome

This is a consequence of chronic uncorrected left-to-right shunt, and it causes right ventricular hypertrophy, increased pulmonary artery pressure, and right ventricular dysfunction. Primary lesion may either be ASD, VSD, or PDA. When pulmonary arterial pressure overwhelms systemic pressure and finally irreversible pulmonary hypertension develops, a reversal of shunt occurs, and at this point the correction of primary lesion does not help. Correction is indicated in arterial hypoxemia and right ventricular failure. The decrease in SVR associated with pregnancy causes an increase in the severity of right-to-left shunt with decreased pulmonary perfusion. Decrease in functional residual capacity leads to hypoxemia. When fixed pulmonary hypertension is present, sudden profound hypoxemia and death may be caused by reduction in right ventricular filling pressure due to hypotension from any cause. Decreased oxygen delivery to the fetus and thus high incidence of intrauterine growth retardation and fetal demise are results of maternal hypoxemia. In such patients, maternal mortality is as high as 30–50%. Pregnant patients with Eisenmenger syndrome should be consulted to terminate pregnancy. For a patient who does not terminate her pregnancy, hospitalization for the duration of pregnancy is often appropriate. About 43% of the maternal deaths are caused by thromboembolic phenomenon, and prophylactic anticoagulation can be favorable [33, 34].

The primary goals of anesthetic management consist of maintaining adequate SVR, intravascular volume, and venous return; preventing pain, hypoxemia, hypercarbia, and acidosis; avoiding aortocaval compression; and also avoiding myocardial depression during general anesthesia.

13.8.3 Cardiac Dysrhythmias and Conduction Defects During Pregnancy

Cardiac dysrhythmia observed during pregnancy is mostly benign in nature. The main causes of serious dysrhythmias are abnormalities in cardiac conducting tissue and rheumatic heart disease. A recent onset of atrial fibrillation during pregnancy is related to a high incidence of congestive heart failure, embolization, and subsequently mortality. Verapamil, digoxin, quinidine, and beta adrenergic blocking agents are frequently used to control the ventricular rate. To terminate supraventricular tachycardia, while IV adenosine is the treatment of choice, direct current cardioversion can be used efficiently with no harm to the fetus [2].

13.9 Others

13.9.1 Coronary Artery Disease

Myocardial infarction is fortunately an uncommon event during pregnancy. Most parturients who have severe cardiac diseases can be medically managed. Ischemia that does not respond to medical treatment may require percutaneous transluminal coronary angioplasty or coronary artery bypass surgery. Clopidogrel, an antiplatelet agent, is avoided in pregnancy for safety issues, but aspirin at a low dose can be used without any contraindication for regional anesthetic technique that may be employed for labor analgesia or cesarean delivery, if platelet count is more than 80,000 mm^{-3} and bleeding time is normal [34].

Excellent pain relief is provided, and maternal concentrations of catecholamines and thus the risk of coronary artery vasoconstriction are reduced by epidural anesthesia. In patients with coronary artery disease, the preferred vasopressor for treatment of hypotension is phenylephrine since maternal heart rate and myocardial oxygen demands are increased because myocardial ischemia is exacerbated by ephedrine. When general anesthesia is performed, a modified rapid sequence induction using etomidate and remifentanil can be performed over 1 or 2 min without any compromises on hemodynamics. Single-shot spinal anesthesia leads to rapid onset of sympathectomy, and thus it carries an increased risk of severe hypotension. For cesarean delivery, epidural anesthesia is the favored technique. General anesthesia should be regarded only in cases where regional anesthesia is contraindicated due to concurrent anticoagulant therapy [38].

Bolus-dose oxytocin should be avoided, as its use can result in profound vasodilatation and compensatory tachycardia resulting in decreased coronary diastolic filling. It may be administered as 5–10 U/100 mL saline over 5 min and then 20 U/500 mL saline over 4 h. The rate should be decreased if there is an increase in the heart rate [39].

The main anesthetic goals cover standard monitoring, and phenylephrine is the preferred vasopressor for avoiding hypotension.

13.9.1.1 Cardiopulmonary Bypass During Pregnancy

A great burden is created on the cardiovascular system due to pregnancy, and it can result in decompensation in women with an underlying cardiac disease. In order to minimize the maternal and fetal risks, medical treatment should be the first choice. However, in cases that are unresponsive to medical treatment, corrective cardiac operations should be performed. As a general principle, surgery requiring cardiopulmonary bypass (CPB) should not be performed until the second trimester or later. In order to detect fetal bradycardia on bypass, continuous intraoperative fetal monitoring is necessary. For the compensation of the lack of autoregulation in the uteroplacental unit, high normal-range perfusion pressures during CPB should be kept at 60 mmHg or more, while hypothermia on bypass is usually maintained at 32 °C and not lowered below as lower temperatures may lead to fetal dysrhythmias and fetal cardiac arrest [40–42].

Even though it would be suitable to avoid such surgery until after pregnancy, no pregnant patient should be denied a definitive operation due to gestation. As long as it is possible, cardiac surgery should be avoided during the period of organogenesis, and the second trimester is preferred. If CPB is required following 28 weeks' gestation, the cesarean delivery immediately prior to the cardiac surgery is suggested as a reasonable and safe procedure [14].

Among the many potential side effects of CPB, alteration of the cellular protein components of blood as well as coagulation, vasoactive substance release from leukocytes, complement activation, particulate and air embolism, nonpulsatile flow, hypotension, and hypothermia can be listed. Uteroplacental perfusion and fetal development can be hindered by all these factors. Moreover, the blood flow can be obstructed, and reduced right ventricular filling and resultant alterations in placental perfusion can be caused by the cannulation of the inferior vena cava. The effects of the pump and perfusate type that are employed during CPB and the duration of perfusion on maternal and fetal outcome are well known. Theoretically, CPB-related factors including nonpulsatile perfusion, hyperoxygenation, and heparinization may have adverse effects on the placenta and the fetus [40, 41].

All in all, to prevent the deleterious effects caused by the reduction in perfusion of the placental intervillous space during CPB, high flow rate (>2.5 L/m^2/min) and high pressure (mean arterial pressure>70 mmHg) are recommended in parallel to the physiologic increase in maternal cardiac output accompanying the increase in gestational age. However, in spite of a perfusion flow rate of 3 L/m^2, permanent fetal bradycardia was reported to indicate fetal acidosis. Short periods of normothermic and pulsatile perfusions, where possible, are considered to be useful as well [40–42].

Even though hypothermia is believed to protect the fetus as it reduces fetal oxygen requirement, the application of normothermic or mild hypothermic perfusion is recommended unless the aortic clamp time is unexpectedly long since the rewarming period can be a risk for premature labor because of the augmentation of the uterine contractions. Despite loss of FHR during CPB, fetal heart sounds were reheard in the intensive care unit as we stated in our previous study, and therefore, we presumed that the loss of fetal heart tones should not always indicate fetal death [40].

To sum up, the appropriate selection and dosage of anesthetic agents and supportive agents; the maintenance of acid-base balance during open-heart operations in pregnant women; the use of high flow rate, high perfusion pressure, and normothermia or mild hypothermia during CPB; the minimization of the duration of CPB and the aortic cross-clamp time; and the continuous cardiotocographic monitoring during and after the entire procedure are suggested.

13.9.2 Primary Pulmonary Hypertension

Primary pulmonary hypertension (PPH) is characterized by significantly increased pulmonary artery pressure in the absence of an intracardiac or aortopulmonary shunt. Pulmonary hypertension is not tolerated well in the parturients. Deterioration typically occurs in the second trimester with fatigue, dyspnea, syncope, and chest pain symptoms. This is because of the physiological increase in CO and blood volume by 40–50%. During labor, uterine contractions effectively add 500 mL of blood to the circulation. Right atrium (RA) pressure, blood pressure, and CO are increased by the pain and expulsive effort of labor [27, 33].

Women who have PPH are advised not to become pregnant. A termination should be considered in early pregnancy as maternal mortality may be as high as 30–40% and a high incidence of preterm delivery and fetal loss is in question. In undiagnosed PPH until late in pregnancy, an elective delivery at 32–34 weeks' gestation is recommended, since premature spontaneous labor is not uncommon. Patients with PPH often have a reactive pulmonary vascularity which is likely to be responsive to vasodilator therapy [43, 44].

The anesthetic management goals are similar to those of Eisenmenger syndrome. As a good pulmonary vasodilator, supplemental oxygen should be administered routinely. Intra-arterial blood pressure as well as central venous pressure monitoring is required. During cesarean delivery, the intraoperative use of TEE has been reported [45]. Among the agents that have been used to treat PPH, inhaled nitric oxide (NO), nitroglycerin, calcium entry blockers, and prostaglandins are listed. Patients with PPH carry a risk of thrombosis and thromboembolism. The outcome in severe pulmonary hypertension can be improved by anticoagulation therapy [43, 46, 47].

Epidural anesthesia does not only render a pain-free first and second stage of labor possible but also helps elective forceps delivery. The successful use of epidural anesthesia for cesarean delivery has been noted. It is essential that epidural anesthesia be induced slowly. The IV fluids should be used to treat hypotension, and ephedrine should be avoided since it can cause an increase in pulmonary artery pressure. Regarding cases where regional anesthesia is contraindicated due to concurrent anticoagulant therapy, IV dexmedetomidine and etomidate have proven to be useful as an adjunct to general anesthesia in order to provide pain relief and hemodynamic stability [48–50].

The main anesthetic goals include supplemental oxygen and invasive hemodynamic monitoring, avoiding pulmonary artery catheter and treating pulmonary hypertension.

13.9.3 Cardiomyopathy

Cardiomyopathy can be classified as hypertrophic, restrictive, or dilated.

13.9.3.1 Hypertrophic Cardiomyopathies

Idiopathic hypertrophic subaortic stenosis (IHSS) or asymmetric septal hypertrophy (ASH) is a disease which does not have a defined etiology. Among the primary features of this cardiomyopathy are significant hypertrophy of the left ventricle and interventricular septum and obstruction of the left ventricular outflow tract during systole by the hypertrophied muscle. In some patients, the possible displacement of the anterior leaflet of the mitral valve may add to obstruction. Depending on both the severity and nature of the disorder, patients with IHSS experience a variable effect of the cardiovascular and hemodynamic changes of pregnancy. The pregnancy-related increase in blood volume yields a useful effect as it increases preload. The usual increase in heart rate and stroke volume in pregnancy as well as the decrease in SVR, beginning during the second trimester, may have a negative effect on cardiac performance. Although there is a potential for LV failure and cardiac arrhythmias during pregnancy, the outcome of patients with IHSS has been notably good [2, 33].

The therapeutic objectives during parturition should include minimization of increases in catecholamine levels associated with pain, maintenance of preload by sufficient IV fluid administration, and also avoidance of the Valsalva maneuver causing a sudden decrease in preload.

The employment of systemic narcotics, inhaled analgesics, or paracervical block is recommended for analgesia in the first stage of labor. Regional analgesia has been considered a substantial risk due to the potential for both venodilation and arterial dilation leading to decreased SVR. Nevertheless, this is likely to be avoided if careful incremental titration of lumbar epidural analgesia is administered. Analgesia at a limited segmental level from T10 to L2 provides adequate analgesia with minimal sympathetic blockade, and thus preload is preserved. Optimal analgesia is obtained with dilute solutions of a local anesthetic agent with the addition of a narcotic, such as fentanyl. The employment of intrathecal narcotics is also possible; thus the risk of sympathetic blockade is eliminated, but the potential side effects of respiratory depression, pruritus, and nausea may be increased; however, all of these can be easily treated [1, 51].

For a patient with IHSS, a combined spinal and epidural analgesic approach has been used successfully. It is possible to accomplish vaginal delivery with pudendal block, epidural analgesia extended carefully, or saddle block. The spinal segments from L2 to S5 are included in the saddle block, and thus the majority of sympathetic nerve elements are avoided. Regional anesthesia is efficient in blocking the uncontrollable urge to bear down. If a vasopressor-requiring hypotension occurs, the use of ephedrine is relatively contraindicated as it causes tachycardia and increased myocardial contractility. Metaraminol or phenylephrine should be administered in the lowest effective dose in order to minimize its effect on the uterine arteries. For hypotension after sympathetic blockade, the treatment of choice is phenylephrine in 50 μg increments; however, larger doses of phenylephrine should not be administered to prevent further reduction in placental perfusion [52, 53].

There are additional challenges related to anesthesia for cesarean delivery. Left uterine displacement must be maintained, and volume requirements must be carefully evaluated in anticipated greater blood loss. General anesthesia is preferred widely, and the use of volatile anesthetic agents is considered advantageous since they reduce myocardial contractility; however, they also cause a decrease in uterine contractility and SVR. The stimulating effects of laryngoscopy and intubation need to be pharmacologically blunted for the preeclamptic patient. Oxytocin must be administered carefully as it may lead to a decrease in SVR and result in tachycardia when it is administered rapidly. The parturient with IHSS requires careful attention through appropriate monitoring and the immediate availability of the necessary vasopressors, beta blockers, and IV volume expanders [1, 53].

13.9.3.2 Restrictive Cardiomyopathies

Restrictive cardiomyopathy is an uncommon entity representing the end stage of myocarditis or an infiltrative process of the myocardium, such as amyloidosis or hemochromatosis. It imitates constrictive pericarditis and is characterized by impaired ventricular filling and poor contractility. At the beginning, CO is maintained by an increase in heart rate and filling pressure, but not by an increase in myocardial contractility. Whether the dominant feature of the disease is restrictive ventricular filling or impaired ventricular function determines the anesthetic management. Therapy focuses on the provision of sufficient ventricular filling, heart rate, and myocardial contractility. Since beta agonists such as isoproterenol or dobutamine do not only increase ejection fraction but also raise heart rate and usually decrease SVR, they are the inotropic agents of choice. Epidural anesthesia is preferred over general anesthesia since myocardial depressants can be avoided and under general anesthesia, venous return can be decreased by positive pressure ventilation [2, 54].

13.9.3.3 Dilated Cardiomyopathies

In pregnant patients, idiopathic dilated cardiomyopathy may be present with a reported incidence of 5–8/100,000 live births per year. This is a poorer outcome in comparison to peripartum cardiomyopathy (PPCM). Diagnostic criteria for PPCM are the development of heart failure within the last month of pregnancy or 5 months' postpartum without any prior heart diseases and with no cause that can be determined. There also has to be an echocardiographical indication of LV failure such as ejection fraction <45% or fractional shortening <30% and end-diastolic dimension >2.7 cm/m^2 body surface area [55].

The incidence of PPCM is approximately between 1/3000 and 1/4000 pregnancies. Dilated cardiomyopathy that is unexplained should be treated as heart failure, regardless of the presence of congestion. Although symptoms may occur abruptly, cardiac failure often develops subtly. In 20–40% of cases, symptoms may resolve spontaneously with little or no treatment. PPCM can be related to pulmonary hypertension; however, in this case, it may result in multiorgan failure. Parturients present with fatigue, dyspnea, edema, and occasionally chest pain with hemoptysis. They often have a raised jugular venous pressure, cardiomegaly, and gallop rhythm. Hypokinetic dilated ventricles with normal valves are reported in echocardiography [33, 56, 57].

In such cases, treatment with diuretics, inotropes, afterload reducers, and anticoagulants is empirical. In women with myocarditis and LV dysfunction, immunosuppressive therapy with oral prednisone and azathioprine for 6–8 weeks has improved LV function and prognosis. Continuous venovenous hemofiltration has proven to be successful in the treatment of severe cardiomyopathy after failure in conventional therapy. Heart transplantation is considered for severe cases that do not respond to all medical therapy [2, 58].

Anesthetic goals include avoiding general anesthesia whenever possible, slow induction of epidural anesthesia has a better outcome, pulmonary artery pressure monitoring, and also reduction of preload and afterload.

13.9.4 Pregnancy Postcardiac Transplant

Cardiac transplantation has become an accepted mode of therapy for many end-stage heart diseases, and thus, a number of parturients with cardiac transplant have successfully come to term and delivered vaginally or by cesarean section. Patients with organ transplants must be maintained on immunosuppressive therapy in order to prevent rejection. This usually includes cyclosporine, steroids, and antibiotics, all of which must be continued during pregnancy. Strict attention to sterile technique is crucial. Before anesthesia and surgery, prophylactic antibiotics and "stress dose" of steroids are indicated [59, 60].

The heart rate is affected only by sympathomimetic agents which act directly (atropine is ineffective, whereas isoprenaline is effective). Unlike the case in normal patients, sympathectomy associated with high central neuraxial blocks will not cause bradycardia. Because of the upregulation of receptors, these patients may be more sensitive to beta-mimetics (adrenaline being clinically significant). It is essential to avoid endogenous catecholamines associated with pain. The optimal choice is the induction of continuous epidural analgesia with low concentration of local anesthetic solution with opioid early in labor. Thus, in the event of an obstetric emergency, it will be possible to bring up the level rapidly, and the need for general or single-shot spinal anesthesia and the uncontrolled hemodynamic changes related to these techniques will be avoided. Epidural or continuous spinal anesthesia techniques allow careful titration and a greater control of cardiovascular parameters. Blood pressure ought to be maintained with volume loading and ephedrine, phenylephrine, or mephentermine. The use of central neuraxial narcotics is advantageous. In cases where general anesthesia is used, thiopental will possibly have exaggerated depressant effects on transplanted heart. Due to the change in beta receptor sensitivity, ketamine may cause excessive tachycardia. The most stable induction will be obtained by a high-dose fentanyl technique or etomidate, though onset time will be longer with narcotics [2, 54].

Eventually, the cooperative efforts of the obstetrician, the cardiologist, and the anesthesiologist involved in peripartum care determine the successful management of the pregnant cardiac patient. With regard to this high-risk group of parturients, a thorough understanding of physiology of pregnancy and pathophysiology of the underlying cardiac disease is essential in obstetric and anesthetic management.

Key Learning Points
- Anesthesiologists should not assume a dogmatic approach regarding the choice of anesthesia for parturients with heart disease.
- Each case should be assessed individually, by paying special attention to the functional damage.
- For the provision of optimal conditions for labor and delivery, an understanding of the hemodynamics associated with the structural lesion and the appropriate use of invasive monitors bears great importance.

References

1. Kuczkowski KM. Anesthesia for the parturient with cardiovascular disease. South Afr J Anaesth Analg. 2014;9:19–25.
2. Luthra A, Bajaj R, Jafra A, Jangra K, Arya VK. Anesthesia in pregnancy with heart disease. Saudi J Anaesth. 2017;11:454–71.
3. Gianopoulos JG. Cardiac disease in pregnancy. Med Clin North Am. 1989;73:639–51.
4. Johnson MD, Saltzman DH. Cardiac disease. In: Dutta S, editor. Anesthetic and obstetric management of high-risk pregnancy. St Louis: Mosby; 1996. p. 200–45.
5. The Criteria Committee of the New York Heart Association. Nomenclature and criteria for diagnosis of diseases of the heart and great vessels. 9th ed. Boston: Little, Brown; 1994. p. 253–6.
6. Kuczkowski KM. Labor analgesia for the parturient with cardiac disease: what does an obstetrician need to know? Acta Obstet Gynecol Scand. 2004;83:223–33.
7. Ramin SM, Maberry MC, Gilstrap LC 3rd. Congenital heart disease. Clin Obstet Gynecol. 1989;32:41–7.
8. Van de Velde M. Nonobstetric surgery during pregnancy. In: Chestnut DH, Wong CA, Tsen LC, Ngan Kee WD, Beilin Y, Mhyre J, editors. Chestnut's obstetric anesthesia principles and practice. 5th ed. Philadelphia: Saunders; 2014. p. 358–79.
9. Ní Mhuireachtaigh R, O'Gorman DA. Anesthesia in pregnant patients for nonobstetric surgery. J Clin Anesth. 2006;18:60–6.
10. Mazze RI, Kallen B. Reproductive outcome after anesthesia and operations during pregnancy: a registry study of 5405 cases. Am J Obstet Gynecol. 1989;161:1178.
11. Ngan Kee WD, Lau TK, Khaw KS, Lee BB. Comparison of metaraminol and ephedrine infusions for maintaining arterial pressure during spinal anesthesia for elective cesarean section. Anesthesiology. 2001;95:307–13.
12. Lee A, Ngan Kee WD, Gin T. A quantitative, systematic review of randomized controlled trials of ephedrine versus phenylephrine for the management of hypotension during spinal anesthesia for cesarean delivery. Anesth Analg. 2002;94:920–6.
13. Steinbrook RA, Bhavani-Shankar K. Hemodynamics during laparoscopic surgery in pregnancy. Anesth Analg. 2001;93:1570–1.
14. Parry AJ, Westaby S. Cardiopulmonary bypass during pregnancy. Ann Thorac Surg. 1996;61:1865–9.
15. Dajani AS, Bisno AL, Chung KJ, Durack DT, Freed M, Gerber MA, et al. Prevention of bacterial endocarditis. Recommendations by the American Heart Association. JAMA. 1990;264:2919–22.
16. Moore RA. Anesthesia for pediatric congenital heart patient for non-cardiac surgery. Anesthesiol Rev. 1981;8:23.
17. Oxorn D, Edelist G, Smith MS. An introduction to transoesophageal echocardiography: II. Clinical applications. Can J Anaesth. 1996;43:278–94.
18. Wong V, Cheng CH, Chan KC. Fetal and neonatal outcome of exposure to anticoagulants during pregnancy. Am J Med Genet. 1993;45:17–21.
19. Barbour LA, Pickard J. Controversies in thromboembolic disease during pregnancy: a critical review. Obstet Gynecol. 1995;86:621–33.
20. Sugrue D, Blake S, MacDonald D. Pregnancy complicated by maternal heart disease at the National Maternity Hospital, Dublin, Ireland: 1969 to 1978. Am J Obstet Gynecol. 1981;139:1–6.
21. Clark SL. Monitoring and anaesthetic management of parturients with mitral stenosis. Can J Anaesth. 1987;34:654.
22. Hemmings GT, Whalley DG, O'Connor PJ, Benjamin A, Dunn C. Invasive monitoring and anaesthetic management of a parturient with mitral stenosis. Can J Anaesth. 1987;34:182–5.
23. WDN K, Shen J, Chiu AT, Lok I, Khaw KS. Combined spinal-epidural analgesia in the management of labouring parturients with mitral stenosis. Anaesth Intensive Care. 1999;27:523–6.

24. Ziskind S, Etchin A, Frenkel Y, Mashiach S, Lusky A, Goor DA, et al. Epidural anesthesia with the trendelenburg position for cesarean section with or without a cardiac surgical procedure in patients with severe mitral stenosis: a hemodynamic study. J Cardiothorac Anesth. 1990;3:354–9.
25. Batson MA, Longmire S, Csontos E. Alfentanil for urgent caesarean section in a patient with severe mitral stenosis and pulmonary hypertension. Can J Anaesth. 1990;37:685–8.
26. Rayburn WF, Fontana ME. Mitral valve prolapse and pregnancy. Am J Obstet Gynecol. 1981;41:9–11.
27. Shaikh SI, Lakshmi RR, Hegade G. Perioperative anesthetic management for cesarean section in patients with cardiac disease. Anesth Pain Intensive Care. 2014;18:377–85.
28. Easterling TR, Chadwick HS, Otto CM, Benedetti TJ. Aortic stenosis in pregnancy. Obstet Gynecol. 1988;72:113–8.
29. Colclough GW, Ackerman WE 3rd, Walmsley PM, Hessel EA. Epidural anesthesia for a parturient with critical aortic stenosis. J Clin Anesth. 1995;7:264–5.
30. Redfern N, Bower S, Bullock RE, Hull CJ. Alfentanil for caesarean section complicated by severe aortic stenosis. A case report. Br J Anaesth. 1988;60:477.
31. Forster R, Joyce T. Spinal opioids and the treatment of the obstetric patient with cardiac disease. Clin Perinatol. 1989;16:955–74.
32. Walker E, Malins AF. Anesthetic management of aortic coarctation in pregnancy. Int J Obstet Anesth. 2004;13:266–70.
33. Maitra G, Sengupta S, Rudra A, Debnath S. Pregnancy and non-valvular heart disease – anesthetic considerations. Ann Card Anaesth. 2010;13:102–9.
34. Vidovich MI. Cardiovascular disease. In: Chestnut DH, Wong CA, Tsen LC, Ngan Kee WD, Beilin Y, Mhyre J, editors. Chestnut's obstetric anesthesia principles and practice. 5th ed. Philadelphia: Saunders; 2014. p. 960–1002.
35. Mangano DT. Anesthesia for the pregnant cardiac patient. In: Shnider SM, Levinson G, editors. Anesthesia for obstetrics. 3rd ed. Philadelphia: Williams & Wilkins; 1993. p. 485.
36. Brickner ME. Cardiovascular management in pregnancy: congenital heart disease. Circulation. 2014;130:273–82.
37. Patton DE, Lee W, Cotton DB, Miller J, Carpenter RJ Jr, Huhta J, et al. Cyanotic maternal heart disease in pregnancy. Obstet Gynecol Surv. 1990;45:594–600.
38. Aglio LS, Johnson MD. Anesthetic management of myocardial infarction in a parturient. Br J Anaesth. 1990;65:258–61.
39. Smith RL, Young SJ, Greer IA. The parturient with coronary heart disease. Int J Obstet Anesth. 2008;17:46–52.
40. Mahli A, Izdes S, Coskun D. Cardiac operations during pregnancy: review of factors influencing fetal outcome. Ann Thorac Surg. 2000;69:1622–6.
41. Chambers CE, Clark SL. Cardiac surgery during pregnancy. Clin Obstet Gynecol. 1994;37:316–23.
42. Rossouw GJ, Knott-Craig CJ, Barnard PM, Macgregor LA, Van Zyl WP. Intracardiac operation in seven pregnant women. Ann Thorac Surg. 1993;55:1172–4.
43. Monnery L, Nanson J, Charlton G. Primary pulmonary hypertension in pregnancy; a role for novel vasodilators. Br J Anaesth. 2001;87:295–8.
44. Weiss BM, Zemp L, Seifert B, Hess OM. Outcome of pulmonary vascular disease in pregnancy: a systematic overview from 1978 through 1996. J Am Coll Cardiol. 1998;31:1650–7.
45. Palmer CM, DiNardo JA, Hays RL, van Maren GA. Use of transesophageal echocardiography for delivery of a parturient with severe pulmonary hypertension. Int J Obstet Anesth. 2002;11:48–51.
46. Decoene C, Bourzoufi K, Moreau D, Narducci F, Crepin F, Krivosic-Horber R. Use of inhaled nitric oxide for emergency cesarean section in a woman with unexpected primary pulmonary hypertension. Can J Anaesth. 2001;48:584–7.
47. Lam GK, Stafford RE, Thorp J, Moise KJ Jr, Cairns BA. Inhaled nitric oxide for primary pulmonary hypertension in pregnancy. Obstet Gynecol. 2001;98:895–8.

48. Khan MJ, Bhatt SB, Kryc JJ. Anesthetic considerations for parturient with primary pulmonary hypertension: review of the literature and clinical presentation. Int J Obstet Anesth. 1996;5:36–42.
49. Toyama H, Wagatsuma T, Ejima Y, Matsubara M, Kurosawa S. Cesarean section and primary pulmonary hypertension: the role of intravenous dexmedetomidine. Int J Obstet Anesth. 2009;18:262–7.
50. Coskun D, Mahli A, Korkmaz S, Demir FS, Inan GK, Erer D, et al. Anaesthesia for caesarean section in the presence of multivalvular heart disease and severe pulmonary hypertension: a case report. Cases J. 2009;22(2):9383.
51. Minnich ME, Quirk JG, Clark RB. Epidural anesthesia for vaginal delivery in a patient with idiopathic hypertrophic subaortic stenosis. Anesthesiology. 1987;67:590–2.
52. Ho KW, Kee WDN, Poon MCM. Combined spinal and epidural anesthesia in a parturient with idiopathic hypertrophic subaortic stenosis. Anesthesiology. 1997;87:168–9.
53. Tessler MJ, Hudson R, Naugler-Colville M, Biehl DR. Pulmonary oedema in two parturients with hypertrophic obstructive cardiomyopathy (HOCM). Can J Anaesth. 1990;37:469–73.
54. Gei AF, Hankins GD. Cardiac disease and pregnancy. Obstet Gynecol Clin N Am. 2001;28:465–512.
55. Yacoub A, Martel MJ. Pregnancy in a patient with primary dilated cardiomyopathy. Obstet Gynecol. 2002;99:928.
56. Kluger MT, Bersten AD. Multi-organ failure in peripartum cardiomyopathy. Anaesth Intensive Care. 1991;19:450–3.
57. Hibbard JU, Lindheimer M, Lang RM. A modified definition for peripartum cardiomyopathy and prognosis based on echocardiography. Obstet Gynecol. 1999;94:311–6.
58. Beards SC, Freebairn RC, Lipman J. Successful use of continuous veno-venous haemofiltration to treat profound fluid retention in severe peripartum cardiomyopathy. Anaesthesia. 1993;48:1065–7.
59. Löwenstein BR, Vain NW, Perrone SV, Wright DR, Boullón FJ, Favaloro RG. Successful pregnancy and vaginal delivery after heart transplantation. Am J Obstet Gynecol. 1988;158(3 Pt 1):589–90.
60. Camann WR, Goldman GA, Johnson MD, Moore J, Greene M. Cesarean delivery in a patient with a transplanted heart. Anesthesiology. 1989;71:618–20.

Anesthesia for Parturient with Human Immunodeficiency Virus

14

Hasan Kutluk Pampal and Gökçen Emmez

14.1 Introduction

Acquired immunodeficiency syndrome (AIDS) is a global health problem especially seen in low and middle income countries. The disease was first described in 1981 in adults, and the causative agent, human immunodeficiency virus (HIV), was first isolated in 1983 [1, 2]. Infection with this virus is accepted to cause "a disease knowing no borders and respecting no moral codes" [3]. The most recent United Nations update declares 34.5 million adults living with HIV with the fact that 51% of these adults are females. The majority of these women are of childbearing age [4]. Also UNAIDS data reveal that everyday nearly 2000 women are newly diagnosed with HIV infection, and half of these women are aged between 15 and 24 years.

With the dramatic success of highly active antiretroviral treatment (ART), disease "with no borders" has evolved from a fatal condition to a chronic condition. Despite the relative decline in HIV infections for the last few years, as the HIV survivors increase by time, it is inevitable for anesthesiologists to come across such patients. When dealing with HIV-infected patients, the anesthesiologists must pay attention to the stage of the disease, comorbidities, antiviral therapy, and its possible interactions with anesthetic drugs. Moreover, it is also important to protect health-care workers and other patients from contamination.

The aim of this chapter is to review the HIV infection and the challenges of anesthetic management particularly for parturient infected with HIV. The preoperative evaluation, the choice of anesthetic technique, and the problems related to ART as well as the prevention of transmission will be discussed briefly in this chapter.

H. K. Pampal (✉) · G. Emmez
Gazi University Faculty of Medicine, Department of Anesthesia, Ankara, Turkey
e-mail: kutlukpampal@gazi.edu.tr

© Springer International Publishing AG, part of Springer Nature 2018   205
B. Gunaydin, S. Ismail (eds.), *Obstetric Anesthesia for Co-morbid Conditions*,
https://doi.org/10.1007/978-3-319-93163-0_14

14.2   Pathophysiology

Human immunodeficiency virus, the causative agent of the disease, is a member of the lentivirus, a subtype of human retroviruses. There are two types of HIV: HIV-1 and HIV-2. Although both of them cause similar clinical problems, HIV-1 is known to be more virulent and infective than HIV-2 and is the major cause of worldwide HIV infections. Human immunodeficiency virus is a single-stranded RNA virus. Upon binding of viral envelope protein GP160 to the specific CD4$^+$ receptors found on T4 lymphocytes with a co-receptor named chemokine co-receptor (CCR5), the virion fuses with host membrane and enters the cell. Viral reverse transcriptase transcribes RNA genome to double-stranded DNA, and the viral DNA imports into nucleus to integrate to host genomic DNA by viral integrase. This integration results in latency of virus and avoids detection of the virus from immune system. The virus can remain silent in the host cells for an indefinite time. Alternatively, the transcription of integrated viral DNA to viral RNA and messenger RNA later forms various viral progeny [5, 6].

14.3   Transmission

Transmission of HIV occurs generally with human secretions and blood. Heterosexual transmission is the most common way of transmission. One important way of transmission is the vertical one, from mother to child, during pregnancy, labor, delivery, and breastfeeding [5, 6].

14.4   Clinical Findings

After transmission, an initial period with acute flu-like symptoms commonly occurs within 2–6 weeks. Following this period, viral levels decrease to and equilibrate at a viral set point. This viral set point helps to predict the speed of progression of the disease. A higher set point is generally related to a rapid progression. In this latent period, the virus can stay dormant in host cells, corresponding to an asymptomatic clinical course for patients lasting for 6–12 years. Thereafter the advanced period of the disease takes place with rising viral loads and declining CD4$^+$ T-lymphocytes counts. This period comes along with quantitative and qualitative T4$^+$ lymphocytes deficiency resulting in opportunistic infections and neoplasms [5, 6].

14.4.1 Seroconversion and Diagnosis

Seroconversion generally occurs within 2–8 weeks but can be prolonged to 12 weeks. A few individuals do not seroconvert until 6 months [5]. There are three types of HIV diagnostic tests: antigen/antibody tests, antibody tests, and nucleic acid tests. Traditional HIV testing is done using enzyme-linked immunosorbent assay (ELISA) to detect antibodies against HIV-1. More specific tests are polymerase chain reaction (PCR), Western blotting, nucleic acid testing, and immunofluorescence assays (IFA). The latest recommendation by CDC is to start with an immunoassay combination test for HIV-1 and HIV-2 antibodies and p24 antigen [7]. The CDC recommends testing for HIV at least once as a part of routine healthcare for individuals between 13 and 64 and annually for those with higher risk. In case of a possible HIV exposure, follow-up testing for HIV is recommended by CDC at 45th and 90th days of exposure if the earlier tests are negative [7].

14.5 Anesthetic Management

14.5.1 Preoperative Evaluation

Preoperative evaluation should involve past medical history, systemic examination, laboratory tests, assessment of the organs involved, and ART including the complications related to drugs. Most of the anesthesiologists do not question about drug abuse which is an important coexisting problem in patients with HIV, and it is also mentioned that the number of anesthesiologist assessing the patients whether they are HIV-positive or not is even fewer [8]. However, possibility of HIV infection, intravenous drug use, and alcohol abuse should always be questioned for safe anesthesia management and for protecting healthcare workers who will deal with the patient.

Detailed history of the patients in terms of multiple organ involvement, drug therapy, and adverse events should also be determined and recorded during preoperative evaluation. Other sexually transmitted diseases such as syphilis and hepatitis B should also be questioned. Detailed neurological examination and documentation are important in patients with syphilis as the disease effects neurological system in later stages [9].

Human immunodeficiency virus infection is a multisystem disease, and nearly all vital organ systems are involved as indicated below:

Cardiovascular system involvement may present as pericardial, myocardial, or vascular lesions. Intravenous drug users may present with infective endocarditis. Pericarditis is the most frequent cardiovascular pathology observed in HIV-positive patients. The pathophysiology of the cardiovascular disease is not clear, but it is thought to be multifactorial. Opportunistic infections, HIV itself, and ART are some of the accused etiological factors [10]. Antiretroviral therapy, especially protease inhibitors, may cause premature atherosclerosis which leads to coronary disease [11].

The respiratory system findings of HIV-positive patients may be related to both the upper and lower respiratory tract. The most important underlying factor for pulmonary disease in these patients is the opportunistic infections. Neoplasms such as Kaposi sarcoma or lymphoma also play a role in the etiology of the HIV-related pulmonary abnormalities. Kaposi sarcoma is the commonest neoplasm found in AIDS patients. It is usually located at the head and neck, and it may present as supraglottic mass without causing stridor which requires vigilance. The most well-known organism in HIV-positive patients responsible for the pulmonary infections is the *Pneumocystis jiroveci* (known as *Pneumocystis carinii* before 1999). It usually occurs when CD4$^+$ count is less than 200 cell/mm^3 [11]. Tuberculosis is a common cause of respiratory failure in HIV-positive patients. Patients with HIV are more prone to acquire infection when they are exposed to infectious environment, and reactivation of latent tuberculosis is more common because of the defective cellular immunity. Pulmonary secretions should be evaluated for *Myocobacterium tuberculosis* in suspected patients. Arterial blood gas analysis and pulmonary function test may also be performed for preoperative assessment of the respiratory functions in HIV-positive pregnant patients. If general anesthesia is planned, maximum attention should be paid to sterility, and the availability of postoperative intensive care and ventilatory support should be considered [12].

Gastrointestinal system abnormalities are common, and almost all the patients with HIV encounter HIV-related gastrointestinal pathology. Pathologies located at the oral cavity or esophagus lead to increased risk of aspiration and difficulties during intubation or mask ventilation. Viral esophagitis, aphthous ulcers, and leukoplakia cause severe pain and difficulty in swallowing. Hepatobiliary disease is common and may lead to elevated liver function tests. Primer infection of the intestinal epithelium with HIV or with the opportunistic agents leads to severe and chronic diarrhea. These patients may have fluid and electrolyte imbalance which should be corrected before the surgery [8, 9].

Renal system involvement may present as acute renal failure. Sepsis, dehydration, and adverse effects of drugs play an important role in HIV-associated renal failure. Besides, deposition of immune complexes also leads to proliferative glomerulonephritis. There is a specific entity known as HIV-associated nephropathy characterized by a focal segmental glomerulosclerosis and leads to renal failure especially in African-American patients [9].

Nervous system manifestations can occur at any time during the course of HIV infection, and clinical findings are specific to the stage of the disease. These findings are important especially if neuraxial anesthesia is planned. Headache, photophobia, cognitive changes, cranial neuropathy, and meningoencephalitis are nonspecific and self-limited signs observed in the initial period of HIV infection [8, 9]. Even isolation of the virions and antibodies in cerebrospinal fluid is possible during this early phase [13]. Demyelinating neuropathy and cerebrospinal fluid abnormalities, even in asymptomatic patients, occur during latent phase of the infection [14]. Late stages of the HIV infection are associated with meningitis, diffuse encephalopathy, focal central nerve system lesions, myelopathy, and peripheral neuropathy seen in almost all patients. AIDS dementia complex is a severe, late-stage neurological manifestation of the disease in which cognitive and motor functions are impaired, but level of alertness is preserved [9]. Postural hypotension, syncope, or diarrhea can be observed in HIV-positive patients as a result of neurological involvement leading to autonomic dysfunction [14]. Both neoplasms such as Kaposi sarcoma, primary central nervous system lymphoma, and neurological adverse effects of ART should be considered during preoperative neurological evaluation of the patients.

The primary target of the anesthetic techniques is either the peripheric or central nervous system. Therefore, full preoperative neurological evaluation and appropriate documentation are of crucial importance.

Hematologic abnormalities associated with HIV infection include anemia, leukopenia, thrombocytopenia, and coagulation disturbances. Anemia is the most common cause of hematologic abnormality in HIV-infected patients, and if untreated it indicates poor prognosis [15]. The major cause of hematologic disturbances in HIV-infected patents is bone marrow suppression as a result of direct HIV infection, secondary opportunistic infections, malignancies, and adverse drug reactions [16]. Coagulation abnormalities are common in HIV-infected patients and occur as a consequence of HIV-related immune activation and vascular disease. Prolonged activated partial thromboplastin time may present because of lupus anticoagulants, and it is related with higher incidence of major thromboembolic events [9]. Hence, assessing the whole blood count and coagulation parameters is essential for preoperative evaluation.

Endocrine and metabolic disturbances observed in HIV-infected patients are lipodystrophy and metabolic syndrome (elevated plasma levels of triglycerides, glucose, and cholesterol) which are associated with ART. Most serious endocrine complication of HIV infection is primary or secondary adrenal insufficiency [17]. Although they are asymptomatic, thyroid function tests of the patients with HIV infection are usually abnormal. Possible causes of endocrine and metabolic disturbances in these patients may be direct effects of HIV on the related gland, opportunistic infections, neoplasms, and ART [18].

A list of various organ-related abnormalities is summarized in Table 14.1.

Table 14.1 Clinical findings of organ involvement of HIV infection

Organ systems	Problems associated with HIV infection	
Cardiovascular system	Pericardial effusion	Acute coronary syndrome
	Dilated cardiomyopathy	Vasculitis
	Endocarditis	Pulmonary hypertension
	Valvular lesions	Kaposi sarcoma
Respiratory system	Obstruction (tumor/infection)	Pneumonia
	Bronchitis	Pneumothorax
	Sinusitis	Atypical infections (Tuberculosis)
Gastrointestinal system	Esophagitis/dysphagia	Biliary disease
	Regurgitation	Malnutrition
	Hepatitis	Diarrhea
Renal system	Drug induced nephrotoxicity	HIV-associated nephropathy
Neurological system	Headache	Meningitis
	Photophobia	Diffuse encephalopathy
	Meningoencephalitis	Focal CNS lesions
	Cognitive changes	Myelopathy
	Demyelinating neuropathy	Peripheral neuropathy
	Abnormal CSF findings	Myopathy
Hematological system	Anemia	Thrombocytopenia
	Leukopenia	Coagulation disturbances
Endocrine and metabolic system	Lipodystrophy	SIADH
	Metabolic syndrome	Hypo/hyperthyroidism
	Adrenal insufficiency	Lactic acidosis

In addition to routine laboratory tests such as full blood count, clotting functions, biochemical tests (glucose, hepatic and renal functions, electrolytes), electrocardiography, and organ-specific advanced investigations may be performed in order to elicit the functions of the various systems that are involved. Determining the viral load and CD4$^+$ count is strongly advised in HIV-positive parturient.

14.5.2 Choice of the Anesthetic Technique: General vs Regional

Regional anesthesia (epidural, spinal, and combined spinal epidural (CSE)) is the preferred way of anesthesia management for cesarean delivery. Recent knowledge reveals a progressive increase in the use of regional techniques, especially spinal anesthesia, both in developed and developing countries [19]. Although regional anesthesia techniques have several advantages in otherwise healthy parturient over general anesthesia, one can ask whether it is safe to use them in HIV-positive patients.

The major concern in HIV-infected patients who will undergo regional anesthesia is spreading the infection into the previously uninfected central nervous system or worsening the preexisting neurological symptoms. However, there is no data in the literature that regional anesthesia accelerates the progression of the disease or increases perioperative complications. In fact it is a well-known fact that HIV is a neurotropic virus and virions and antibodies of HIV can be isolated even at the early phase of the disease [20].

Hughes et al. evaluated the effects of regional anesthesia on 30 HIV-infected parturient of whom 18 received neuraxial anesthesia for labor. They followed up 30 patients who received regional anesthesia for labor analgesia and cesarean delivery [21]. They followed up the patients for 4–6 months postpartum and did not observe any neurologic complication or alterations in immune functions. A review by Avidan et al. comparing the effects of spinal anesthesia in 44 HIV-infected parturient with 45 healthy patients undergoing cesarean section confirmed the findings of the above study as they found no difference between the two groups in terms of intraoperative hemodynamic stability or postoperative complications [22].

Another question is whether it is a malpractice to perform regional anesthesia in a patient who has neurologic involvement with or without clinical signs. Considering the benefits of regional anesthesia and other possible organ system involvements such as pulmonary or cardiac and the aforementioned clinical evidence about the early neurologic involvement of the disease, it seems logical to use neuraxial techniques in HIV-infected parturient.

Finally epidural and CSE anesthesia have the advantage of a catheter for effective postoperative pain control. However, placing and holding a catheter in the epidural space for some time after surgery may increase the risk of infection. Therefore, spinal anesthesia with local anesthetic and opioids for postoperative analgesia seems to be safer than the techniques that a catheter is placed.

When administrating general anesthesia for HIV-infected parturient, the most important factors that should be considered are possible immunomodulatory effects of anesthetic drugs, organ system involvement and drug interactions, and adverse effects of ART. Possible immunodepressant effects of any drug or condition in immunosuppressed HIV-infected patients should be a great concern. Therefore, the immunomodulatory effect of general anesthetics is an important issue in parturient who will have general anesthesia.

The effects of various anesthetic agents on immune system have been widely investigated, but the debate on the topic still goes on. The data is derived mostly from in vitro studies rather than clinical studies. It is hard to investigate the sole role of anesthetics on human studies because various variables such as type and duration of the surgery and patient-dependent variables contribute to the total effect on patient's immune system.

Recent knowledge on this issue reveals that general anesthesia may lead to transient immune depression, but no study was able to show that this depression is of clinical significance in healthy patients [23]. Pregnancy also suppresses patient's cell-mediated immune system [24]. However, no increase in complication rate and worsening of the HIV infection related to general anesthesia were shown in a retrospective study by Gershon and Manning-Williams [25].

It is not possible to recommend general or regional anesthesia in terms of the effects on the immune system in HIV-infected parturient. Further studies assessing the effects of anesthetic drugs and techniques on immune system in HIV-infected parturient are needed. In the light of recent literature, anesthesiologist should also consider the fact that the immune suppression related to general anesthesia could be clinically significant in HIV-infected parturient. The argument for choosing the better anesthetic technique should focus on the stage of the disease, affected organ systems, and drug interactions rather than immunomodulatory effects or neurological spread.

If general anesthesia is preferred, endotracheal intubation should be performed with a strict sterile technique. Prolonged postoperative mechanical ventilation should be avoided in order to prevent ventilator-associated pneumonia [9].

Although both general anesthesia and regional anesthesia seem safe for HIV-infected parturient, potential immunomodulatory effects of general anesthesia, additional risk factors due to organ involvement, drug interactions between general anesthetics and ART, and evidence for the safety of regional anesthesia lead us to recommend regional techniques unless there is a contraindication.

Another concern about the parturient receiving regional anesthesia is the possibility of postdural puncture headache (PDPH). Despite all precautions and using a careful technique, pregnancy remains as a risk factor for PDPH. If PDPH is diagnosed, the initial treatment should be conservative usually pharmacological and noninvasive. Recumbent bed rest and aggressive hydration are common methods. Bed rest can relieve headache but it is not therapeutic. Although hydration is the most common therapeutic regimen for PDPH, there is no evidence in the literature that has showed its effectiveness. Pharmacological treatment of the PDPH includes methylxanthines (caffeine, theophylline, and aminophylline), sumatriptan, adrenocorticotropic hormone and corticosteroids, gabapentin, and pregabalin [26]. If the symptoms of PDPH do not resolve despite the conservative and pharmacological therapies, then epidural blood patch should be performed. It should be mentioned that the concern about spreading the virus to the central nervous system is unnecessary because no serious complications have been reported to date [5]. Although they are not effective as autologous epidural blood patch, epidural infusion of normal saline or colloidal solutions are alternative invasive methods [26]. Other proposed alternatives are epidural patch with fresh allogeneic whole blood and platelet-rich plasma or epidural injection of fibrin glue. However, these methods need further investigation [9, 26, 27].

14.5.3 Drugs Used for HIV-Infected Parturient and Anesthesia

Drugs used by HIV-infected parturient can be classified into two groups: antiretroviral drugs which are used to treat the primary disease and the drugs used for prophylaxis or treatment of opportunistic infections. The use of ART during pregnancy has the goal of reducing or eliminating mother to child transmission besides the treatment of the maternal HIV infection. All parturients with HIV infection should be treated with combination ART regardless of the CD4+ cell count. Extensive use of ART during pregnancy has led the incidence of mother to child transmission to decrease to levels less than 2% [28, 29]. Although adverse event rates are elevated, mother to child transmission is prevented better with combination therapy than single-drug therapy [30]. When ART is initiated earlier in an HIV-infected parturient, effective reduction in mother to child transmission is achieved [31]. The study by Hoffman et al. showed that each additional week of highly active ART in an HIV-infected parturient reduced the incidence of mother to child transmission by 8% [32]. Therefore, strategies should be developed to facilitate earlier initiation of the combination ART in especially low resource settings. Moreover the treatment should not be limited to antepartum or intrapartum period. A strategy including ART during antepartum, intrapartum, and also postpartum periods for infant prophylaxis is more effective in preventing mother to child transmission [28, 33].

Recent developments in the treatment of HIV infection improved the outcome of the HIV-infected patients. Six groups of antiretroviral drugs which are usually used in combination are listed in Table 14.2. The treatment plan includes different groups of antiretroviral drugs in order to minimize the development of resistance pattern [34]. Human immunodeficiency virus treatment with a combination of three or more antiretroviral drugs is called highly active ART. Usually one or two nucleoside reverse transcriptase inhibitors (NRTI) are combined with one nonnucleoside reverse transcriptase inhibitors (NNRTI) and/or protease inhibitors (PI). If a patient exhibits drug resistance than a fourth agent can be added to the treatment regimen.

Anesthesiologists should be aware of the adverse effects of the ART and question the patient during the preoperative assessment. The adverse effects related to ART can be classified into four groups. Lactic acidosis, hepatic toxicity, pancreatitis, and peripheral neuropathy are related to mitochondrial dysfunction. Fat maldistribution and change in body composition, dyslipidemia, hyperglycemia, and insulin resistance are the result of metabolic disturbances. Bone marrow suppression leads to anemia,

Table 14.2 Classification of anti-retroviral drugs with mechanism of action and side effects

Drug class	Mechanism of action	Examples	Side effects
Protease inhibitors	Prevents cleavage of viral precursor proteins into the subunits required for the formation of new virions	Saquinavir	Nephrolithiasis, diarrhea, enzyme inhibition, elevated triglycerides
		Ritonavir	
		Indinavir	
		Nelfinavir	
Nucleoside reverse transcriptase inhibitors	Inhibiting viral DNA synthesis by preventing reverse transcription Also inhibits human mitochondrial DNA polymerase	Zidovudine	Bone marrow suppression, myopathy, neuropathy, diarrhea, headache, lactic acidosis, pancreatitis
		Lamivudine	
		Emtricitabine	
		Abacavir	
		Didanosine	
Nonnucleoside reverse transcriptase inhibitors	Inhibiting viral DNA synthesis by preventing reverse transcription Do not require phosphorylation/do not inhibit human DNA polymerases	Nevirapine	Rash, dizziness, teratogenicity, enzyme induction
		Delavirdine	
		Efavirenz	
Integrase inhibitors	Inhibit incorporation into cellular genome	Raltegravir	Hepatotoxicity
Fusion inhibitors	Interfere with HIV binding to cells, preventing entry	Enfuvirtide	Headache, bacterial pneumonia
CCR5 antagonists		Maraviroc	

neutropenia, and thrombocytopenia. Finally skin rashes and hypersensitivity responses are related to allergic reactions. Risk of cardiovascular disease is associated with long-term use of the antiretroviral drugs. Premature atherosclerosis which is a characteristic cardiovascular pathology in HIV-infected patients worsens with the use of PI due to further impairment of endothelial function. Hyperlipidemia and insulin resistance occur after PI exposure and they further increase cardiovascular risks. Lipodystrophy is a syndrome of fat redistribution characterized with central fat accumulation and peripheral fat loss [11]. The appearance of the patient may mimic Cushing's disease, but the hypothalamic-pituitary-adrenal axis is normal. Lipodystrophy causes redistribution of fat to the neck, back of the neck, and abdomen. Thus, airway management which may be a potential problem in pregnant patients may be more difficult, and intraabdominal pressure further increases [11]. Drug interaction is an important concern especially for HIV-infected parturient who will have surgery under general anesthesia as anesthetic drugs may interact with antiretroviral medications.

Protease inhibitors are metabolized by cytochrome P450 system and they are inhibitors of CYP3A [35]. However, ritonavir is also a potent inducer of P450 isoenzymes.

Potential drug interactions with PI and opioids, benzodiazepines, local anesthetics, neuromuscular blockers, and antiarrhythmic drugs should be kept in mind during anesthetic management of the HIV-infected parturient.

Impairment in metabolism of opioids, especially fentanyl and alfentanil, has been observed which leads to respiratory depression because of higher serum levels.

Drug interaction with fentanyl occurs both with enzyme induction and inhibition: enzyme inhibition leads to reduction in clearance of fentanyl, and enzyme induction increases its metabolism to active metabolites. Remifentanil is not dependent on P450 metabolism; therefore it can be the safest choice of opioid in these patients.

Administering benzodiazepines to patients using PI may also lead to prolonged sedation and respiratory depression. Dose reduction of midazolam and diazepam is advised in parturient using PI. Amiodarone, calcium channel blockers, digoxin, and quinidine should be used carefully because of the cardiovascular toxicity caused by the interaction with PI [35].

Opioids may also interact with NNRTI. This group of antiretroviral drugs leads to both cytochrome enzyme induction and inhibition depending on the specific drug being administered. They affect the plasma concentration of methadone and opioids. Nevirapine and efavirenz reduce plasma concentration of methadone by 50%. It is recommended to increase the dose of fentanyl and alfentanil in patients using NNRTI [36].

Nucleoside reverse transcriptase inhibitors are prodrugs, and activation requires intracellular phosphorylation. They are main drugs for combination therapy. Fortunately they do not interact through the P450 enzyme system [37]. Interaction with metronidazole may lead to peripheral neuropathy, and combination of zidovudine and corticosteroids is reported to cause severe myopathy and respiratory muscle dysfunction [11].

14.5.4 Role of Anesthesiologist in Preventing Transmission of HIV

Anesthetists play an important role in preventing or decreasing the risk of transmission of HIV infection to uninfected patients. Transfusion of infected blood is the most common cause of transmission of blood-borne infections. Not only HIV but also coinfections frequently found in HIV-infected patients such as HBV and HCV can also be transmitted. Anesthesiologists can reduce the risk of transmission by minimizing allogenic blood transfusion. This is possible by having an adequate knowledge on blood transfusion practices and following the updated guidelines.

Other route of transmission is contamination of the devices used during anesthesia practice. Most of the devices are reusable, but laryngoscope blades, face masks, and endoscopes can be the source of transmission. Human immunodeficiency virus may survive up to 7 days outside the body; however, it is quite sensitive to disinfectants such as sodium hypochlorite and heat [38]. Therefore, ASA Subcommittee on Infection Control Policy recommends that such equipment with visible blood on it should be washed as soon as possible. Routine hospital sterilization techniques are usually enough to eradicate the HIV, but ASA recommends high level of sterilization or disinfection methods [8, 39]. Apart from blood-borne infections, tuberculosis may also be transmitted as a result of inhalational exposure. A filter that protects the anesthesia machine from contamination should be used in the circuit to avoid exposure of the machine to mycobacterium tuberculosis. Internal components of the anesthesia machine should be cared for according to the manufacturer's recommendations. Unidirectional valves, carbon dioxide absorbent chambers, and bellows should be cleaned and disinfected.

Human Immunodeficiency virus can also be transmitted to healthcare workers as a result of exposure to infected body fluids. Universal safety precautions should be used during anesthesia management of the HIV-infected patients regardless of the HIV status.

Not only anesthesiologists but also all healthcare providers should wear gloves in order to avoid direct contact of infected fluids to open lesions of the hands. Double gloving or using virus-inhibiting gloves are extra safety precautions that can be easily practiced [40]. Sharp objects should be handled carefully for preventing penetrating injuries. Needles should not be recapped and discarded properly in the appropriate containers. If there is a risk of exposure of blood or other body fluids to the eye, eye shields should be used [41].

It is impossible to eliminate the risk of exposure although all precautions have been used. Once the percutaneous exposure to HIV-infected blood has occurred, the transmission of HIV is approximately 0.3% [42]. All healthcare workers with needlestick injury should take ART as soon as possible. This is called postexposure prophylaxis, and drugs should be taken maximum of 72 h, at least for 4 weeks [43]. Postexposure prophylaxis usually includes combination of three or even four antiretroviral drug. Group of drugs preferred for PEP are usually NRTI, integrase inhibitors, PI, and NNRTI [44]. According to the guidelines in pregnant healthcare workers, the PEP procedure is the same with any other person, but certain drugs such as efavirenz, stavudine, didanosine, and indinavir should be avoided because of teratogenicity, lactic acidosis, or hyperbilirubinemia in newborns [45].

Modern ART prolongs the lives of the patients with HIV infection. Most of the HIV-infected patients are at the childbearing age which means that anesthesiologist will face with parturient during the perioperative period. The unique properties of the disease such as immunosuppression and multiple organ involvement, adverse effects, and interactions of the drugs make the anesthetic management of these pregnant patients more complex. Possibility of transmission of the virus to newborn or healthcare providers is another important concern in these patients. Therefore, the anesthesiologist must have adequate knowledge of the disease, clinical manifestations, treatment, and complications in order to provide patient safety during anesthetic management.

Key Learning Points
- HIV infection is accepted as a chronic condition rather than a fatal condition due to the success of ART.
- The anesthesiologist encounters HIV-positive parturients more frequently.
- Either general or regional anesthesia can be the choice of anesthetic technique in a HIV-positive parturient.
- Preventing transmission of the disease to newborn and healthcare workers is an important concern when dealing with an HIV-positive parturient.
- It is essential for the anesthesiologist to have adequate knowledge of the disease, clinical manifestations, treatment, and complications in order to provide patient's and healthcare workers' safety.

References

1. Gottlieb MS, Schroff R, Schanker HM, Weisman JD, Fan PT, Wolf RA, et al. Pneumocystis carinii pneumonia and mucosal candidiasis in previously healthy homosexual men: evidence of a new acquired cellular immunodeficiency. N Engl J Med. 1981;305:1425–31.
2. Barré-Sinoussi F, Chermann JC, Rey F, Nugeyre MT, Chamaret S, Gruest J, et al. Isolation of a T-lymphotropic retrovirus from a patient at risk for acquired immune deficiency syndrome (AIDS). Science. 1983;220:868–71.
3. Hughes SC. AIDS: the focus turns to women. Int J Obstet Anesth. 1993;2:1–2.
4. UNAIDS data 2017. http://www.unaids.org/sites/default/files/media_asset/20170720_Data_book_2017_en.pdf. Accessed 20 Feb 2018.
5. Hignett R, Fernando R. Anesthesia for the pregnant HIV patient. Anesthesiol Clin. 2008;26:127–43.
6. Bajwa SJS, Kulshrestha A. The potential anesthetic threats, challenges and intensive care considerations in patients with HIV infection. J Pharm Bioallied Sci. 2013;5:10–6. https://doi.org/10.4103/0975-7406.106554.
7. HIV testing. https://www.cdc.gov/hiv/testing/index.html. Accessed 20 Feb 2018.
8. Kuczkowski KM. Human immunodeficiency virus in the parturient. J Clin Anesth. 2003;15:224–33.
9. Wlody DJ. Human immunodeficiency virus. In: Chestnut DH, Wong CA, Tsen LC, Kee WDN, Beilin Y, Mhyre JM, Nathan N, editors. Chestnut's obstetric anesthesia: principles and practice E-book. Amsterdam: Elsevier Health Sciences; 2014.
10. Ntusi N, O'Dwyer E, Dorrell L, Wainwright E, Piechnik S, Clutton G, et al. HIV-1-related cardiovascular disease is associated with chronic inflammation, frequent pericardial effusions, and probable myocardial edema. Circ Cardiovasc Imaging. 2016;9:e004430.
11. Conte AH. Infectious disease. In: Hines RL, Marschall KE, editors. Stoelting's anesthesia and co-existing disease. 7th ed. Philadelphia: Elsevier; 2018.
12. Prout J, Agarwal B. Anaesthesia and critical care for patients with HIV infection. Contin Educ Anesth Crit Care Pain. 2005;5:153–6.
13. Denning DW, Anderson J, Rudge P, Smith H. Acute myelopathy associated with primary infection with human immunodeficiency virus. Br Med J (Clin Res Ed). 1987;294:143–4.
14. Evron S, Glezerman M, Harow E, Sadan O, Ezri T. Human immunodeficiency virus: anesthetic and obstetric considerations. Anesth Analg. 2004;98:503–11.
15. Leelanukrom R. Anaesthetic considerations of the HIV-infected patients. Curr Opin Anaesthesiol. 2009;22:412–8.
16. Vishnu P, Aboulafia DM. Haematological manifestations of human immune deficiency virus infection. Br J Haematol. 2015;171:695–709.
17. Eledrisi MS, Verghese AC. Adrenal insufficiency in HIV infection: a review and recommendations. Am J Med Sci. 2001;321:137–44.
18. Lo JC, Schambelan M. Adrenal, gonadal, and thyroid disorders. In: Dolin R, Masur H, Saag MS, editors. AIDS therapy. 3rd ed. St. Louis: Churchill Livingstone; 2008.
19. Caton D. Cesarean delivery. In: Chestnut DH, Wong CA, Tsen LC, Kee WDN, Beilin Y, Mhyre JM, Nathan N, editors. Chestnut's obstetric anesthesia: principles and practice. 5th ed. Philadelphia: Elsevier Saunders; 2014.
20. García F, Niebla G, Romeu J, Vidal C, Plana M, Ortega M, et al. Cerebrospinal fluid HIV-1 RNA levels in asymptomatic patients with early stage chronic HIV-1 infection: support for the hypothesis of local virus replication. AIDS. 1999;13:1491–6.
21. Hughes SC, Dailey PA, Landers D, Dattel BJ, Crombleholme WR, Johnson JL. Parturients infected with human immunodeficiency virus and regional anesthesia. Clinical and immunologic response. Anesthesiology. 1995;82:32–7.
22. Avidan MS, Groves P, Blott M, Welch J, Leung T, Pozniak A. Low complication rate associated with cesarean section under spinal anesthesia for HIV-1-infected women on antiretroviral therapy. Anesthesiology. 2002;97:320–4.

23. Cruz FF, Rocco PR, Pelosi P. Anti-inflammatory properties of anesthetic agents. Crit Care. 2017;21:67.
24. Barnett MA, Learmonth RP, Pihl E, Wood EC. T helper lymphocyte depression in early human pregnancy. J Reprod Immunol. 1983;5:55–7.
25. Gershon RY, Manning-Williams D. Anesthesia and the HIV infected parturient: a retrospective study. Int J Obstet Anesth. 1997;6:76–81.
26. Katz D, Beilin Y. Review of the alternatives to epidural blood patch for treatment of postdural puncture headache in the parturient. Anesth Analg. 2017;124:1219–28.
27. Gunaydin B, Acar M, Emmez G, Akcali D, Tokgoz N. Epidural patch with autologous platelet rich plasma: a novel approach. J Anesth. 2017;31:907–10.
28. Townsend CL, Cortina-Borja M, Peckham CS, de Ruiter A, Lyall H, Tookey PA. Low rates of mother-to-child transmission of HIV following effective pregnancy interventions in the United Kingdom and Ireland, 2000–2006. AIDS. 2008;22:973–81.
29. European Collaborative Study. Mother-to-child transmission of HIV infection in the era of highly active antiretroviral therapy. Clin Infect Dis. 2005;40:458–65.
30. Fowler MG, Qin M, Fiscus SA, Currier JS, Flynn PM, Chipato T, et al. Benefits and risks of antiretroviral therapy for perinatal HIV prevention. N Engl J Med. 2016;375:1726–37.
31. Townsend CL, Byrne L, Cortina-Borja M, Thorne C, de Ruiter A, Lyall H, et al. Earlier initiation of ART and further decline in mother-to-child HIV transmission rates, 2000–2011. AIDS. 2014;28:1049–57.
32. Hoffman RM, Black V, Technau K, van der Merwe KJ, Currier J, Coovadia A, et al. Effects of highly active antiretroviral therapy duration and regimen on risk for mother-to-child transmission of HIV in Johannesburg, South Africa. J Acquir Immune Defic Syndr. 2010;54:35–41.
33. Tubiana R, Le Chenadec J, Rouzioux C, Mandelbrot L, Hamrene K, Dollfus C, et al. Factors associated with mother-to-child transmission of HIV-1 despite a maternal viral load <500 copies/ml at delivery: a case-control study nested in the French perinatal cohort (EPF-ANRS CO1). Clin Infect Dis. 2010;50:585–96.
34. Menéndez-Arias L. Targeting HIV: antiretroviral therapy and development of drug resistance. Trends Pharmacol Sci. 2002;23:381–8.
35. de Maat MM, Ekhart GC, Huitema AD, et al. Drug interactions between antiretroviral drugs and comedicated agents. Clin Pharmacokinet. 2003;42:223–82.
36. Schulenburg F, Le Roux PJ. Antiretroviral therapy and anaesthesia. SAJAA. 2008;14:31–8.
37. Piscitelli SC, Gallicano KD. Interactions among drugs for HIV and opportunistic infections. N Engl J Med. 2001;344:984–96.
38. Coates TJ, Collins J. Preventing HIV infection. Sci Am. 1998;279:96–7.
39. American Society of Anesthesiology subcommittee on infection control policy recommendations for infection control for the practice of anesthesiology. https://asahq.org/~/media/sites/asahq/files/public/resources/asa%20committees/recommendations-for-infection-control-for-the-practice-of-anesthesiology-(1).pdf?la=en. Accessed 20 Feb 2018.
40. Bricout F, Moraillon A, Sonntag P, Hoerner P, Blackwelder W, Plotkin S. Virus-inhibiting surgical glove to reduce the risk of infection by enveloped viruses. J Med Virol. 2003;69:538–45.
41. Baluch A, Maass H, Rivera C, Gautam A, Kaye AD, Frost EA. Current perioperative management of the patient with HIV. Middle East J Anaesthesiol. 2009;20:167–77.
42. Diprose P, Deakin CD, Smedley J. Ignorance of post-exposure prophylaxis guidelines following HIV needlestick injury may increase the risk of seroconversion. Br J Anaesth. 2000;84:767–70.
43. Panlilio AL, Cardo DM, Grohskopf LA, Heneine W, Ross CS, US Public Health Service. Updated U.S. Public Health Service guidelines for the management of occupational exposures to HIV and recommendations for postexposure prophylaxis. MMWR Recomm Rep. 2005;54:1–17.
44. Guidelines for the use of antiretroviral agents in HIV-1-infected adults and adolescents. https://aidsinfo.nih.gov/contentfiles/lvguidelines/adultandadolescentgl.pdf. Accessed 20 Feb 2018.
45. Parthasarathy S, Ravishankar M. HIV and anaesthesia. Indian J Anaesth. 2007;51:91–9.

Anesthesia for Pregnant Patients with Eisenmenger Syndrome

15

Ahmet Mahli and Demet Coskun

15.1 Introduction

Eisenmenger syndrome is a complex combination of cardiovascular abnormalities. It involves pulmonary hypertension, a right-to-left extra-cardiac shunt, and arterial hypoxemia [1]. Pregnancy is not tolerated very well by patients who have this condition. When pregnancy occurs in women with Eisenmenger syndrome, medical termination is considered to be safer than any delivery mode [2]. Because these patients have little or no cardiac reserve and need a normal sinus rhythm to meet the increased workload, acute arrhythmias are particularly dangerous. Therefore, maternal mortality rate is estimated to be 30–50% [3].

A typical example of what is known as Eisenmenger complex was first described by Dr. Victor Eisenmenger [4] in 1897. Necroscopy findings suggested the presence of a 2–2.5 cm ventricular septal defect (VSD), a large right ventricle, and substantial atherosclerosis of the pulmonary artery and its branches while there was none in the aorta. Secondary to multiple thrombosis, there was extensive hemorrhagic infarction of the lungs. Wood's definition of Eisenmenger complex was pulmonary hypertension at systemic level due to a high pulmonary vascular resistance (PVR) with reversed or bidirectional shunt through a large VSD. It was also noted by Wood that when any communication between the two circulations is complicated by a raised PVR that is sufficient to cause reverse (right-to-left) shunting, a similar physiological situation occurred [5].

A. Mahli
Yuksek Ihtisas University School of Medicine, Department of Anesthesiology and Reanimation, Ankara, Turkey
e-mail: amahli@gazi.edu.tr

D. Coskun (✉)
Gazi University School of Medicine, Department of Anesthesiology and Reanimation, Ankara, Turkey
e-mail: dcoskun@gazi.edu.tr

© Springer International Publishing AG, part of Springer Nature 2018
B. Gunaydin, S. Ismail (eds.), *Obstetric Anesthesia for Co-morbid Conditions*,
https://doi.org/10.1007/978-3-319-93163-0_15

15.2   Pathophysiology

Eisenmenger syndrome is described as a chronic, uncorrected right-to-left shunt, produces right ventricular hypertrophy, elevated pulmonary artery pressure, and right ventricular dysfunction. Atrial septal defect (ASD), VSD, or patent ductus arteriosus (PDA) may be the primary lesion [6]. As a result of the chronic pulmonary volume overload, the pulmonary and the right ventricle musculature goes through remodeling; flow through the pulmonary vasculature is limited by the high fixed pulmonary artery pressure; and when the level of systemic pressure is exceeded by pulmonary artery pressure, reversal of shunt flow occurs. The initial left-to-right shunt then becomes a right-to-left shunt and conclusively leads to the Eisenmenger syndrome, which involves the sequelae of arterial hypoxemia and right ventricle failure [7].

In the Eisenmenger syndrome, there is decreased cross-sectional area of the pulmonary arteriolar bed with commonly irreversible, pulmonary hypertension. The pulmonary hypertension precludes corrective surgery because after surgical closure of the defect, the elevated PVR persists or worsens. However, this is not the case with patients who have obligatory right-to-left shunts such as Fallot's tetralogy when, even in adulthood, the hemodynamic status may be improved by corrective surgery. Sometimes, in patients who have Eisenmenger syndrome, the increased resistance is not fixed and an attempt for the correction of the underlying pulmonary-systemic connection may result in an improved hemodynamic status. In Eisenmenger syndrome, PVR and systemic vascular resistance (SVR) are approximately the same, and the shunt is balanced. A sudden increase in the right-to-left shunt, which is clinically associated with an increase in cyanosis, can occur due to either an increase in PVR or a fall in SVR. The factors that are known to be in favor of the development of pulmonary hypertension are hypercarbia, acidosis, hypoxia, high left atrial pressure, and a high pulmonary blood flow. Despite the fact that the attempts made in order to decrease PVR in the case of Eisenmenger syndrome are generally ineffective, SVR remains either normal or low and responds to physiological and pharmacological influences. Any fall that occurs in SVR will be adverse, as such a fall causes an increase in the right-to-left shunt and, thus, arterial hypoxemia. An increase in SVR will increase the left-to-right shunt and pulmonary blood flow, which is detrimental as it causes a further increase in pulmonary arterial blood pressure [8–11].

15.3   Clinical Manifestations

The pregnant women who have Eisenmenger syndrome may present with cyanosis or differential cyanosis, dyspnea, fatigue, dizziness, and even right heart failure [12]. Cyanosis and clubbing of the fingers may be observed during physical examinations [13]. Hemorrhagic tendency like epistaxis and hemoptysis has been documented [14]. Auscultation may disclose an inspiratory crepitation [15] and a loud P2 and a systolic murmur at the pulmonary area. Jugular venous distention and mild lower

extremity edema can be observed [13]. Patients may suffer from a low oxygen saturation [16] and polycythemia [17]. Severe complications, such as heart failure, endocarditis, and thromboembolic accidents, may develop in case of pregnancy. Delivery
by a pregnant woman who has Eisenmenger syndrome represents an increased risk
of pulmonary thromboembolism and sudden death, which often occurs within the
first few days of postpartum [16]. Cardiomegaly with bilateral pulmonary congestion
may be seen in a chest X-ray [15]. Right ventricular hypertrophy and sometimes left
ventricular hypertrophy is revealed by electrocardiogram [18].

Patients may present for any elective and emergent surgery. Among the more
common indications for elective surgery are dental procedures, gynecologic procedures, left and right heart catheterization, transesophageal echocardiogram, appen-
dectomy, cholecystectomy, etc. Additionally, anesthetic management should be
planned depending on which trimester of pregnancy the mother is in.

15.4 Anesthetic Considerations

The primary goals of anesthetic management for pregnant patient with Eisenmenger
syndrome are maintaining adequate SVR, intravascular volume, and venous return,
avoiding aortocaval compression and myocardial depression perioperatively, and
preventing pain, hypoxemia, hypercarbia, and acidosis, which may cause an increase
in PVR [19]. Anesthetic considerations focus on avoiding any decrease in
SVR. Hypotension due to any cause results in insufficient right ventricular pressure
required to perfuse the hypertensive pulmonary arterial bed, which may result in
sudden death of the patient [20].

Particularly regarding obstetric or surgical procedures in the lower abdomen, a
choice between a general or regional anesthetic technique may be required. General
and regional anesthesia techniques have yielded satisfactory results in patients with
Eisenmenger syndrome. Any anesthetic technique chosen for a patient who has
Eisenmenger syndrome should be based on the principle of avoiding a decrease in
arterial blood pressure which requires the maintenance of both cardiac output and
SVR [21–23].

Regarding patients that present for noncardiac surgery and have Eisenmenger
syndrome, the induction and maintenance of anesthesia should center on the maintenance of preoperative baseline hemodynamics, avoidance from hypotension to
prevent the worsening of right-to-left shunt, and provision of adequate gas exchange
via the lungs so as to reduce shunting, acidosis, and cardiac decompensation. The
objective of pharmacologic management of patients who have Eisenmenger physiology is the attenuation of the increased PVR [19].

In order to avoid the hazard of paradoxical air embolism, particular attention
should be paid by the anesthetist regarding infusion lines, as well as by the surgeon
regarding the opening of large veins or venous sinuses when the patient is in a position in which vascular air entrainment is possible. Fluid replacement requires meticulous attention since a loss in extracellular fluid is not tolerated well. On the other
hand, an overload of volume may cause an increase in right-to-left shunt, or right

ventricular failure, or even both. Additionally, current medical therapies (phospho-diesterase-5 inhibitors, prostanoids, and endothelin-1 receptor antagonists) should be continued perioperatively [24, 25].

Regarding the choice of anesthesia, the anesthetic technique that is least likely to decrease the patient's systemic blood pressure and SVR should be chosen since such changes cause an increase in the magnitude of right-to-left shunting and cyanosis. Myocardial function is depressed, and SVR is reduced by many anesthetic agents that are used for induction and maintenance of general anesthesia [26].

Induction of anesthesia presents the time when a fall in SVR and hypotension are likely to occur. Right-to-left shunt results in a short arm-brain circulation time, and thus, agents that are given intravenously will act very quickly. As barbiturates reduce cardiac output and decrease the tone of the systemic capacitance vessels, they lead to hypotension, which is an effect that is dose-dependent. Ketamine has advantages as it does not reduce SVR and has been used to induce anesthesia in patients with the Eisenmenger syndrome. Etomidate and midazolam are other alternatives since they have minimal cardiovascular effects [8, 27]. Opioids are quite effective in blunting sympathetic discharges during anesthesia and surgery causing minimal or no myocardial depression [28]. Since remifentanil is known to be rapidly metabolized by nonspecific plasma esterases, it has a very short context-sensitive half-life. Remifentanil has been reported to provide safe anesthesia in Eisenmenger syndrome patients undergoing noncardiac surgery [22]. Ketamine and etomidate with supplemental opioids to attenuate the sympathetic surge during stimulation and intubation are among the frequently used drugs. In order to avoid periods of hypoventilation, general anesthesia should be induced rapidly, but the occurrence of significant hypotension should not be allowed. A bolus of a vasopressor during induction was shown to be beneficial in reducing hypotension in patients receiving general anesthesia, and thus, it should be considered. An infusion of vasopressor may be ideal to maintain SVR both during induction and maintenance of anesthesia. In order to decrease the catecholamine surge that is present in patients with poorly controlled pain, pain management is required, and multimodal analgesia may be considered [29].

Either volatile agents or total intravenous anesthesia (TIVA) can be used to maintain general anesthesia. It is known that volatile agents decrease SVR with less effect on the pulmonary system. The decreased response to hypoxemia via the hypoxic pulmonary vasoconstrictive response, which is blunted by volatile anesthetics, is a potential benefit. Although N_2O has little effect on pulmonary blood flow, it leads to pulmonary vasoconstriction, which results in an increase in PVR. The effects of TIVA on hypoxic pulmonary vasoconstriction are less than those of volatile agents. SVR decrease during TIVA may be more common than it is with volatile agents, and drug concentration could be titrated successfully using bispectral index. For any method of maintenance, opioids need to be discreetly given in order to reduce significant effects on respiration (hypoventilation, hypercarbia, decreased ventilatory responsiveness to hypoxia, etc.) [30].

Because of insufflation with CO_2 under pressure, general anesthesia with laparoscopic surgery presents a particular increased risk in Eisenmenger syndrome. This may lead to hypercapnia which is difficult to manage and results in respiratory acidosis, potential worsening of the right-to-left shunt with subsequent hypotension, arterial deoxygenation, and ultimately cardiac decompensation. Trendelenburg positioning can exacerbate these intraoperative events to a further degree and result in acute decompensation. If the patient does not tolerate any portion of the laparoscopic procedure, open surgical procedures may be required, and the surgical team should be ready to reduce the intra-abdominal pressure rapidly to achieve hemodynamic compensation [31, 32].

Regional anesthesia has been successfully used in noncardiac surgery in addition to parturients which offers an alternative to general anesthesia. In order to provide surgical anesthesia, selective nerve blocks can be used under judicious sedation. Regarding neuraxial blocks, epidural anesthesia is preferred over subarachnoid block as it allows for slow titration of the anesthetic level as well as close monitoring of hemodynamics. In this patient population, spinal anesthesia is contraindicated because of the rapid and often unpredictable block level. Significant hypotension and cardiac decompensation potential can dramatically lead to the worsening of the shunt fraction. Epidural anesthesia should be slowly topped up, and preparations that contain epinephrine should be avoided since encountering an intravascular injection may affect PVR significantly [33, 34]. Nevertheless, the successful use of spinal anesthesia during cesarean delivery in patients who have Eisenmenger syndrome has been reported [35, 36].

Regardless of anesthetic technique, oxygen desaturation and potential refractory hypotension may be the indicators of acute hemodynamic decompensation [31, 32]. Hypotension is frequently followed by oxygen desaturation as the worsening of the shunt is in question. For the treatment or prevention of hypotension, phenylephrine is usually the drug of choice for many anesthetists, though the effect on the pulmonary vasculature with a pure alpha-agonist may require mixed agents, such as ephedrine or norepinephrine. Vasopressin is another potential effective vasopressor owing to its reduced effect on the pulmonary vascular bed while maintaining SVR [37]. Further treatment in addition to vasopressor delivery includes the correction of hypercarbia, hypoxia, acidosis, and hypothermia, since they all trigger worsening of pulmonary hypertension. Moreover, as excessive sympathetic response can increase PVR, inadequate anesthesia or analgesia should be reevaluated and managed [38, 39].

In the postoperative period, a rapid return to consciousness and avoidance of hypoxia, which would cause an increase in PVR, are essential. Avoidance of extreme changes in heart rate, oxygen therapy, and early mobilization are also recommended. Monitoring of such patients closely during the postoperative period up to a week is essential, looking out for worsening of the shunt and thromboembolic phenomenon since these are complications that can occur as late as third postoperative day [8, 40].

Finally, anesthetic management of patients who have Eisenmenger syndrome is challenging. If the patient reaches full term, a multidisciplinary approach including close communication between obstetrician, cardiologist, and anesthesiologist is crucial. No matter what the anesthetic technique is, the principle always remains the same. The cardiac output must be maintained, and SVR must not be allowed to fall at all times. Thus, minimal change in the amount of right-to-left shunt will be ensured.

Key Learning Points

- The anesthetic goal in patients who have Eisenmenger syndrome should be to provide a stable cardiac output without causing any exacerbation in the intracardiac shunt.
- In case of a requirement for an operation, either regional or general anesthesia is used very cautiously.
- Both regional and general anesthesia can potentially cause an increase in the right-to-left shunt: regional anesthesia results in such an increase by reducing SVR, while general anesthesia increases PVR due to catecholamine release particularly during laryngoscopy, intubation, and surgical stimulation.
- The general principle of anesthesia should always be based on the maintenance of cardiac output and avoidance of a fall in SVR.

References

1. Kuczhowski KM. Labour analgesia for parturient with cardiac disease – what does an obstetrician need to know? Acta Obstet Gynecol Scand. 2004;83:223–33.
2. Ghai B, Mohan V, Khetarpal M, Malhotra N. Epidural anaesthesia for C section in patients with Eisenmenger syndrome. Int J Obstet Anesth. 2002;11:44–7.
3. Avila WS, Grinberg M, Snitcowsky R, Faccioli R, Luz PL, Bellotti G, et al. Maternal and fetal outcome in pregnant women with Eisenmenger's syndrome. Eur Heart J. 1995;16:460–4.
4. Eisenmenger V. Die angeborenon Defete der Kammerscheiderwand des Herzeas. Z Klin Med. 1897;32:1–28.
5. Wood P. The Eisenmenger syndrome or pulmonary hypertension with reversed central shunt. Br Med J. 1958;2:701–709, 755–762.
6. Laura L, Klein MD, Henry L, Galar MD. Cardiac diseases in pregnancy. Clin Obstet Gynecol N Am. 2004;31:429–59.
7. Blanchard DG, Shabetai R. Cardiac diseases. In: Creasy RK, Resnik R, Iams JD, editors. Maternal-fetal medicine. 5th ed. Philadelphia: Saunders; 2004. p. 823–4.
8. Foster JMG, Jones RM. The anaesthetic management of the Eisenmenger syndrome. Ann R Coll Surg Engl. 1984;66:353–5.
9. Jones A, Howitt G. Eisenmenger syndrome in pregnancy. Br Med J. 1965;1:1627–31.
10. Yuan S-M. Eisenmenger syndrome in pregnancy. Braz J Cardiovasc Surg. 2016;31:325–9.
11. Asling J, Fung D. Epidural anesthesia in Eisenmenger's syndrome: a case report. Anesth Analg. 1974;53:965–8.
12. Wang L, Liu YN, Zhang J. Analysis of the pregnancy outcome of 7 pregnant women with Eisenmenger's syndrome. Clin Med. 2010;30:3–5.
13. Fang G, Tian YK, Mei W. Anaesthesia management of caesarean section in two patients with Eisenmenger's syndrome. Anesthesiol Res Pract. 2011;2011:972671.
14. Mukhopadhyav P, Bhattacharya P, Begum N. Successful pregnancy outcome with Eisenmenger syndrome. J Obstet Gynaecol India. 2012;62:68–9.
15. Bazmi S, Malhotra S, Zaman F. A rare case of pregnancy with Eisenmenger syndrome. Int J Obstet Gynaecol Res (IJOGR). 2015;2:151–4.
16. Kahn ML. Eisenmenger's syndrome in pregnancy. N Engl J Med. 1993;329:887.
17. Borges VT, Magalhaes CG, Martins AM, Matsubara BB. Eisenmenger syndrome in pregnancy. Arq Bras Cardiol. 2008;90:e39–40.

18. Miller LD. Eisenmenger's syndrome and the pregnant patient. JOGN Nurs. 1983;12:175–80.
19. Vidovich MI. Cardiovascular disease. In: Chestnut DH, Wong CA, Tsen LC, Ngan Kee WD, Beilin Y, Mhyre J, editors. Chestnut's obstetric anesthesia principles and practice. 5th ed. Philadelphia: Saunders; 2014. p. 960–1002.
20. Chohan U, Afshan G, Mone A. Anaesthesia for caesarean section in patients with cardiac disease. J Pak Med Assoc. 2006;56:32–8.
21. Duman A, Sarkilar G, Dayioglu M, Ozden M, Görmüs N. Use of remifentanil in a patient with Eisenmenger syndrome requiring urgent cesarean section. Middle East J Anaesthesiol. 2010;20:577–80.
22. Kopka A, McMenemin IM, Serpell MG, Quasim I. Anaesthesia for cholecystectomy in two non-parturients with Eisenmenger's syndrome. Acta Anaesthesiol Scand. 2004;48:782–6.
23. Ghai B, Mohan V, Khetarpal M, Malhotra N. Epidural anesthesia for cesarean section in a patient with Eisenmenger's syndrome. Int J Obstet Anesth. 2002;11:44–7.
24. Raines DE, Liberthson RR, Murray JR. Anesthetic management and outcome following non-cardiac surgery in nonparturients with Eisenmenger's physiology. J Clin Anesth. 1996;8:341–7.
25. Baum VC, Perloff JK. Anesthetic implications of adults with congenital heart disease. Anesth Analg. 1993;76:1342–58.
26. Jones P, Patel A. Eisenmenger's syndrome and problems with anaesthesia. Br J Hosp Med. 1995;54:214.
27. Tweed W, Minuck M, Mymin D. Circulatory responses to ketamine anesthesia. Anesthesiology. 1972;37:613–9.
28. Hanouz JL, Yvon A, Guesne G, Eustratiades C, Babatasi G, Rouet R, et al. The in vitro effects of remifentanil, sufentanil, fentanyl, and alfentanil on isolated human right atria. Anesth Analg. 2001;93:543–9.
29. Bennett JM, Ehrenfeld JM, Markham L, Eagle SS. Anesthetic management and outcomes for patients with pulmonary hypertension and intracardiac shunts and Eisenmenger syndrome: a review of institutional experience. J Clin Anesth. 2014;26:286–90.
30. Slinger PD, Campos JH. Anesthesia for thoracic surgery. In: Miller RD, Miller's anesthesia. 8th ed. Philadelphia: Saunders; 2015. p. 1942–2006.
31. Ammash NM, Connolly HM, Abel MD, Warnes CA. Noncardiac surgery in Eisenmenger syndrome. J Am Coll Cardiol. 1999;33:222–7.
32. Teo YW, Greenhalgh DL. Update on anaesthetic approach to pulmonary hypertension. Eur J Anaesthesiol. 2010;27:317–23.
33. Martin JT, Tautz TJ, Antognini JF. Safety of regional anesthesia in Eisenmenger's syndrome. Reg Anesth Pain Med. 2002;27:509–13.
34. Tsutsumi Y, Mizuno J, Takada S, Morita S. Paracervical block for dilatation and curettage in a parturient with Eisenmenger's syndrome. Masui. 2010;59:379–82.
35. Minicucci S, Segala V, Verdecchia C, Sismondi P, Casabona R, Sansone F. Safe management of cesarean section in a patient of Eisenmenger syndrome. Ann Card Anaesth. 2012;15:296–8.
36. Cole PJ, Cross MH, Dresner M. Incremental spinal anaesthesia for elective caesarean section in a patient with Eisenmenger's syndrome. Br J Anaesth. 2001;86:723–6.
37. Currigan DA, Hughes RJ, Wright CE, Angus JA, Soeding PF. Vasoconstrictor responses to vasopressor agents in human pulmonary and radial arteries: an in vitro study. Anesthesiology. 2014;121:930–6.
38. Benedict N, Seybert A, Mathier MA. Evidence-based pharmacologic management of pulmonary arterial hypertension. Clin Ther. 2007;29:2134–53.
39. Galie N, Manes A, Palazzini M, Negro L, Marinelli A, Gambetti S, et al. Management of pulmonary arterial hypertension associated with congenital systemic-to-pulmonary shunts and Eisenmenger's syndrome. Drugs. 2008;68:1049–66.
40. Kandasamy R, Koh KF, Tham SL, Reddy S. Anaesthesia for caesarean section in a patient with Eisenmenger's syndrome. Singapore Med J. 2000;41:356–8.

Anesthesia for the Pregnant Patient with Intrathoracic Tumor

16

Bülent Serhan Yurtlu and Derya Arslan Yurtlu

16.1 Introduction

Intrathoracic tumors can be divided into subclasses as either primary or secondary lung tumors or pleural or mediastinal tumors. Among these lung cancers, the most frequent type of tumor group is the intrathoracic tumor. Pleural and mediastinal masses are relatively rare. The frequency of lung cancer increased throughout the twentieth century, and it has become the most common cancer type among all cancers. Lung cancer is also the leading cause of cancer-related mortality worldwide which is typically diagnosed in the late decades of life. However, its frequency is also increasing in people younger than 40 years, thus including the woman of childbearing age. The aim of this chapter is to focus and give a compiled information on the pregnants with lung/thoracic tumors. Hereby, typical sources of problems in the management of these patients, anesthetic challenges, and experiences are summarized.

16.2 Lung Tumors in Pregnancy and Treatment Approach

Cancer in pregnancy is a rare occasion affecting about 17–38 of every 100,000 births. Most common cancers diagnosed during pregnancy are breast cancer, cervical and ovarian cancer, Hodgkin and non-Hodgkin lymphomas, leukemias, and malignant melanoma [1]. Lung tumor in the pregnant patient is an exceedingly rare

B. S. Yurtlu (✉)
Dokuz Eylül University, School of Medicine, Anesthesia and Reanimation
Department, İzmir, Turkey

D. A. Yurtlu
Katip Celebi University, Atatürk Education and Research Hospital, Anesthesia
and Reanimation Department, İzmir, Turkey

© Springer International Publishing AG, part of Springer Nature 2018
B. Gunaydin, S. Ismail (eds.), *Obstetric Anesthesia for Co-morbid Conditions*,
https://doi.org/10.1007/978-3-319-93163-0_16

occasion, and it is not possible to give out a true frequency of it. There are about 60 reported cases of lung cancer during pregnancy in the last two decades [2].

Reasons of this gradual increase possibly might be related to increased awareness, increased chance of diagnosis, increasing trend of smoking among young women, and the advanced maternal age. Majority of the lung tumors are non-small cell lung cancer type in the nonpregnant population; similarly, the pregnant patients share the same diagnosis distribution [3]. Non-small cell lung cancer diagnosis constitutes approximately 80% of the lung cancers, and the rest of the cases are mainly small cell cancers [3].

In case of confirming lung tumor diagnosis in the early stages of a pregnancy, therapeutic choices depending on the gestational week, tumor type, and patient's preferences are considered. There is no definitive knowledge on how pregnancy affects the prognosis of lung tumor or how the lung tumor affects pregnancy. It is wise to terminate pregnancy if the patient is diagnosed in early weeks and expected to get high benefit from chemotherapy. Almost all of chemotherapeutics are known to be teratogenic. However, most of the patients have grade III or IV lung tumors at the time of their diagnosis, and the efficiency of terminating pregnancy is not known [4, 5]. Therapeutic options for pregnant patients with lung cancer are chemotherapy, targeted agents, and radiotherapy [5, 6]. Both chemotherapy and radiotherapy carry significant risks for the fetus. Radiotherapy is generally reserved for the palliation of symptoms during pregnancy and for the treatment of distant lesions such as brain or bone metastases. Chemotherapy is the cornerstone of therapy in pregnancy for malignancies during gestation. Due to the teratogenic effects of chemotherapeutics, physicians must respect to the preferences of an individual patient [7].

In a case series of eight parturients with thoracic tumors, authors noted that the patients who underwent surgery, radiation, and chemotherapy had good maternal neonatal outcomes [6]. Patients in this report had both malignant and benign tumor diagnoses with multiple types of tumors in origin. These authors recommended an aggressive approach for these patients [6]. Unfortunately such successful similar case series are lacking in the literature.

Utilization of targeted agents is an evolving issue with a yet unknown results and safety concerns [7]. They are not recommended until any evidence of safety appears.

The remaining option of therapy in pregnant patients with lung cancer is surgery. There is a paucity of literature about thoracic surgery for lung cancer during gestation probably because majority of the cases are at advanced stage of the disease at the time of diagnosis [8]. There is at least one successful case of video-assisted thoracoscopic surgery (VATS) in a pregnant patient [9]. In this case report, a parturient at 24 weeks' gestation having a thoracic mass in her right lower lobe underwent a successful surgery including right lower lobectomy and lymph node dissection. Both maternal and fetal outcomes were uncomplicated in this report. There were no details of anesthesia, but it is well known that VATS necessitates one lung ventilation using double-lumen endotracheal intubation or endobronchial blockers. Airway edema in pregnant patient may preclude the use of smaller-size double-lumen endotracheal tubes. Another concerns for the anesthesiologist is the position of the patient and monitoring of fetal well-being during surgery. Right lateral position for a left-sided thoracic intervention would probably increase the pressure on inferior vena cava of a term pregnant which should be best avoided. Theoretically, periods of decreased oxygen partial pressures during one-lung ventilation may compromise fetal status and lead to changes in fetal heart rate. Continuous monitoring of fetal heart rate would be wise in such cases.

The second case underwent surgical intervention for treatment of a tracheal carcinoma [10]. The parturient was at 27 weeks' gestation when admitted to the emergency department for hemoptysis. The first endobronchial intervention for this patient was for urgent control of bleeding, and the second attempt was for the resection of the tumor, where both procedures were performed under general anesthesia. Argon plasma laser coagulation with cycling 30–100% FiO_2 periods was used for tumor resection. Patient and fetus well tolerated the procedure, and tracheal resection was completed. Remaining of pregnancy was uneventful, and healthy newborn was delivered with cesarean section. At 3 years follow-up, the patient had no signs of recurrence, and no neonatal anomaly developed. This case represents the second successful intervention for an intrathoracic mass during pregnancy. It is possible that with the evolution of surgical and anesthetic techniques, more cases will be witnessed in the following years.

16.3 Anesthesia Challenges

In principle, all preoperative patients with pre-existing comorbidities are consulted with the appropriate medical specialties, and physicians aim to operate these patients at the best medical situation that can be achieved. The same principles are applied to those pregnant patients having a thoracic mass or lung cancer diagnosis. It is well known that pulmonary complications are observed in patients who underwent anesthesia even in those without pre-existing pulmonary disorders. If there is an inadequately treated pulmonary disorder preoperatively, frequency of pulmonary complications increases. Pregnancy leads to certain well-known physiologic changes in the respiratory system. One of the most important of these changes for the anesthesiologists is the 20% decrease in functional residual capacity in the pregnant [11]. Supine position during the surgery further decreases the functional residual capacity. Secondly, oxygen consumption in the pregnant rises about 75% in the second trimester, and metabolic oxygen need exceeds maternal supply in the laboring woman. Associated medical diseases such as preeclampsia may further increase the airway edema in the term pregnant. Coupling these changes with pulmonary functional losses in pregnant woman with lung tumor makes the parturient more susceptible to periods of apnea and concomitant oxygen reserve depletion. Moreover, these group of patients may present within a severe medical condition to the anesthesiologists. Despite the increased rate of diagnosis of lung tumors in the last few decades, physicians may be reluctant to use valuable diagnostic tests in pregnant patients with respiratory symptoms mainly for the concerns about fetal radiation exposure. This approach may delay the diagnosis of the cases, and anesthesiologist may face with an

untreated term pregnant in a severe medical condition [12, 13]. Especially bronchogenic tumors and mediastinal masses challenge anesthesiologists. Regional
anesthesia seems a rational choice in these patients, but it is not without problems
[8, 11]. If the regional anesthesia reaches to middle or upper thoracic dermatomes,
spinal or epidural anesthesia may interfere with respiratory muscle functions.
Normally well-functioning respiratory system in upright position of daily life
might become inefficient with combination of supine position and the added
effects of partially anesthetized respiratory muscles. Then, special caution should
be taken for exclusion of high thoracic dermatomal involvement under regional
anesthesia. Since epidural block provides segmental anesthesia which might be
titrated to the desired dermatomal level by administration of fractional doses, it
can be easier to control the sensory block height. Precise determination of highest
dermatomal level of anesthesia is somewhat more difficult with spinal anesthesia
in comparison to epidural, although spinal anesthesia has the advantage of providing dense block and full sacral anesthesia. Alternatively, combined spinal epidural
technique provides both dense block with sufficient sacral involvement, and anesthesia might be advanced to higher dermatomes if needed [14]. Other features of
parturients presenting with mediastinal masses are the potential of these intrathoracic tumors to compress nearby structures such as trachea, left or right bronchus,
anterior aspect of heart, lung, pulmonary arteries, or superior vena cava. In a
spontaneously breathing parturient, the effect of mass on the trachea may not collapse the airway; her respiratory symptoms such as dyspnea might be easily over-
looked. Dyspnea in a parturient extending beyond the second trimester of
pregnancy which worsens with the progression of the pregnancy should alert the
clinician about the possibility of mediastinal mass. Other symptoms depend on
the place where the tumor tissue compresses on. If the tumor depresses one of the
main bronchi or tracheas, then airway's circumferential area may decrease and
wheeze, and/or tachypnea might be seen in the parturient [15]. Atelectasis or pleural effusion might be detected on X-ray examinations [16]. Mediastinal mass may
also compress on the superior vena cava or brachiocephalic trunk. The superior
vena cava may easily be compressed as intramural pressure inside the veins is
lower in this region compared to the nearby heart chambers and great vessels [17,
18]. Bilateral swelling of the neck, upper extremities, head, and upper body parts
can be observed. Pleural and pericardial effusion and pulmonary edema may also
complicate the presentation of parturients [15, 19].

   True frequency of mediastinal masses during pregnancy is not known. In a literature search with PubMed interface (2017), we have encountered only ten cases during pregnancy with the search terms as anesthesia, cesarean, and mediastinal mass.
Majority of the mediastinal masses during pregnancy are lymphomas with predomi-
nant Hodgkin's lymphoma. Preoperative evaluation of these patients should be performed with a multidisciplinary team since the lesion severely effects multiple
systems. This team should involve cardiologists, cardiovascular surgeons, obstetricians, and anesthesiologists. A preoperative echocardiogram would be useful for
detection of pericardial effusions and evaluation of cardiac output. Ideally,

cardiovascular surgeons should be ready to start an immediate cardiopulmonary bypass in case of a sudden cardiac deterioration. It is advised that femoral veins should be cannulated before the surgery under local anesthesia in case of emergency need for cardiopulmonary bypass [16, 20].

However, even cannulation of femoral veins in pregnant patients may not be a sufficient precaution since aortocaval compression exists in the term parturients. Placement of multiple intravenous cannulas with large bores both from upper and lower extremities is necessary. Invasive arterial measurement of blood pressure is mandatory in such cases. In a few reports, prior to application of anesthesia, patients were cannulated through femoral arteries and veins as a precautionary measure for the possibility of sudden cardiopulmonary or tracheobronchial collapse during surgery [17, 21, 22]. All of these reports were uneventful without the need for emergent cardiopulmonary bypass. There is at least one review/opinion in the literature indicating that cardiopulmonary bypass on standby is unnecessary in the management of such cases [23]. It is speculated that in the event of a cardiopulmonary deterioration, either at the induction or maintenance of anesthesia, initiation of a cardiopulmonary bypass will necessitate at least 5–10 min to start, which will lead to neurologic injuries [26]. It is advised to have rigid bronchoscope and the presence of a staff in the operation room ready to manipulate it in case of airway collapse or loss of spontaneous ventilation. Appropriate readiness for such surgery depends on the condition of individual patient and the center's preferences. Another consideration point for the anesthesiologist in patients with intrathoracic tumor is the possibility of brain, vertebral, or distant metastases presence in the parturient. Lung tumors frequently make metastases to brain tissue [3–6]. In a parturient with advanced stage of the disease, a metastatic possibility is important for the anesthesiologist. Obviously most of the anesthesiologists would prefer regional anesthesia for a parturient with lung/thoracic tumor, but a raised intracranial pressure is a contraindication for neuraxial blocks. In addition such metastases might be found at the thoracic, lumbar vertebral levels of patients with lung carcinoma. There is at least one report in the literature describing a lung cancer parturient presenting with seizures discovered later to have brain metastases [24]. Initially seizures were attributed to eclampsia; in this case, cesarean section was performed under regional anesthesia. Postoperatively they have discovered the presence of brain metastases with signs of raised intracranial pressure (midline shift) together with a large bronchogenic adenocarcinoma [24]. Such a coincidence of metastases in the lung and brain in a pregnant patient has also been reported for a primary alveolar sarcoma tumor [25]. Regional anesthesia was performed for cesarean section, and 3 days later neurosurgical removal of brain metastases was performed with uneventful general anesthesia. Initial clinical presenting feature of this patient was headache and vomiting history which was attributed to other reasons that could occur during pregnancy. Therefore, a headache, seizure, vomiting, or other neurologic manifestations should be carefully evaluated in a parturient with lung tumor, and a multidisciplinary team approach involving neurosurgeons should be instituted for these patients.

16.4 Anesthesia Practice in Pregnant Patients with Lung Tumor

The available information about the lung/thoracic tumors and pregnancy comes from occasional case reports. According to a study of Burlacu et al. [26], only 35 cases of pregnant patients with lung tumors were identified starting from 1953 until 2007. According to his study, only 11 of the cases delivered vaginally, and the rest of them underwent cesarean section. Anesthetic technique was documented in only five of these cases that underwent cesarean. One patient had spinal, three had epidural, and one had general anesthesia [26].

When key words such as "lung cancer," "pregnancy," and "mediastinal mass" were searched in PubMed interface between 2008 and the end of 2017, additional 34 parturients with lung cancer were identified within this period. Since we have determined almost identical number of cases within 10 years of duration, it seems that thoracic/lung cancer reports during pregnancy are increasing gradually. After eliminating 5 out of 34 reports written in languages other than English, 29 of them were reviewed. One of the reports was a case series including nine cases, but it was focused on the therapeutic choices in these patients and data about surgery/anesthesia without presenting outcome data [2]. On one occasion the mode of delivery was not indicated, whereas the remaining 27 of the cases had cesarean delivery.

In other reports, maternal age of the parturients was between 19 and 42 years, and the gestational age of delivery was varying between 30 and 42 weeks. There were three reports describing general anesthesia management for cesarean section [25, 27, 28]. The first case [27] was already intubated in the intensive care unit to control pulmonary bleeding, the second case [28] was an emergency cesarean section, and the third case who was a term parturient [25] had an intracranial tumor metastases at the time of diagnosis. In one of these reports, anesthesia-related complications were presented. In 8 of the 27 cases, method of anesthesia was regional anesthesia. There are at least five cases with epidural anesthesia [19, 21, 29–31]: two of the cases had combined spinal-epidural anesthesia [15, 32], and one case had spinal anesthesia [33]. The type of anesthesia for cesarean section was not documented in the remaining reports. Fortunately, except for a single case described earlier, all of the mothers have survived [34].

In summary, clinicians prefer cesarean delivery in parturients with intrathoracic tumors because of already increased intra-abdominal pressure and possible negative effects of increased intrathoracic pressure during pushing efforts in labor. Anesthesiologists already prefer regional anesthesia in parturients who are candidates for cesarean section because of increased risk of airway and respiratory problems due to general anesthesia. Therefore, regional anesthesia techniques are commonly offered to parturients with thoracic/lung tumor. Sudden cardiorespiratory deterioration at induction of anesthesia for a mediastinal mass had been described before. A special cautious multidisciplinary approach is very valuable particularly in the parturients with mediastinal masses. This approach should include a second plan in case of failed regional anesthesia, difficult airway, or development of a sudden intraoperative catastrophe [31].

Key Learning Points
- Anesthesia in a pregnant with intrathoracic tumor is a great challenge for anesthesiologists.
- Neuraxial anesthesia is the preferred method of delivery in pregnants with thoracic mass, but anesthesiologist should have extra precautions other than routine in order to manage unexpected intraoperative events.

Conflict of Interest None
Funding None

References

1. Howdeshell KL, Shelby MD. Epidemiology of cancer during pregnancy. In: Azim Jr HA, editor. Managing cancer during pregnancy. Basel: Springer; 2016. p. 3–16.
2. Boussios S, Han SN, Fruscio R, Halaska MJ, Ottevanger PB, Peccatori FA, et al. Lung cancer in pregnancy: report of nine cases from an international collaborative study. Lung Cancer. 2013;82:499–59.
3. Pavlidis N, Zarkavelis G. Managing thoracic tumours during pregnancy. In: Azim Jr HA, editor. Managing cancer during pregnancy. Basel: Springer; 2016. p. 185–91.
4. Pavlidis NA. Coexistence of pregnancy and malignancy. Oncologist. 2002;7:279–879.
5. Sarıman N, Levent E, Yener NA, Orki A, Saygı A. Lung cancer and pregnancy. Lung Cancer. 2013;79:321–3.
6. Dieter RA Jr, Kuzycz GB, Dieter RA 3rd. Malignant and benign thoracic tumors during pregnancy. Int Surg. 2006;91:S103–6.
7. Azim HA Jr, Peccatori FA, Pavlidis N. Lung cancer in the pregnant woman: to treat or not to treat, that is the question. Lung Cancer. 2010;67:251–6.
8. Whang B. Thoracic surgery in the pregnant patient. Thorac Surg Clin. 2018;28:1–7.
9. Kim JW, Kim JS, Cho JY, Lee DH. Successful video-assisted thoracoscopic lobectomy in a pregnant woman with lung cancer. Lung Cancer. 2014;85:331–4.
10. Kesrouani A, Dabar G, Rahal S, Ghorra C. Treatment of tracheal mucoepidermoid carcinoma by argon plasma coagulation during pregnancy. Int Surg. 2015;100:927–9.
11. Alaily AB, Carrol KB. Pulmonary ventilation in pregnancy. Br J Obstet Gynaecol. 1978;85:518–4.
12. Yurtlu S, Hakimoğlu S, Hancı V, Ayoğlu H, Erdoğan G, Özköçak I. Epidural anesthesia for a parturient with superior vena cava syndrome. Turk J Anesth Reanim. 2012;40:52–7. https://doi.org/10.5222/jtaics.2012.052.
13. Reddy YN, Sundaram V, Stamler JS. An unusual case of peripartum pulmonary oedema. BMJ Case Rep. 2013;2013:bcr2013200150. https://doi.org/10.1136/bcr-2013-200150.
14. Tyagi A, Sharma CS, Kumar S, Sharma DK, Jain AK, Sethi AK. Epidural volume extension: a review. Anaesth Intensive Care. 2012;40:604–3.
15. Lee CY, Izaham A, Zainuddin K. Anaesthetic management of a parturient with a mediastinal mass for caesarean delivery. Int J Obstet Anesth. 2013;22:356–8. https://doi.org/10.1016/j.ijoa.2013.03.017.
16. Chiang JC, Irwin MG, Hussain A, Tang YK, Hiong YT. Anaesthesia for emergency caesarean section in a patient with large anterior mediastinal tumour presenting as intrathoracic airway compression and superior vena cava obstruction. Case Rep Med. 2010;2010:708481. https://doi.org/10.1155/2010/708481.

17. Chan YK, Ng KP, Chiu CL, Rajan G, Tan KC, Lim YC. Anesthetic management of a parturient with superior vena cava obstruction for cesarean section. Anesthesiology. 2001;94:167–9.
18. Buvanendran A, Mohajer P, Pombar X, Tuman KJ. Perioperative management with epidural anesthesia for a parturient with superior vena caval obstruction. Anesth Analg. 2004;98:1160–3.
19. Shastri U, Slinger P, Nguyen E, Carvalho JC, Balki M. Pulmonary edema during cesarean delivery in a patient with a mediastinal mass. Can J Anaesth. 2011;58:285–9. https://doi.org/10.1007/s12630-010-9431-0.
20. Erdös G, Tzanova I. Perioperative anaesthetic management of mediastinal mass in adults. Eur J Anaesthesiol. 2009;26:627–32. https://doi.org/10.1097/EJA.0b013e328324b7f8.
21. Roze des Ordons AL, Lee J, Bader E, Scheelar L, Achen B, Taam J, et al. Cesarean delivery in a parturient with an anterior mediastinal mass. Can J Anaesth. 2013;60:89–90. https://doi.org/10.1007/s12630-012-9815-4.
22. Bevinaguddaiah Y, Shivanna S, Pujari VS, Chikkapillappa MA. Anesthesia for cesarean delivery in a patient with large anterior mediastinal tumor presenting as intrathoracic airway compression. Saudi J Anaesth. 2014;8:556–8. https://doi.org/10.4103/1658-354X.140901.
23. Slinger P, Karsli C. Management of the patient with a large anterior mediastinal mass: recurring myths. Curr Opin Anaesthesiol. 2007;20:1–3.
24. Innamaa A, Deering P, Powell MC. Advanced lung cancer presenting with a generalized seizure in pregnancy. Acta Obstet Gynecol Scand. 2006;85:1148–9.
25. Wang Y, Cui J, Yan X, Jin R, Hong X. Alveolar soft part sarcoma with multiple brain and lung metastases in pregnancy: a case report and literature review. Medicine (Baltimore). 2017;96:e8790. https://doi.org/10.1097/MD.0000000000008790.
26. Burlacu CL, Fitzpatrick C, Carey M. Anaesthesia for caesarean section in a woman with lung cancer: case report and review. Int J Obstet Anesth. 2007;16:50–62.
27. Chhajed PN, Kate A, Chaudhari P, Tulasigiri C, Shetty S, Kesarwani R, et al. Massive hemoptysis during pregnancy. J Assoc Physicians India. 2011;59:660–2.
28. Ceauşu M, Hostiuc S, Sajin M, Roman G, Nicodin O, Dermengiu D. Gestational lung adenocarcinoma: case report. Int J Surg Pathol. 2014;22:663–6. https://doi.org/10.1177/1066896914531816.
29. Zambelli A, Prada GA, Fregoni V, Ponchio L, Sagrada P, Pavesi L. Erlotinib administration for advanced non-small cell lung cancer during the first 2 months of unrecognized pregnancy. Lung Cancer. 2008;60:455–7.
30. Kim JH, Kim HS, Sung CW, Kim KJ, Kim CH, Lee KY. Docetaxel, gemcitabine, and cisplatin administered for non-small cell lung cancer during the first and second trimester of an unrecognized pregnancy. Lung Cancer. 2008;59:270–3.
31. Kanellakos GW. Perioperative management of the pregnant patient with an anterior mediastinal mass. Anesthesiol Clin. 2012;30:749–8. https://doi.org/10.1016/j.anclin.2012.07.010.
32. Kashif S, Saleem J. Anaesthetic management of caesarean section in a patient with large mediastinal mass. J Coll Physicians Surg Pak. 2015;25:143–5.
33. Kojima M, Yoshie K, Shimazaki A, Ohtsuka N, Otake H, Koide K, et al. Anesthetic management of cesarean section in a pregnant woman with advanced tongue cancer. Masui. 2016;65:632–5.
34. Said M, Migaw H, Hafsa C, Braham R, Golli M, Moussa A, et al. Imaging features of primary pulmonary liposarcoma. Australas Radiol. 2003;47:313–7.

Anesthesia for the Pregnant Patient with Obstructive Sleep Apnea

Tülay Özkan Seyhan and Dilan Büyük

17.1 Introduction

Obstructive sleep apnea (OSA) is the most common form of sleep-related breathing disorders [1]. Repetitive blockage of upper airway causes hypopnea (partial obstruction) or apnea (complete obstruction) during sleep with oxygen desaturation. Characteristic symptoms of OSA are snoring, periods of awakening by gasping or choking during night, and excessive daytime sleepiness. OSA is a widespread problem due to increased obesity prevalence. The diagnosis and management during pregnancy are important as OSA is related to increased fetal and maternal morbidity. This chapter aims to point out the interaction between OSA and pregnancy, as well as the problems related to the diagnosis and current knowledge about the management of pregnant patient with OSA.

17.2 Pregnancy and Obstructive Sleep Apnea

Pregnancy-induced alteration of sleep, physiological changes including weight gain, fluid retention, mucosal hyperemia and edema, and hypersecretion may result in snoring and OSA or even in an increase in the severity of OSA.

In the United States, the prevalence of OSA with different severity is reported to be between 6.5 and 21% among pregnant population, with the highest prevalence among the obese gravidas [1, 2]. The prevalence is increased with the growing problem of obesity in recent decades. During pregnancy, most of the cases with OSA are undiagnosed, and therefore the actual prevalence is still unknown.

During pregnancy, minute ventilation and the sensitivity of respiratory center to carbon dioxide increase due to elevated progesterone levels. The resulting mild

T. Ö. Seyhan (✉) · D. Büyük
Istanbul University, Istanbul Faculty of Medicine, Department of Anesthesiology,
Capa Clinics, 34093 Istanbul, Turkey

© Springer International Publishing AG, part of Springer Nature 2018
B. Gunaydin, S. Ismail (eds.), *Obstetric Anesthesia for Co-morbid Conditions*,
https://doi.org/10.1007/978-3-319-93163-0_17

respiratory alkalosis is assumed to cause instability in respiratory control pathways [3]. Oxygen reserves in pregnant patients are decreased due to reduced functional residual capacity and increased oxygen consumption in addition to small airway closure at the lung volumes greater than the functional residual capacity in supine position. Episodic hypoxia by OSA coupled with low maternal oxygen reserves risks oxygen delivery to the fetus.

Obstructive sleep apnea causes inflammation, sympathetic activation, insulin resistance, and oxidative stress resulting in increased vascular resistance, diabetes mellitus type II, metabolic syndrome, and cardiac insufficiency. Increased inspiratory effort against an obstructed airway results in a negative intrathoracic pressure gradient leading to cardiac dysfunction over a period of time [4, 5]. Several studies suggest that OSA increases maternal and fetal morbidity and mortality. Maternal OSA is associated with increased rates of both chronic and gestational hypertension, pulmonary hypertension, preeclampsia, gestational diabetes, depression, asthma, fetal growth retardation, preterm birth, fetal distress, lower Apgar scores at birth, and cesarean delivery [2, 6–11].

17.3 Diagnosis of Obstructive Sleep Apnea

The diagnosis of OSA is determined by polysomnography (PSG), which measures several sleep variables including the apnea-hypopnea index [12]. The apnea-hypopnea index is the sum of respiratory events, detected as apnea and hypopnea, during 1 h of sleep. Apnea is defined as the absence of airflow for ≥ 10 s, whereas hypopnea is defined as reduction in respiratory effort with $\geq 4\%$ oxygen desaturation. An apnea-hypopnea index of ≥ 5 per hour is defined as mild OSA, whereas ≥ 15 and ≥ 30 per hour are designated as moderate and severe OSA, respectively. The diagnosis by an overnight laboratory PSG is time consuming and expensive. Portable home polysomnography is a reasonable alternative among the general population, but the data supporting its use for pregnant women is currently inadequate. Many screening tools and questionnaires have been developed for daily clinical practice which are highly sensitive and specific for the identification of nonpregnant patients at high risk for OSA. Out of the different screening tools, shown in Tables 17.1, 17.2 and 17.3, STOP-BANG Questionnaire is the most validated one for surgical patient populations and in the sleep clinic population [13]. Lockhart et al. compared six OSA screening tools with overnight portable polysomnography in pregnant women at the third trimester [9]. Although none of the tools could accurately detect OSA, STOP-BANG Questionnaire had the highest specificity with a high negative predictive value. A score of 0–2 shows that OSA is unlikely and may reduce the need for PSG during pregnancy. Facco et al. screened pregnant women at high risk for sleep apnea (women with chronic hypertension, pregestational diabetes, obesity, and/or a prior history of preeclampsia) using the Berlin Questionnaire, the Epworth Sleepiness Scale, and overnight portable polysomnography [14]. Whereas Berlin Questionnaire and Epworth Sleepiness Scale were inaccurate in predicting sleep apnea, a model incorporating frequent snoring, chronic hypertension, age, and body mass index predicted more accurately sleep apnea [14].

Table 17.1   STOP-BANG Questionnaire

Snoring? Do you **Snore Loudly** (loud enough to be heard through closed doors or your bed-partner elbows you for snoring night)?	☐ Yes	☐ No
Tired? Do you often feel **Tired, Fatigued or Sleepy** during the daytime (such as falling asleep during driving or talking to someone)?	☐ Yes	☐ No
Observed? Has anyone **Observed** you **Stop Breathing** or **Choking/Gasping** during your sleep?	☐ Yes	☐ No
Pressure? Do you have or are being treated for **High Blood Pressure**?	☐ Yes	☐ No
Body Mass Index more than 35kg/m²?	☐ Yes	☐ No
Age older than 50?	☐ Yes	☐ No
Neck size large? (Measured around Adams apple) For male, is your shirt collar 17 inches / 43cm or larger? For female, is your shirt collar 16 inches / 41cm or larger?	☐ Yes	☐ No
Gender = Male ?	☐ Yes	☐ No

Adapted from the official STOP-BANG questionnaire website at http://www.stopbang.ca/osa/screening.php
For general population
OSA: Low Risk: Yes to 0–2 questions
OSA: Intermediate Risk: Yes to 3–4 questions
OSA: High Risk: Yes to 5–8 questions
or Yes to 2 or more of 4 STOP questions + male gender
or Yes to 2 or more of 4 STOP questions + BMI >35 kg/m²
or Yes to 2 or more of 4 STOP questions + neck circumference 17 in./43 cm in male or 16 in./41 cm in female

Table 17.2 Berlin Questionnaire

Height (m) _____ Weight (kg) _____
Age _____ Male / Female

Category 1

1. **Do you snore?**
   _a. Yes *(1 point)*
   _b. No
   _c. Don't know

If you snore:
2. **Your snoring is:**
   _a. Slightly louder than breathing
   _b. As loud as talking
   _c. Louder than talking *(1 point)*
   _d. Very loud – can be heard in
   adjacent rooms *(1 point)*

3. **How often do you snore?**
   _a. Nearly every day *(1 point)*
   _b. Three to four times a week *(1 point)*
   _c. One to two times a week
   _d. One to two times a month
   _e. Never or nearly never

4. **Has your snoring ever bothered other people?**
   _a. Yes *(1 point)*
   _b. No
   _c. Don't know

5. **Has anyone noticed that you quit breathing during your sleep?**
   _a. Nearly every day *(2 point)*
   _b. Three to four times a week *(2 point)*
   _c. One to two times a week
   _d. One to two times a month
   _e. Never or nearly never

Category 2

6. **How often do you feel tired or fatigued after your sleep?**
   _a. Nearly every day *(1 point)*
   _b. Three to four times a week *(1 point)*
   _c. One to two times a week
   _d. One to two times a month
   _e. Never or nearly never

7. **During your waking time, do you feel tired, fatigued or not up to par?**
   _a. Nearly every day *(1 point)*
   _b. Three to four times a week *(1 point)*
   _c. One to two times a week
   _d. One to two times a month
   _e. Never or nearly never

8. **Have you ever nodded off or fallen asleep while driving a vehicle?**
   _a. Yes *(1 point)*
   _b. No

If yes:
9. **How often does this occur?**
   _a. Nearly every day
   _b. Three to four times a week
   _c. One to two times a week
   _d. One to two times a month
   _e. Never or nearly never

Category 3

10. **Do you have high blood pressure?**
    _a. Yes *(1 point)*
    _b. No
    _c. Don't know

From https://www.sleepapnea.org/assets/files/pdf/berlin-questionnaire.pdf

The screening tools in current form cannot be validated for pregnant patients [1]. Some questions in the screening tools are not applicable. Tiredness and daytime sleepiness are common in pregnancy, so they cannot be distinguished as risk factors. High body mass index (BMI) and higher prepregnancy BMI are clearly risk factors without clear cutoff value. Another problem is the dynamic process of pregnancy, which leads to a progressive change in the airway anatomy, so that OSA may develop over the course of pregnancy [15]. The appropriate timing for OSA screening is yet unknown; an earlier screening may overlook patients. Reducing OSA-related maternal and fetal complications with early screening and treatment is the current topic of investigations.

Table 17.3 Epworth Sleepiness Scale

Use the following scale to choose the most appropriate number for each situation:
0 = would never doze
1 = slight chance of dozing
2 = moderate chance of dozing
3 = high chance of dozing

Situation	Chance of Dozing
Sitting and reading _____	___
Watching TV _____	___
Sitting, inactive in public place (e.g. a theatre or a meeting) ____	___
As a passenger in a car for an hour without a break _____	___
Lying down to rest in the afternoon when circumstances permit ___	___
Sitting and talking to someone _____	___
Sitting quietly after a lunch without alcohol _____	___
In a car, while stopped for a few minutes in the traffic _____	___

From https://www.sleepapnea.org/assets/files/pdf/ESS%20PDF%201990-97.pdf
Score:
0–5 lower normal daytime sleepiness
6–10 higher normal daytime sleepiness
11–12 mild excessive daytime sleepiness
13–15 moderate excessive daytime sleepiness
16–24 severe excessive daytime sleepiness

17.4 Management of Pregnant Women with Obstructive Sleep Apnea

17.4.1 Management of Patient During Pregnancy

Multidisciplinary approach involving the obstetrician, anesthesiologist, neonatologist, and sleep physician is recommended to decrease OSA-related problems during peripartum period. Pregnancy-specific management of OSA is lacking because of the insufficient evidence in terms of reducing maternal and fetal morbidity. In patients with severe OSA, upper airway surgery and significant weight loss may be good therapy alternatives in indicated patients and have to be done before a planned pregnancy. However, during pregnancy a well-controlled weight gain can be beneficial.

Options, including continuous positive airway pressure (CPAP) and positional therapy, used in general OSA population can be adapted and safely applied along the pregnancy. In preeclamptic patients, OSA causes decrease in heart rate, stroke volume, and cardiac output during sleep, which has been shown to be minimized with the use of nocturnal nasal CPAP [16]. Readjustment of CPAP pressure may be necessary according to the patients' requirements over the course of pregnancy. Although early application of CPAP may relieve sleep-related breathing disturbances, it cannot prevent negative pregnancy outcomes but may aid to reduce their severity [17, 18].

Lateral recumbent or head-elevated positions should be encouraged to avoid the aggravating effect of supine position on OSA as known from general population [19]. Furthermore in postpartum patients with OSA, 45° upper body elevation has to be demonstrated to increase upper airway cross-sectional area and reduce apnea-hypopnea index [19].

17.4.2 Anesthetic Management

17.4.2.1 Preoperative Assessment
Pregnant OSA patients should be counseled by the anesthesiologist during the early phases of pregnancy. Patient's history should be evaluated for difficult or failed intubations and postoperative course of previous operations. Routine preoperative evaluation is sufficient in asymptomatic or mild OSA patients. Patients with moderate or severe OSA need optimization of comorbid conditions prior to labor or a planned cesarean delivery. Patients, who are on CPAP, should be informed to bring their devices while coming for delivery.

17.4.2.2 Labor Analgesia
Neuraxial analgesia is the technique of choice during labor. Most of the OSA patients are obese, which is related to increased risk of fetal macrosomia, dysfunctional or prolonged labor, instrumental delivery, or even emergency cesarean delivery. The pain intensity is also positively correlated with body mass index [20]. Therefore, the insertion of a functioning epidural catheter during the early phase of labor is mandatory. Combined techniques like combined spinal epidural (CSE) or dural puncture epidural (DPE) can also be chosen as they offer a faster onset of analgesia [18]. An untested epidural catheter in CSE was a subject of discussion for many years and was assumed to be a risk factor for epidural catheter failure. But a recent retrospective cohort study revealed a significantly lower incident of catheter failure with a CSE compared to straight epidural (6.6% vs. 11.6%) without a significant delay in recognition of it [21]. In DPE, dura is punctured with a spinal needle similar to CSE technique without injecting drugs into subarachnoid space while epidural catheter can be tested as well. Beside faster analgesia onset by intrathecal spread of epidural drug, DPE also offers a better sacral analgesia than a straight epidural technique. The identification of bony landmarks and midline may be facilitated by ultrasound imaging. To avoid the catheter dislodgement in obese patients, catheters should be fixed at the skin after changing the posture given during epidural puncture [22].

In case of contraindication of neuraxial techniques, opioid-based systemic analgesia may be used under closed control with monitoring of oxygen saturation and respiratory rate.

17.4.2.3 Anesthesia for Cesarean Section
Neuraxial anesthesia should be preferred also for cesarean delivery while avoiding high doses of long-acting neuraxial opioids. Spinal anesthesia may be an inappropriate choice in obese patients with previous abdominal operations as operation

times may be prolonged. Epidural or CSE technique allows titrating the drugs according to the patient's needs [18].

When general anesthesia is justified, short-acting anesthetics and analgesics with careful titration are recommended. Patients with OSA are sensitive to sedatives, opioids, and inhaled anesthetics. Head-up position and CPAP are helpful for pre-oxygenation prior to anesthetic induction in obese parturient. Anesthetic team should be prepared for difficult intubation. Oxygen insufflation during apnea may avoid hypoxia during airway management. The trachea should be extubated after full reversal of neuromuscular blockade while the patient is awake and positioned semi-upright or lateral. In addition to standard monitoring, an arterial line is advisable for accurate blood pressure monitoring as well as frequent blood sampling in patients with severe OSA or OSA-related comorbidities. Pulmonary hypertension or conditions with decreased cardiac output may necessitate more sophisticated noninvasive or invasive monitoring [18, 23].

17.4.3 Postpartum Care

Postpartum care of a patient with moderate to severe OSA requires high dependency care unit with monitoring and cardiorespiratory support facilities. Labor and delivery cause narrowing of the airway resulting in a decrease of oral and pharyngeal volume, which can objectively be observed as an increase of Mallampati class [24]. This change in airway diameter is reported both in normal and preeclamptic parturient, which may persist for 48 h postpartum in both groups of patients. Therefore, careful monitoring, including respiratory rate, pulse oximetry, and capnography, is essential in the postpartum period especially in cases with moderate to severe OSA or suspicious for undiagnosed OSA, in the postpartum period [23, 25]. CPAP reduce airway obstruction, but evidence is lacking for its use to decrease major postoperative complications [23]. Patients could be discharged to an unmonitored position when they are able to maintain oxygen saturation on room air especially during sleep.

Following operative delivery, analgesia without interfering the respiration is very important. Epidural technique allows excellent postoperative analgesia via epidural catheter utilizing local anesthetics and lipophilic opioid combinations. Local anesthetics are effective against both visceral and somatic pain. They should be used in low concentrations to avoid muscle weakness resulting from neuraxial analgesia. The more hydrophilic morphine has to be applied with care as it may result in a biphasic respiratory depression: Intravascular absorption may lead to an early depression after 30–90 min, whereas a late one may appear due to its rostral migration into the respiratory center, which necessitates monitoring for 24 h following intrathecal morphine injection [26]. Intrathecal morphine up to 0.15 mg offers a relatively safe alternative for postoperative analgesia following single-shot spinal anesthesia [27]. But data for its use in parturients with OSA is lacking.

Following general anesthesia, multimodal analgesia, utilizing non-opioid analgesics like paracetamol and nonsteroidal anti-inflammatory drugs supported with peripheral nerve blocks, is challenging because of the opioid-induced respiratory depression risk following opioid analgesics [28–30]. Bilateral transversus abdominis plane (TAP) block may reduce opioid consumption and opioid-related side effects by providing pain control and improving patient satisfaction [31]. However, TAP blocks do offer any additional benefit if patients have received intrathecal morphine [32]. Local anesthetic wound infiltration in the form of an infusion or single-injection technique is used also for postoperative analgesia [33]. But despite reduction in opioid requirements, no clear benefits can be shown in terms of reducing opioid-related side effects following cesarean delivery.

A reevaluation of patients for OSA 2–3 months postpartum is suggested, because after this period of time most of the gestational weight gain would have been lost. There is not sufficient data about the risk of developing OSA in subsequent pregnancies with previously diagnosed pregnancy-related OSA. It is advisable to follow up the patient for possible OSA development.

In conclusion, OSA during pregnancy is related to higher maternal and fetal morbidity. Therefore special attention should be paid for the detection of pregnant patients with OSA. Validated diagnostic tools and specific management options for pregnant population are still lacking. The adaptation of current knowledge to the dynamic process and progressive change of pregnancy and postpartum period is a challenge for anesthesiologist in this particular group of patients.

Key Learning Points
- Pregnancy-related physiological changes make pregnant patients prone to OSA or increase the severity of previously existing OSA.
- Maternal OSA is associated with increased rates of systemic and pulmonary hypertension, preeclampsia, gestational diabetes, depression, asthma, fetal growth retardation, preterm birth, fetal distress, and lower Apgar scores at delivery.
- Currently there are no screening tools for accurate diagnosis of OSA during pregnancy. However STOP-BANG Questionnaire had the highest specificity with a high negative predictive value. Portable home polysomnography may also be used, but the data supporting its application for pregnant women is currently inadequate.
- Pregnancy-specific management of OSA is lacking. A well-controlled weight gain, continuous positive airway pressure, and positional therapy may be beneficial.
- Neuraxial blocks are the technique of choice for labor and cesarean delivery. Short-acting anesthetics and analgesics with careful titration are recommended for general anesthesia.
- Postpartum care of a patient with moderate to severe OSA requires high dependency care unit with monitoring and cardiorespiratory support facilities. Multimodal analgesia including neuraxial or regional local anesthetics is challenging to avoid respiratory depression risk following opioid analgesics.

References

1. Abdullah HR, Nagappa M, Siddiqui N, Chung F. Diagnosis and treatment of obstructive sleep apnea during pregnancy. Curr Opin Anaesthesiol. 2016;29:317–24.
2. Louis JM, Mogos MF, Salemi JL, Redline S, Salihu HM. Obstructive sleep apnea and severe maternal-infant morbidity/mortality in the United States, 1998-2009. Sleep. 2014;37:843–9.
3. Contreras G, Gutiérrez M, Beroíza T, Fantín A, Oddó H, Villarroel L, et al. Ventilatory drive and respiratory muscle function in pregnancy. Am Rev Respir Dis. 1991;144:837–41.
4. Louis JM, Auckley D, Sokol RJ, Mercer BM. Maternal and neonatal morbidities associated with obstructive sleep apnea complicating pregnancy. Am J Obstet Gynecol. 2010;202:261. e1–5.
5. Campos-Rodriguez F, Martinez-Garcia MA, de la Cruz-Moron I, Almeida-Gonzalez C, Catalan-Serra P, Montserrat JM. Cardiovascular mortality in women with obstructive sleep apnea with or without continuous positive airway pressure treatment; a cohort study. Ann Intern Med. 2012;156.115–22.
6. Louis J, Auckley D, Bolden N. Management of Obstructive Sleep Apnea in pregnant women. Obstet Gynecol. 2012;119:864–8.
7. Sahin FK, Koken G, Cosar E, Saylan F, Fidan F, Yilmazer M, et al. Obstructive sleep apnea in pregnancy and fetal outcome. Int J Gynaecol Obstet. 2008;100:141–6.
8. Chen YH, Kang JH, Lin CC, Wang IT, Keller JJ, Lin HC. Obstructive sleep apnea and the risk of adverse pregnancy outcomes. Am J Obstet Gynecol. 2012;206:136.e1–5.
9. Lockhart EM, Ben Abdallah A, Tuuli MG, Leighton BL. Obstructive sleep Apnea in pregnancy: assessment of current screening tools. Obstet Gynecol. 2015;126:93–102.
10. Ding X-X, Wu Y-L, Xu S-J, Zhang SF, Jia XM, Zhu RP, et al. A systematic review and quantitative assessment of sleep-disordered breathing during pregnancy and perinatal outcomes. Sleep Breath. 2014;18:703–13.
11. Xu T, Feng Y, Peng H, Guo D, Li T. Obstructive sleep apnea and the risk of perinatal outcomes: a meta-analysis of cohort studies. Sci Rep. 2014;4:6982.
12. Health Quality Ontario. Polysomnography in patients with obstructive sleep apnea: an evidence-based analysis. Ont Heal Technol Assess Ser. 2006;6:1–38.
13. Nagappa M, Liao P, Wong J, Auckley D, Ramachandran SK, Memtsoudis S, et al. Validation of the STOP-Bang questionnaire as a screening tool for obstructive sleep Apnea among different populations: a systematic review and meta-analysis. PLoS One. 2015;10:e0143697.
14. Facco FL, Ouyang DW, Zee PC, Grobman WA. Development of a pregnancy-specific screening tool for sleep apnea. J Clin Sleep Med. 2012;8:389–94.
15. Pien GW, Pack AI, Jackson N, Maislin G, Macones GA, Schwab RJ. Risk factors for sleep-disordered breathing in pregnancy. Thorax. 2014;69:371–7.
16. Blyton DM, Sullivan CE, Edwards N. Reduced nocturnal cardiac output associated with pre-eclampsia is minimized with the use of nocturnal nasal CPAP. Sleep. 2004;27:79–84.
17. Guilleminault C, Palombini L, Poyares D, Takaoka S, Huynh NT-L, El-Sayed Y. Pre-eclampsia and nasal CPAP: part 1. Early intervention with nasal CPAP in pregnant women with risk-factors for pre-eclampsia: preliminary findings. Sleep Med. 2007;9:9–14.
18. Booth JM, Tonidandel AM. Peripartum management of obstructive sleep Apnea. Clin Obstet Gynecol. 2017;60:405–17.
19. Zaremba S, Mueller N, Heisig AM, Shin CH, Jung S, Leffert LR, et al. Elevated upper body position improves pregnancy-related OSA without impairing sleep quality or sleep architecture early after delivery. Chest. 2015;148:936–44.
20. Melzack R, Kinch R, Dobkin P, Lebrun M, Taenzer P. Severity of labour pain: influence of physical as well as psychologic variables. Can Med Assoc J. 1984;130:579–84.
21. Booth JM, Pan JC, Ross VH, Russell GB, Harris LC, Pan PH. Combined spinal epidural technique for labor analgesia does not delay recognition of epidural catheter failures: a single-center retrospective cohort survival analysis. Anesthesiology. 2016;125:516–24.
22. Hamilton CL, Riley ET, Cohen SE. Changes in the position of epidural catheters associated with patient movement. Anesthesiology. 1997;86:778–84. discussion 29A.

23. Ankichetty SP, Angle P, Joselyn AS, Chinnappa V, Halpern S. Anesthetic considerations of parturients with obesity and obstructive sleep apnea. J Anaesthesiol Clin Pharmacol. 2012;28:436–43.
24. Kodali B-S, Chandrasekhar S, Bulich LN, Topulos GP, Datta S. Airway changes during labor and delivery. Anesthesiology. 2008;108:357–62.
25. Ahuja P, Jain D, Bhardwaj N, Jain K, Gainder S, Kang M. Airway changes following labor and delivery in preeclamptic parturients: a prospective case control study. Int J Obstet Anesth. 2018;33:17–22.
26. Carvalho B. Respiratory depression after neuraxial opioids in the obstetric setting. Anesth Analg. 2008;107:956–61.
27. Kato R, Shimamoto H, Terui K, Yokota K, Miyao H. Delayed respiratory depression associated with 0.15 mg intrathecal morphine for cesarean section: a review of 1915 cases. J Anesth. 2008;22:112–6.
28. Gupta K, Prasad A, Nagappa M, Wong J, Abrahamyan L, Chung F. Risk factors for opioid-induced respiratory depression and failure to rescue: a review. Curr Opin Anaesthesiol. 2018;31:110–9.
29. Corso R, Russotto V, Gregoretti C, Cattano D. Perioperative management of obstructive sleep apnea: a systematic review. Minerva Anestesiol. 2018;84:81–93.
30. Lam KK, Kunder S, Wong J, Doufas AG. Obstructive sleep apnea, pain, and opioids: is the riddle solved? Curr Opin Anaesthesiol. 2016;29:134–40.
31. Fusco P, Scimia P, Paladini G, Fiorenzi M, Petrucci E, Pozone T, et al. Transversus abdominis plane block for analgesia after Cesarean delivery. A systematic review. Minerva Anestesiol. 2015;81:195–204.
32. Champaneria R, Shah L, Wilson MJ, Daniels JP. Clinical effectiveness of transversus abdominis plane (TAP) blocks for pain relief after caesarean section: a meta-analysis. Int J Obstet Anesth. 2016;28:45–60.
33. Adesope O, Ituk U, Habib AS. Local anaesthetic wound infiltration for postcaesarean section analgesia: a systematic review and meta-analysis. Eur J Anaesthesiol. 2016;33:731–42.

4   81452   25845   2